Ethnopsychiatry

SUNY Series in Medical Anthropology
Setha M. Low, editor

Ethnopsychiatry

The Cultural Construction
of Professional and Folk Psychiatries

Edited by Atwood D. Gaines

State University of New York Press

Published by
State University of New York Press, Albany

For information, address State University of New York
Press, State University Plaza, Albany, NY 12246

Production by Cathleen Collins
Marketing by Lynne Lekakis

Library of Congress Cataloging-in-Publication Data

Ethnopsychiatry : the cultural construction of professional and folk
    psychiatries / Atwood D. Gaines, editor.
        p.   cm. — (SUNY series in medical anthropology)
    Includes index.
    ISBN 0–7914–1022–6 (pbk.) — ISBN 0–7914–1021–8
    1. Cultural psychiatry. 2. Medical anthropology.
I. Gaines, Atwood., 1945–   . II. Series.
[DNLM: 1. Cross-Cultural Comparison.
2. Ethnopsychology. 3. Medicine Traditional.
4. Mental Disorders—ethnology. WM 31 E84 1986]
RC455.4.E8E85   1992
616.89—dc20
DNLM/DLC
for Library of Congress   91–5076
                                                                                 CIP

10 9 8 7 6 5 4 3 2 1

*To the memory of
George Devereux;
scholar, friend,
and inspiration,*

*and
for my son, Woody;
rock on.*

Contents

One must ask, why should a discipline whose roots are so deeply planted in Western culture, whose major figures are almost entirely European and North American (and male), and whose data base is largely limited to the mainstream population in Western societies, why should so strongly Western-oriented a discipline regard cross-cultural research among the more than 80 percent of the world's people who inhabit non-Western societies as marginal? Is not cross-cultural research essential to establish the universality of mental illness and the international validity of psychiatric categories? Are not comparative studies an antidote to professional ethnocentrism? *Can psychiatry be a science if it is limited to middle-class whites in North America, the United Kingdom and Western Europe?*

Arthur Kleinmen
Rethinking Psychiatry:
From Cultural Category to Personal Experience

Preface

Borrowing Kleinman's words, I pose a question for anthropology in general and ethnopsychiatry in particular. Can anthropology be a science if it is limited in its normative ideology to middle-class Anglos in North America and Western Europe? In this volume, the reader will find united a variety of perspectives from a variety of sciences and life worlds. The articles focus on a range of professional and popular psychiatric systems around the world. The contributors include veritable novices in their first publishing ventures (Nomura, Oths and Blue), junior scholars (Farmer, Nuckolls, Hershel), scholars in or near mid-career (Csordas, Dwyer, Katz, Gaines, Jenkins, Rhodes, Swartz), and a senior scholar (Maretzki). The authors are from a variety of national, religious and cultural backgrounds including South African, German, Cosmopolitan, Japanese, Eastern and Western European-American Protestant, Catholic and Jewish. The scholars represent origins in both rural and urban areas as well.

The disciplines represented and more or less reflected in the authors' work include history, sociology, psychology, public health, psychoanalysis, medicine and psychiatry, as well as what I regard as the umbrella discipline, anthropology. In terms of the meeting of disciplines, it may be noted that many of the authors are trained in several fields; and a number apply at least one of their fields. Our accounts, then, come from scholars and practitioners of a variety of mainstream and alternative healing arts, from clinical and counseling psychology, medicine, public and international health to musculoskeletal massage. The inclusion of a range of vantage points is intended to provide the greatest possible view of our subject in order to overcome what has been in the past implicit, narrow andro- and Eurocentric perspectives in our field in general and in earlier noteworthy volumes in ethnomedicine, including, to a certain extent, several of my own done with Robert Hahn. In this we here take greater cognizance of the culturally situated nature of knowledge and the impact of age, gender, ethnic, disciplinary and national identities on knowledge, its production and reproduction and on its voice.

The volume's discourse is not necessarily radically different nor even remotely exhaustive. But the inclusion of a plethora of voices rather than one can help us gain some assurance that, after all, we are beginning to get the darn thing right; that our findings are less likely reproductions of one ethos, one cultural form of conventional wisdom or one ethnopsychology. We seemed headed in the right direction several decades ago with the very multicultural East West Center books in ethnopsychiatry. Unfortunately, those volumes, edited by Caudill and Lin (1969) and Lebra (1972, 1976), appear to have marked a moment, rather than a trend, in the direction of ethnopsychiatric research. It is a moment worthy of a renaissance.

The emphasis on professional ethnopsychiatries in this volume is intentional. Such psychiatric systems are, it is assumed by critics and proponents, set apart and distinct from their surrounding societies; their ideologies ontologically distinct from local popular ethnopsychiatries and ethnopsychologies. In the Western world, practitioners assume a scientific status of their ethnopsychiatry. They regard it as universal in its scientific bases and in its objects of concern, mental diseases. Until recently, this view was held within anthropology with respect to psychiatry and other fields of medicine. However, by including work on both folk and professional ethnopsychiatries, the volume metacommunicatively shows that both are cultural constructions. The volume symbolizes fully for the first time the observations of the last decade that folk and professional psychiatries are epistemologically comparable. As cultural constructions all, one is no more, nor less, privileged than another.

The selections in this volume seek to characterize various ethnopsychiatric ideologies and practices and place them in their respective and generative cultural contexts. My intent, and that of some of the contributors, is to present ethnopsychiatries from modern, interpretive social science perspectives as these seem appropriate to each. The interpretive stance for my own work is *cultural constructivism,* hence the subtitle of the volume. As is explained in the first chapter, cultural constructivism is a useful new paradigm for ethnopsychiatric and ethnomedical research. And, it is a critique of the various extant "critical medical anthropologies." Toward that end, the book is intended for the ethnopsychiatric and medical anthropological audiences, certainly. But it is hoped also that the focus on professional ethnopsychiatries will suggest to members of those bodies that something might be learned from our discipline, if only that they are now to be considered in the same discourse as shamans and medicine persons! While there is much of theoretical interest in the chapters, these studies of the reality and implications of practice and institutions can also serve as mirrors for professional healers who all too often assume that abstract ideals are real.

The present volume grew out of a 1986 symposium presented at the American Anthropological Association Meetings entitled, Ethnopsychiatry: Professional and Folk Knowledge and Practice. Three original participants appear in this volume, Oths, Farmer and Nuckolls, though their papers have changed greatly in the interim. As I set about finding other contributions for the projected volume, I realized that business as usual would not assemble the diverse group, in terms of gender, age, experience, etc., I felt was needed for a reformulated, new ethnopsychiatry, one which considers popular and professional ethnopsychiatries as a single domain in a multitude of voices. A 1987 American Anthropological Association Symposium on psychiatric institutions proved to be a rich vein. There, I found three excellent contributors, Dwyer, Hershel and Nomura. Because his conference paper already was committed, Dr. Nomura was kind enough to write a new chapter for inclusion here. I was fortunate that all agreed to participate in this venture. I have profited from their ideas.

I am also grateful to a number of others who do not appear in the volume, at least they do not appear in person. Nonetheless, I want to express my gratitude for the stimulation of my former colleague Allan Young, now of McGill University. Ever the great inquisitor, his probing always leads to new thoughts. I must give a thousand thanks to Allan and his wife, Roberta, for their support and generosity in Cleveland and in Montréal. A hard act to follow, Allan's large shoes are now ably filled by Janis Jenkins and Thomas Csordas whose stimulating company I have just begun to enjoy at Case Western Reserve University and whose work I am pleased to include in the present volume.

While I had intended to dedicate the volume to George Devereux, I was pleasantly surprised to find his presence in many of the papers that were submitted. The volume gives voice to my personal and professional appreciation of this great scholar, and adds to the recognition of his contributions to the field. This collection, and the specific articles employing his ideas, together constitute a veritable, if small, chorus in his honor. (See R. H. Hook, ed. *Fantasy and Symbol.* New York: Academic Press, 1979 and E. Schröder and D. Friessen, eds. *George Devereux zum 75 Geburtstag. Eine Festschrift.* Wiesbaden: Vieweg und Sohn Verlag, 1984, for *Festschriften* for Devereux.)

I want also to give my thanks to my alma mater, the University of California at Berkeley, where I spent much of my sabbatical in 1990 working on this volume. The Department of Anthropology kindly extended to me use of the considerable resources of the Department and the University. Special acknowledgement to Bill Simmons and Gerry Berreman there for help and friendship. And to the members of Humanities and Social Studies in Medicine at McGill University I express my appreciation for their collegiality and use of institutional resources as I put the final touches on this work. I acknowledge my debt to Lawrence Kirmayer of Psychiatry at McGill for his hospitality, library and his computer which helped me to update references. Finally, I must express my appreciation to Sue Wasserkrug, my graduate assistant, for her work on this and other projects over the last year.

Atwood D. Gaines
Montréal
August 1991

Section I

Orientations

1

Ethnopsychiatry:
The Cultural Construction of Psychiatries

Atwood D. Gaines

It doesn't matter whether your
sunglasses are off or on;
you only see the world you made[*]
  Bonnie Raitt

...we see the lives of others through
lenses of our own grinding and...they
look back on ours through ones of
their own[**]
  Clifford Geertz

Introduction: Ethnopyschiatry and the New Ethnopsychiatry

Psychiatric systems, like religions, kinship systems, or political systems, are culturally constructed. Each mirrors a culturally constructed reality, as Raitt (with John Hiatt's words) and Geertz suggest; but each sees itself as a reflection of an ultimate one. As such, folk and professional psychiatries are equally cultural, or ethnopsychiatries, the psychiatric edifices expressive of particular cultures. In this volume the reader will find a variety of ethnopsychiatric studies focusing on their actors, ideologies and institutions. Serving as foci of the papers are professional, scientific psychiatric systems of Europe, the Caribbean, South Africa, the United States and Asia, as well as the folk systems of those and other areas such as India, the U.S., Mexico and France. In the present chapter I will: 1) introduce the reader to the "new ethnopsychiatry," 2) provide an overview of the vol-

---

[*]"Thing Called Love" (John Hiatt), From: *Nick of Time*, Bonnie Raitt. Capital Compact Disc 7912682, (1989).
[**]Clifford Geertz, Anti-anti-relativism (1984).

ume's contributions, 3) briefly describe "cultural constructivism," a new paradigm for ethnopsychiatry and other ethnomedical research, and 4) briefly consider the future of the new ethnopsychiatry in terms of traditional and nascent topics of research.

Ethnopsychiatry: Old and New

Our field of study was first delineated by Hungarian-born, French and U.S.-trained anthropologist-psychoanalyst-classicist George Devereux (d. 1985). While Devereux should be credited as the architect of our field of study, its name-giver is Dr. Louis Mars, Haitian psychiatrist extraordinaire (see Farmer, this volume). As Devereux saw it, the field of ethnopsychiatry is, properly speaking, one of two forms of research. First, as he states in his groundbreaking book, *Mohave Ethnopsychiatry* (original 1961), ethnopsychiatry is:

> ...the systematic study of the psychiatric theories and practices of a primitive (sic) tribe. Its primary focus is, thus, the exploration of (a) culture that pertains to mental derangements, as (locally) understood. In this sense, (it) is comparable in its orientation to monographs entitled, e.g., "Ethnobotany" or "Ethnogeography" that deal respectively, with the botanical or geographical ideas, beliefs, and practices of some aboriginal group, but *are primarily contributions to anthropology rather than to botany or to geography*. (1969:1) (emphasis added)

And, in this sense, *Mohave Ethnopsychiatry* could be seen as:

> ...in simplest terms...a kind of "Mohave textbook of psychiatry," dictated by Mohave "psychiatrists" to the anthropological fieldworker. (1969:1

The second focus of work properly labeled ethnopsychiatry is:

> ...the recording of all obtainable information on psychiatric illnesses in the Mohave tribe and an analysis of their social and cultural setting. In this sense this work is a contribution to the study of "culture and the abnormal personality," or, as this field of inquiry is presently called, ethnopsychiatry. (Devereux 1969:1)

This second approach I refer to as "cross-cultural" or "transcultural psychiatry." It uses Western categories and looks for what are believed to be local permutations, but assumes that Western categories and nosologies are universally applicable (e.g., Simons and Hughes 1985). I take the field ethnopsychiatry to have as its focus mental derangements as locally understood, treated, managed, and classified. Traditionally, the field focused on folk psychiatry almost exclusively. Here, however, a "new ethnopsychiatry" is proposed. It takes as its subject all forms of ethnopsychiatric theory and practice whether folk or professional. The perspective of the present volume, then, represents an updating of Devereux's original conception(s) of the field.

As an example of the old versus the new ethnopsychiatry, one may consider the application of U.S. or French or English psychiatric knowledge to other cultures. In the new ethnopsychiatry, such would be seen as providing insight and data *both* on the psychiatric system from whose perspective(s) the study is conducted as well as that system or systems serving as the object(s) of study. We differ from Devereux in that all medicines and their psychiatries are seen here as cultural medicines, one no less culturally constructed than another. As a consequence, the distinction between folk and professional medicine is here seen as one of (culturally constructed) degree, not of kind. The term *folk psychiatry*, then, refers not to one kind of system relating to abnormal ethnopsychology and its treatment(s), but simply to a less formalized system than those represented by professional ethnopsychia- tries. Professional, "scientific" ethnopsychiatries of the United States, France, Japan or Germany are, then, to be seen as formalized, professional- ized, folk systems; they are epistemological siblings of their respective folk psychiatries. As such, all forms of psychiatry, whether formal or informal, professional or popular, are equally ethnopsychiatries. All may be consid ered and encompassed in the same discourse. Within specific cultural tradi- tions, popular and professional ethnopsychiatries represent the same cultur- al discourse with different voicings. This is the distinctive, emergent position I term the new ethnopsychiatry and which is reflected in the volume before the reader. The new ethnopsychiatry, unlike the old, has relevance not only for anthropology, but for professional (ethno)psychiatries as well.

In reading these essays, the reader quickly will discover that there is no universal psychiatric reality, no firm external base beyond culture on which stands a given ethnopsychiatry or upon which it reflects. The knowl- edge and practice of none are privileged. Rather, each professional and folk system is recognized as a reflection of a constructed world. With this view, we can begin to understand our own and others' systems for we will know enough of lenses and sunglasses to seek understandings in terms of the local knowledge that generates, validates, and perpetuates ethnopsychi- atric systems in their ontological, epistemological, and social dimensions.

Each ethnopsychiatric system of beliefs and practices may be seen as a historical dynamic process ever under construction, with its building blocks deriving from key local conceptions. These conceptions are local versions of reality related to "mental derangements" and their loci. Mem- bers of Western society (and others) and its medical professions commonly assume that their medical knowledge and practice are "scientific," neutral, and set apart from the conventional beliefs and practices of the society in which they are found. This same point of view is argued by various political economic writers, albeit for slightly different reasons. Nonetheless, they demonstrate their epistemological kinship with European scientistic thought. However, here we argue, and present much evidence to demonstrate the view, that both folk and professional systems are equally culturally constructed, equally cultural forms of psychological medicine. In this, we recognize and affirm that sciences and medicines (e.g., of the United States, China, India) are preeminently cultural constructions.

This volume serves a dual purpose. First, it presents the ethnopsychiatric knowledge and practice of a number of cultures, as one might expect in a volume on ethnopsychiatry. Second, since the contributors to the volume recognize the culturally constructed realities of professional ethnopsychiatries, the volume simultaneously serves as a "cultural critique" (Marcus and Fischer 1986), of popular and professional ethnopsychiatries. Interpretive approaches provide the means by which these ethnopsychiatries can be *deconstructed*, exposing the made nature of that which appears to be natural and independent of human constructive action. The contributors reflect upon the constructed nature of such systems and demonstrate their formative cultural contexts. Largely as studies of scientific psychiatric medicines, this collection additionally provides an opportunity to reflect upon our own discipline of anthropology, one of the key rationales for the study of these scientific medical systems (Gaines and Hahn 1985).

The articles in the present volume do not stereotype professional or folk psychiatries by assuming or asserting homogeneity or the primacy of one form over another. Rather, these essays show that discussions of scientific, *cosmopolitan* or traditional, local psychiatries belong to the same interpretive discourse on cultural systems. In this sense the present volume serves to update the founding conceptualizations of the field and forthrightly presents a new ethnopsychiatry. In doing so, it should be noted that since the essays in this volume were not commissioned, but rather represent independent work, we are really recognizing a presence rather than creating one.

While updating, even reinventing, his founding conceptions, the present works also recall Devereux's formative studies. Many contributions focus on institutions as did some of his early work (e.g., 1944, 1949). Also recalled is the classic study of Caudill's (1958). However, the present volume largely uses interpretive perspectives while the early studies of Caudill, Devereux, and others (e.g., Goffman 1961), were more concerned with institutions as stable systems and with their maintenance and their effect on patients (see Hershel, this volume). In contrast, this collection generally evidences a concern for the diachronic interpretive apprehension of psychiatric knowledge and action. Professional knowledge and action are considered as problematic, to be interpreted as cultural constructions, thus to be "deconstructed" (the disassembly and revelation of their constituent cultural elements). There is also room in these studies for consideration of both healers and patients as parts of the *same* wider cultural dramas and fields.

Although contributors do not necessarily address causes of illness, their critical view of biological, and other empirical, explanations is fairly clear, if sometimes unstated. The essays in the present volume eschew the universalist, synchronic and positivist forms of explanation characteristic of so-called "critical medical anthropology" (CMA) (e.g., Baer, Singer and Johnson 1986; Singer 1986; Frankenberg 1988; Morgan 1987). Because there are in fact a number of distinct approaches under this rubric (Morgan 1987), the plural acronym will be used (CMAs). Like medicine itself, such approaches produce understandings of sickness that are "thin" indeed (Gaines 1991; Press 1990).

While seeing folk ethnomedicines as cultural (and dominated by biomedicine), CMAs argue that there is a single (Western) professional medicine and psychiatry set apart and opposed to society. Its knowledge is said to be ideology, in the pejorative sense, and is held to be distinct from that of society. Psychiatric (and medical) ideology and practice are asserted to be consciously (sometimes unconsciously) constructed to serve solely as a means of social control, i.e., CMAs commonly propose varieties of functionalist equilibrium theory. Such perspectives suggest that the ideology, the beliefs, and knowledge of psychiatry are not problematic. Rather, they portray all medical and psychiatric knowledge as interest-generated rationalizations, consciously constructed fictions employed to control society (e.g., Baer 1982; Frankenberg 1988; Ingleby 1980, 1983; Singer, Baer and Lazarus 1990; Waitzkin 1979, 1981). Questionable, too, are the reified notions of power found in CMAs (see Rhodes 1991, this volume; Gaines 1991).

Were such assertions accurate, one would not expect to find cultural conceptions and formulations encoded in professional or popular ethnopsychiatric knowledge and practice that are hundreds, in some cases, thousands of years old. However, such demonstrably *is* the case with respect to U.S., Chinese, German, French or other ethnopsychiatric system one might care to investigate (see Foucault 1965; Gaines 1992; Gilman 1988a; Kirmayer 1988; Kleinman 1986; Menninger et al. 1963; Simon 1978). And, any close look at folk or professional psychiatric practice clearly demonstrates the extraordinarily complex webs of significance and meaning that are woven into both thought and practice. Analyses reveal the constructed nature of knowledge and praxis and their local cultural genesis (DelVecchio Good 1988; Gaines 1982a,b,c; Lock 1987; Lock and Gordon 1988; Ohnuki-Tierney 1984; Townsend 1978; Turkle 1978; Weisberg and Long 1984; Young 1988, 1991). But the constructions and their bases are to be seen as shared with the wider society of a particular ethnopsychiatry except when imposed (see Swartz, this volume, for an imposed colonial ethnopsychiatry). CMAs will be critiqued further below.

Ethnopsychiatric beliefs and practices appear under the anthropological gaze as complex, historically constructed cultural tapestries which both
cloak *and* reveal fundamental understandings about life, disorder, experience, person and cultural voice (Conner 1982; Devereux 1969, 1980a,b;
Gaines 1985a, 1989, 1992; Kirmayer 1988). Although, it is not their specific
primary intent, the essays in this volume demonstrate the inadequacy of
CMAs' views and their misrepresentations of professional medicines and
psychiatries. While the studies here focus on the realities of ideology and
praxis of folk and professional ethnopsychiatries, critical medical anthropological perspectives are grounded in nineteenth-century ideology that is
and was, on the theoretical level, deductivist positivism, usually of the functionalist sort. And, on the level of fundamental assumptions, such perspectives also may be seen to be andro- and/or Eurocentric (Tomm and Hamilton 1988; see Morsy [1978, 1991] for a CMA view of the latter point).

Ethnopsychiatries are properly considered as demonstrations of
modal realism for they reflect their respective underlying ethnopsychologies
focused on the domain(s) of abnormal (ethno)psychology. This should seem
obvious, but oddly, while most researchers now accept the fact that culture
shapes normal human behavior, even many culturally cognizant authors
explicitly or implicitly, and contradictorily, assert that abnormal behavior
is somehow exempt from the impress of socialization, training, and experience. That is, they suggest that while normality is cultural, abnormality is
acultural and universal. Such is the basis for the biological approaches to
mental illness (e.g., Simons and Hughes 1985; Yap 1974; and Prince and
Tcheng-Laroche 1987).

As the essays collected here show, illness varies in its nature and seri-
ousness with each culture, as do the criteria determining the nature of the
problematic ideation and/or behavior (e.g., Westermeyer and Wintrob
1979). In line with a new paradigm in medical anthropology, "embodiment," advocated by Csordas (1990),[1] there needs to be a recognition that
ethnopsychiatric systems are embodiments of their respective ethnopsychologies' concerns for, and delineations of, the normal and abnormal self
and the Other (Devereux 1969, 1980a; Gaines 1992; Lutz 1985; Obeyesekere 1985).

Boundaries and Representations

The papers in this volume were selected to represent a variety of
places and topics, but also a variety of voices in terms of characteristics
generally excluded from consideration but which, nonetheless, greatly
affect our representations of cultural and social realities. That is, the contributors represent various ethnopsychiatries from a variety of vantage
points in terms of sex, ethnic and national origin, native language, disci-

plinary training, age, stage in career, type, or lack, of institutional affiliation, and in terms of clinical/healer experience. In this sense, the contributors "traverse boundaries" (Good, Gordon and Pandolfi 1990) not only in their research but also in their being-in-the-world.[2] This heterogeneous group extends our vantage points beyond the usual "intellectual niches" of normal (i.e., customary) academic research and thought (see Geertz 1983). This diversity works against the andro- and Eurocentric norms and the academy-centeredness and is seen here as a crucial component of the new ethnopsychiatry, an aspect of the social organization of its work. Here it is perhaps more brought to consciousness than fully realized; we can say we have made but a second beginning in the normalization of a multicentered, multivocal professional discourse. Twenty years ago, in ethnopsychiatry, we had a series of studies from Hawai'i exemplary in this respect (see Caudill and Lin 1969; W. Lebra 1972, 1976)

In addition, the new ethnopsychiatric discourse presented here in a substantial way considers issues of communalism (e.g., racism) and gender as part of its normal discourse. Usually, such considerations lead to a separate, i.e., segregated, discourse with separate publications, audiences, reviews, and the like. Such work should appear unexceptionally as part of normative, diversified, disciplinary discourse. Communalism is an aspect, not the central concern of many of our contributions. While this is merely as it should be, an integration of concerns in a single focal discourse is strangely uncommon.

The contributors are united by their interests and, to a certain extent, in their approaches. While most contributors were not aware of the formulation of cultural constructivism, which is presented below and which emphasizes culture, meaning and history in medical anthropology, appropriately absent are the contrasting functionalist paradigms and totalizing ideologies of positivist social science. In their stead, we find here sensitive treatments of history, persons, and processes. The studies not only begin to unravel the extraordinarily complex webs of meaning and significance which constitute particular ethnopsychiatries, but they also portray the culturally constitution of knowledge and experience of actors (patients *and* healers).

Overview of the Volume

The contributions to this volume offer a variety of studies of ethnopsychiatric ideologies and institutions around the world. The first section, "Orientations," contains the present chapter and a second by anthropologist Lorna Rhodes. Her work considers the notion of power in medical anthropology. The two chapters of the section focus largely on theoretical issues, but the second embeds this in the context of an ethnographic study.

Specifically, Rhodes's contribution analyzes power in psychiatric and medical anthropological theory and in a particular clinical setting on the East Coast of the United States. Her chapter continues her work on U.S. psychiatric institutions (e.g., Rhodes 1986), and is drawn from her recently published book (1991). She finds that the diagnosis and disposition of a particular patient becomes problematic and in so doing exposes for us the nature of power, its limitations, and the outlines of the local system. Rhodes critiques CMA perspectives on power using Foucault's insights as important tools. But she sees these very tools as needing some modification. Rhodes shows the problematic nature of critical medical anthropologists' view of power. They see "it" as an external and autonomous force wielded by psychiatrists and their associates. In her sensitive portrayal of the case of "the Judge," Rhodes shows that many forces are at work. Most of these are clearly local and impinge not only on patients, but on healers as well. The article clearly shows that the simple dichotomy, however implicit, of controllers and controlled, poorly represents clinical, or other, realities.

Rhodes's paper contributes to further questioning of Foucault's body of work as it relates to medical and state power (Gilman 1988a; Skultans 1979). His work on the state and its omnipotence and his *panopticon* are in fact based on French culture and history. Salient features of French culture include its historically, extraordinarily centralized and authoritarian state organization, with a religious tradition to match. Given these cultural realities, one could regard Foucault's work on the state, and its control of bodies and spaces between them (1973, 1975, 1979), as largely ethnographic rather than as of general applicability to other countries lacking France's level of centralization.

The first paper in "Section II: Illness, Experience and the Problematics of Ethnopsychiatric Knowledge," is by anthropologist Charles Nuckolls. He focuses on the standard of sanity and insanity in an Indian village. He shows the importance of cultural models of insanity as standards against which deviations are measured. As has been noted earlier by Devereux (1980b), ethnopsychiatric judgements in point of fact are not based upon the observation and measurement from an abstract, absolute standard of normalcy. Rather, they are made by comparison to (cultural) models of disorder/disease.

Naidu, the central figure of the article, is found to possess "social mass," after Devereux's formulation, but is without the expected dynamics of authority, i.e., appropriate kinship affiliations, political power, religious position or wealth. We find that Naidu serves as a standard allowing the calibration of the crucial local diagnostic domain of psychopathology; he is the embodied model of madness. Nuckolls concludes by comparing South Indian and U.S. diagnostic practices, showing the similar use of cognitive models build from remembered experiences in Indian folk and United States professional ethnopsychiatry to make diagnostic judgements.

The second paper in section II, Kathryn Oths's study of Chiropractic,

is the first of two contributions focusing on seemingly ancillary ethnopsychiatric figures; the second is Dwyer's study of nineteenth-century women
attendants in New York. In this chapter, anthropologist Oths gives us a
detailed account of the ethnopsychiatric aspects of Chiropractic in the
United States. Her ethnographic research in the office of a U.S. chiropractic healer shows the use, unintentional and intentional, of psychotherapeutic techniques. She compares *spiritist* healing with Chiropractic, to highlight the latter, and compares both with U.S. psychiatry, especially its
biological forms. She shows how the care of chronic problems allows for the
development of a (psycho)therapeutic relationship. Oths's paper, from a
practitioner of musculoskeletal manipulation, takes a biocultural view
unique to the volume. Her paper contributes to our understanding of Chiropractic and to its role in the total ethnopsychiatric system of the United
States. The paper is included here to oppose the tendency of CMAs, and
others interested in professional ethnopsychiatry, to focus on these presumably high status and powerful professionals to the exclusion of other formal
or informal ethnopsychiatric resources. These forms, in fact, overlap with
both professional medicine and popular society, thereby demonstrating
their kindred epistemological spirits.

Anthropologist Thomas Csordas extends his 20 years of work on ritual and charismatic religion, suffering, and embodiment (Csordas 1983,
1990) in "The Affliction of Martin" (chapter 5). Csordas is concerned to
elucidate the relationship between religious and secular clinical embodiments of human suffering in a case of demonic oppression. He first presents
an extended account of Martin's condition and the knowledge and practices
of a charismatic healer, "Peggy," who cares for him. After this presentation, he contrasts critiques elicited from mental health professionals and
charismatic healing ministers of Martin's affliction and of Peggy's healing
strategy and ideology.

Csordas's work provides a critique of the work and beliefs of the
charismatic healer who took on the task of healing Martin. The critique is
provided not by the anthropologist, but by a group of charismatic healers
and a group of secular professional clinicians that are asked to interpret the
case. The paper demonstrates how all three accounts are forms of the objectifications of meanings inherent in sensory experience. As well, the affliction
of Martin embodies and reflects local cultural, as well as idiosyncratic,
meanings. In this, Csordas enlarges upon his notion of embodiment as a
paradigm for medical anthropology, including ethnopsychiatry, presented
in his Stirling Award-winning paper (the award is given by the Association of
Psychological Anthropologists) (Csordas 1990) (see also M. Johnson 1987).

Chapter 6, by the editor, an anthropologist with public health training, considers medical psychiatric knowledge in France and the United
States. Extending his earlier work in those countries on professional

ethnopsychiatry and on social classification, Gaines's chapter initiates an examination of the ontological status of "biology" in the two psychiatric medicines. It considers biology as a cultural system. As one of several explicitly ethnological papers in the volume (the others are those of Nuckolls and Hershel), the paper suggests that biology is a central symbol rather than an external, discoverable reality. As a consequence, very different meanings and referents of "the biological" are discernable in French and U.S. psychiatry. Central to the analysis presented is his notion of "Sickness History." A sickness history is a culture's historical experience with particular diseases/illness and with the perceived social context thereof (e.g., women, "minorities"). The notion specifically refers to cultural categories of thought established over historical time which frame both folk and professional interpretations of and responses to contemporary sickness experiences (see Gaines 1991).

In chapter 7, Stirling Award-winning (Jenkins, 1991a) anthropologist Janis Hunter Jenkins considers schizophrenia and emotional overinvolvement of family members in the life of an afflicted person within the context of Mexican families. Her work not only shows us the family situation of and response to disorder in this cultural context, but also the folk ethnopsychological constructions of what biomedicine terms "schizophrenia." Her methodology includes the use of locals' critiques of other's behavior as the basis of the definition of the "overinvolvement" of particular family members. Her paper extends her work on *Mexicanos* and Expressed Emotion (1988, 1991a) which foreshadowed her work with Salvadoran refugees (see Jenkins 1991b).

In the papers by Csordas, Jenkins, and Swartz, we see the critical evaluation of the behavior of culture mates. These papers recall the editor's suggestion of the need for an "anthropology of cultural competence" (Gaines 1987a). Such an enterprise would not assume a homogeneous view of cultural enactment, i.e., that all people in a particular culture enact it equally well. In every culture, those who know the tradition, implicitly or explicitly, make judgements about themselves and others; that is, they critique the cultural competence/appropriateness of others' (and their own) beliefs and/or actions within the context of their common culture. Using the differences of opinion and/or perspectives within a culture, a critique of culture can be generated from *within* a cultural tradition. This renders moot the anti-relativist argument (see Geertz 1984) that construes cultural relativism as a barrier to the cross-cultural application of critical or ethical judgement(s) (e.g., Dan Gordon 1991; and see Morsy, 1991, for a fine critique of this sort of problematic humanitarianism, constructed biomedical pragmatism and implicit Orientalism).

In the first chapter in section III, "Professional Ethnopsychiatric Ideologies and Institutions," South African clinical psychologist Leslie Swartz analyzes professional ethnopsychiatry in his native country and its misuses of the notion of relativism. Here relativism conceals racism, albeit not very well. Swartz provides a consideration of the sociopolitical uses of the concept. South African psychiatry, as an expression of institutionalized racism, distorts the notion of relativism to legitimize and support "white" minority authority and ideology. The concept of relativism is not invoked as a means of understanding cultural difference and developing a cross-cultural or culturally appropriate psychiatry, as is the case in Haïti (Farmer, this volume).

The psychiatry is, then, an expression of its South African context and attempts to justify a colonial elite, an imposed culture and ideology. We see also that South African psychiatric logic follows local cultural assumptions about social classification ("black, white, Indian and coloured"), as is also the case, but with a different and even less logical system, in the United States (see Gaines, this volume). Swartz cogently argues, as does this volume as a whole, that researchers should pay attention to hidden cultural ideologies (cultural assumptions, including "race" and gender assumptions/roles) of apparently rational and pragmatic expressions in professional psychiatric theory and practice. While closest to a reality asserted to be common by Critical Medical Anthropologies' notions of medicine and psychiatry, South Africa's situation is obviously a local cultural creation and is not typical. It is also a case where the ethnopsychology of one group is imposed on several others.

U.S. physician-anthropologist Paul Farmer provides us with an account of the "Birth of the *Klinik*" (chapter 9), Haitian *patois* (and a pun *in re* Foucault) for a history of Haitian professional ethnopsychiatry. In this poor land, where Farmer for years has been volunteering his medical and anthropological skills, we find a sophisticated professional ethnopsychiatry, not an impoverished one. It is cognizant of and pays attention to the cultural construction of illness, cultural variations in the conception of the person, and to the cultural shaping of the expression of psychopathology. It is likewise cognizant of the cultural biases of Western nosologies (see also Farmer 1980).

This professional ethnopsychiatric reality contrasts sharply with the characterizations of professional medicine from political economic or world systems approaches found in critical medical anthropologies. There, a unitary, culturally irrelevant ethnopsychiatry is seen as exerting hegemony and is said to have been created by extra-local economic forces (Frankenberg 1988; Ingleby 1980, 1983). One would expect these views to be presented in high relief in Haïti, but they are not. In Haïti, we also find irony; the local construction of professional ethnopsychiatric reality is substantially derived from George Devereux himself, through his roles as teacher, friend, and colleague of several of Haïti's psychiatrists. Not the least of these is Haitian psychiatry's founder, Dr. Louis Mars.[3] Perhaps uniquely, we here find a case wherein the cultural history, and clinical and theoretical present, of a professional ethnopsychiatry embodies and expresses aspects of the very discipline for which it is now an object of study; a rare instance of truly reflexive anthropology. The role of racism is also considered central there.

Naoki Nomura presents an account of psychiatrist and patient interaction in Japan (chapter 10). Nomura, a Japanese-born and United States-trained anthropologist, finds that cultural and psychological factors reported by researchers are useful points of departure for a consideration of the cultural bases of ethnopsychiatric interactions. This study considers only a segment of the total range of psychiatric interactions, specifically focusing on a psychiatrist interacting with patients in the outpatient clinic of pseudonymous Hiraoka Mental Hospital. The goal of the paper, and well met it is, is to elucidate cultural and interactional factors embedded in verbal and nonverbal exchanges between the doctor and his patients by analyzing actual interactions. The paper's interactional perspective recalls the earliest work on folk and professional psychiatry done from an interpretive perspective which incorporated aspects of interaction theory (see Good [1977] on Iranian and Gaines [1979] on the U.S.'s professional ethnopsychiatry, both also owing debts to V. Turner [e.g., 1964] and Geertz [1973]).

In chapter 11, U.S. historian Ellen Dwyer opens the section on "Ethnopsychiatric Ideologies and Institutions." Dwyer's chapter focuses on female attendants in several New York asylums of the nineteenth century. She explores their social roles and experiences, including their conditions of hiring, work, and discharge. She shows how the institutional roles were modeled on the Victorian family with the superintendent as the father and patriarch. The largely female attendant staff was defined as sorts of governesses, thus showing the projection of popular social ideals of gender and social roles into the asylum.

In their role(s), a result of sexist stereotyping of the time, attendants, while part parent, part domestic, and part caregiver, were nevertheless completely underpaid and underappreciated. Dwyer provides a fine institutional culture history focusing on overlooked but key ethnopsychiatric figures. In addition to providing excellent material on women and work from the last century, the chapter also allows us to see how the cultural context generates the roles in professional ethnopsychiatric institutions. This represents a tie to the anthropologically informed "new culture history" (see Hunt 1989), also called "anthropological " or "ethnological history" (see Le Goff 1980) but which we have seen in the earlier historical works by George Homans and A.F.C. Wallace in anthropology.

Chapter 12 presents results of a participant-observational study of several French and American mental institutions. Using Weber's notion of ideal types, sociologist and psychotherapist Helena Jia Hershel develops a schema for classifying mental institutions. Case studies of four institutions are presented. She shows that variation in treatment ideology, in the match of institutional norms with those of the larger culture, and patient-staff power relations determine specific rule structures. In turn, these structures engender particular levels of patient expressiveness, including aggressive behavior.

Hershel sees her findings as generating a scheme for analyzing problems in different institutions. While the closest to a functionalist study, Hershel's work acquires depth through the use of the concept of culture and her recognition of the importance of cultural context for institutional behavior. This is something also noted in Dwyer's (11) and Nomura's (10) chapters. These studies of the structure of hospitals and the wards within them demonstrate the validity of seeing psychiatries and their institutions in and of their cultural context(s). In Hershel's study, the French institutions, as do those in the U.S., reflect local cultural context, not universal ideological or organizational hegemony.

Anthropologist Amy Blue's chapter (13) represents one of the first anthropological accounts of professional ethnopsychiatry in Greece. Her study provides a historical account of the development of the profession of ethnopsychiatry. Her recent dissertation (1991) adds considerable detail on both history and current organization and practice. Here, Blue pays attention to the development of institutions which, after a fashion, serve the mentally afflicted. She also considers the development of the psychiatric profession itself in the context of Greek socio/political history. As an autonomous branch of medicine, psychiatry in Greece is only a little over a decade old. Its current organization is found to be a *potpourri* of elements borrowed from, and its psychiatrists trained in, other countries. From an outsider's viewpoint, it is ironic that the land that gave so many psychological conceptions to folk and professional medicines and psychiatries in the Old and New Worlds (see Menninger et al. 1963) should itself be so late in the development of an autonomous psychiatric profession, and that only with considerable pushing from other European Economic Community (EEC) countries (Blue 1991).

Pearl Katz's chapter (14) examines cultural conflicts within a state mental health system in the United States. An anthropologist with psychoanalytic training, Katz considers both the local and the state levels and their mutual influences. Bureaucratic institutional processes at the state level, such as the development of state mental health organizations and policies, and the evolution of two distinct psychiatric training subcultures are sketched. Also examined are the local-level institutional processes and structures in one state mental hospital. With reference to the latter, attention is paid to structural and organizational rigidity. Both local- and state-level forces of change are examined. Katz interprets cultural conflicts enacted on the local level in the context and under the influence of the wider, extra-local, state level which itself is seen as historical process.

In this chapter, we discern bureaucratic conflicts that are actually cultural and gender conflicts. That is, the hospital is staffed by Middle Eastern men and operates in terms of a Mediterranean family-centered, personalistic and androcentric ethos, seen briefly in chapters 6 and 13 and discussed below (also see Gaines 1982; Gaines and Farmer 1986). This ethos conflicts with the Northern European (Protestant) tradition that constitutes the ethos of the state, represented in Katz's article by a female psychiatrist placed in charge of the institution. We see here a conflict of cultures, ethnic and gender, such as we will surely encounter more of in the future in this, or the reversed, form.

In chapter 15, a senior medical anthropologist, Thomas Maretzki continues his work on the professional medicine of his natal land, Germany (also see Maretzki 1988; Maretzki and Seidler 1985). In his contribution, Maretzki describes the integrative therapies of Georg Groddeck who combined *psyche* and *soma* and developed somatic and psychotherapies (under the influence of Freud himself) tailored to individual patients in his private sanatorium which opened in 1900.

Maretzki's account clearly shows how creativity and innovation, as well a personal history, shape clinical reality and therapeutic practices in the context of a professional psychiatry. This historical paper adds to our understanding of demonstrated complexity and wide variations within a professional ethnopsychiatry even in a single place (Gaines 1979; Johnson 1985; Light 1980). The fact of this wide variation is increasingly clear in professional ethnopsychiatries, but it is also noteworthy, though often overlooked, in traditional ethnopsychiatries (see Gaines 1987b; Grim 1983; Devereux 1957). It is also evident that demonstrated personal variations as well as local resistance, creativity, and innovation, are not explainable by "macrocentric" critical medical anthropological views.

The last section, "Sources and Resources," contains the volume's final chapter by Blue and Gaines. It reviews and comments briefly on a large number of ethnopsychiatric and ethnopsychiatrically relevant studies. We hope to be extensive but cannot hope to be exhaustive. Some works are given special consideration while others are simply noted in passing. The chapter provides the reader unfamiliar with ethnopsychiatry an overview of the field and a substantial bibliography. And, it is hoped that some new, less available or well-known, material is provided for those familiar with the field.

Because the new ethnopsychiatry does not privilege any one professional or popular ethnopsychiatric knowledge, the number of works which could be included is virtually limitless. We could justify inclusion of every article or book ever published in psychiatry, clinical psychology, counseling, pastoral counseling and clinical social work as well as all social science works related to or on these and all other, popular, ethnopsychiatric forms.

The recognition in the new ethnopsychiatry of the direct relationship to psychiatric phenomena of nonpsychiatric phenomena, i.e., person concepts, forms of conflict resolution, terrorism, stress, etc., also contribute to the potentially infinite number of relevant works. Our primary interest there is to include studies by anthropologists, sociologists, historians, psychiatrists, and psychologists who are contributing or have contributed to the cultural and cross-cultural debates along with those works by others which are of use to such exchanges.

II. Cultural Constructivism

In this section, I wish to consider in more detail problems with certain approaches found in medical anthropology which are applied to medical and psychiatric issues. Historically, in sociology and in anthropology, the focus was on macrosystems, economy or notions of professionalization and the like. The focus on knowledge and experience, the means by which they are constituted, conveyed, and lived, may be said to be a new turn in the social science of medicine which is of cardinal importance. It leads directly from interpretive, here termed cultural constructive, research emphases. Contrasting with this are the critical forms of research which lead us away from human experience to attributions of needs, desires, and motives to extra-human, nonsentient economic systems, structures, and forces.

Research from critical perspectives seeks to attribute causes to higher order realities. In doing so, it produces a macrocentric view which excludes history, persons, meanings, and local-level realities. As a consequence, investigations of local-level realities do not bear out the predictions or expectations of critical medical anthropology (e.g., Castel, Castel and Lovell 1982; Gaines 1991; Morgan 1987). The contributions to this volume further demonstrate the discrepancy between critical medical anthropological views and local ethnopsychiatric realities while not neglecting extra-local phenomena.

The articles of this volume reflect perspectives I have elsewhere grouped under the rubric cultural constructivism (1991). The term both summarizes key distinctive ideas and serves as a convenient contrast to the various critical medical anthropologies (see Morgan 1987). Below, the perspective is briefly delineated for medical anthropology, and its points of difference with critical medical anthropologies are presented. (For an earlier account, see Gaines [1991].)

Cultural constructivism has a related perspective in sociology called "social constructionism" (Wright and Treacher 1982a, b). The term cultural constructivism is preferred for I am concerned to distinguish an anthropological enterprise from a sociological one and to stress the importance of the key concept of culture. Culture is seen from a historical, interactionist, and semantic perspective. I suggest that theoretical paradigms developed before, or independently of, the modern notion of culture (i.e., "precultural" theories) have greatly limited, if any, utility for modern social science. These precultural forms of social science represent archaic, ethno- and Eurocentric forms and moments of Western social science.

Cultural constructivism (and much social constructionism) provides the basis for important critiques of Western beliefs, practices, and institutions, including those of its professional ethnomedicines. Subjects of these critiques are their systems of knowledge, that is, their classificatory systems (e.g,, the Diagnostic and Statistical Manuals of U.S. Psychiatry (American Psychiatric Association (APA) 1952, 1968, 1980, 1987) (Gaines 1992; Nuckolls 1992; Lock 1987), as well as education, organization and practice.

The constructivist approach allows for the understanding of medical knowledge as an expression of culture rather than as elite knowledge set apart and opposed to society in the form of some putative class (as in Marxist approaches) or "scientific" (as in medicine's view) ideology. While Marxisms and medicine construe medical knowledge in their own way, both agree that is an acultural ideology (Gaines and Hahn 1985).

Critical medical anthropology says, if it says anything at all about peoples' sickness experiences, that sickness is *caused* by "capitalism," "the modern world capitalist system," "social structure," "class" or "power relations," and or other hypothesized structures, processes or systems (e.g., Baer 1982, 1986; Baer, Singer and Johnson 1986; Frankenberg 1980, 1988; Navarro 1976; Scheder 1988; Scheper-Hughes 1988; Susser 1988). It is apparent to others, however, that such putatively causal entities/forces are the positivist constructs of the writers, not extant realities. "Classes," "social control," "hegemony" (Singer, Baer and Lazarus 1990:vi) are but analysts' unexamined and uncritically adopted scientistic (and Eurocentric) conceptions (Gaines 1991; Morgan 1987; Young 1982). As a consequence, while CMAs' advocates present their approaches as new and improved for the study of medical issues, they fail to note that the same conceptions have been tried and rejected in the wider domain of modern social science (not to mention those of European society and politics) (see Rabinow and Sullivan 1979; 1987). Indeed, Ortner (1984) shows how such deductive scientism remade itself in the anthropology of the '70s and '80s such that currently the differences between such positions and interpretive, i.e., cultural constructivist, social science can be quite slight. The shift to interpretive perspectives was forced by inherent weaknesses in the materialist positions, but CMAs' perspectives, presented as remedies, are analogues of models current *prior* to the shift to incorporate interpretive tenets.

Critical views implicitly reaffirm the theory of universal diseases and medicine's perception, labeling, and classification thereof. They differ with medicine only in their attribution of the *causes* of putatively empirical dis-

eases. Ignoring culture, history, meaning, and human agency, critical medical perspectives merely propose other materialist theories of disease etiology
(market position, class, economy) and attribute rationalist, albeit malevo-
lent, motives to healers as social actors. These motives are somehow induced
by external, experience-distant, economic systems. Contradictorily, professional physicians are seen as autonomous and somehow personally responsible for society's medical problems (Waitzkin, Navarro, Frankenberg).

Unlike the political economy of health, constructivist research pays
attention to and, indeed, focuses attention on, meaning, human frailty and
suffering. Important are human agency and responsibility, and ethical considerations of theory and practice (e.g., Jenkins 1991b; Kleinman 1988b;
Ots 1988; Young 1990). Human experience, and how local cultural history,
context, and knowledge construct and shape it, are focal concerns. Ethnomedical research needs to remain cognizant of the cultural nature and
context, for medical systems are not autonomous, isolated sociocultural
strata (Elkana 1981). They represent moments of historical social and cultural processes including borrowing. Given instances are but moments of a
culture-in-the-making, and as such provide one of many windows in the
house of culture into which one might choose to gaze.

Critical researchers ignore the common bases of lay and professional
medical ideologies which are essential to their credibility and utility for a
society's people. As well, CMAs' views conceal, rather than illuminate, the
very real and profound differences among the professional medicines of
various countries. This concealment is accomplished by defining *a priori*
the object of study as economic, acultural and universal.

The cultural constructivist rubric subsumes forms of interpretive
social science in medicine that draw from different theoretical traditions
and which are referred to under a variety of labels. These include: "interpretive," "hermeneutic," "cultural/symbolic studies," "Kleinman's school,"
"meaning-centered," "anthropology of biomedicine" and "semantic"
approaches. Various of these approaches have been subsumed under the
label "microlevel" and "explanatory model approach" (or "EM theorists")
by critical medical anthropologists. The latter designations represent constructivist approaches as being concerned narrowly with definitions of individuals' illness only in the clinical context. It is asserted that the critical
concerns are with "wider issues" i.e, putatively autonomous economic or
political forces at the state or world level (e.g., Baer, Singer and Johnson
1986; Lazarus 1988; Navarro 1976; Singer 1986).

However, constructivist research has never so narrowly defined its
scope of work, nor could it have. Constructivist interests are and have been
medical knowledge and social action in its cultural and social context.
These interests have been reflected in all such studies since the field began
to attract attention and to flourish. Interpretive work continues to fruitful-

ly focus on specific issues far outside of the local clinical setting, as Low notes (1988). These include an interest in and delineation of the "local health care system," ethnomedical efficacy, help-seeking, culture- and society-wide networks of illness meaning and theories, professional medical ideology, medical status, social organization and structure (hierarchy, interactions, status, relationships), and medical history, medical education, and clinical and research practices (e.g., Comaroff 1982; Eisenberg and Kleinman 1981; Gaines and Hahn 1982; Hahn and Gaines 1985; Good, Good and Fischer 1988; Kleinman 1980, 1986; Kleinman, Eisenberg and Good 1978; Lock 1980; Lock and Gordon 1988; Latour and Wolgar 1979; Young 1988, 1990, 1991). The contributions gathered here likewise show concern for the total social context.

Failing to recognize the unique and novel perspective represented by constructivist approaches as parts of a larger interpretive social science (see Marcus and Fischer 1986; Geertz 1973, 1983, 1984; Rabinow and Sullivan 1979, 1987), critical medical anthropologists argue that their approaches are new and will provide greater insights into medical issues. However, we recognize in them the same nineteenth-century acultural, scientistic assumptions that underlie and govern normal science and biomedicine itself (Geertz 1984; Gaines 1991; Gordon 1988; Mendelsohn and Elkana 1981).

Critical approaches cannot provide new understandings of things ethnomedical because their research is based upon the same assumptions as the object of study. Their criticisms actually serve as affirmations of the Eurocentric, rationalist scientism of biomedicine itself. As well, such approaches generally do not consider actual professional medical behavior and experiences, preferring to characterize them as internally undifferentiated and homogeneous (e.g., Ingleby 1980; Frankenberg 1988). Constructivism suggests a different set of fundamental assumptions to lead us to an understanding of the cultural constructions of medicines and psychiatries.

Five central assumptions occur to me now as necessary frames for cultural constructivist medical anthropological research in complex or simple societies (see Gaines 1991, for the first outline with four assumptions.) It is clear that many of these ideas are implicitly shared with the contributors. I do not attempt here to present some of the deeper level notions underlying cultural constructivism (e.g., anti-atomism, modal realism), but rather emphasize the more operational notions which frame my own work and at least some aspects of those views I have grouped under the term.

Cultural Constructivism: Some Key Assumptions

1. ETHNOMEDICAL KNOWLEDGE IS PROBLEMATIC

The first assumption of a constructivist approach is that medical knowledge is problematic. Such a notion was doubtless axiomatic for early researchers of popular and folk (or "primitive") medicines. However, recent research, including that contained in the present volume, clearly demonstrates the cultural bases of knowledge and practice in professional ethnomedicines, including biomedicines (note plural). Biomedicines may thus be seen as representing "many medicines," not one. Biomedicines are professional ethnomedicines and constitute "cultural systems" and are "cultural artifacts" (Gaines and Hahn 1985:4–5). The same may be said of all professional ethnomedicines whether of Asia, Africa, Europe, the Middle East, Latin and North America. As such, the cultural nature, and therefore, the problematic nature of professional medial knowledge is made clear. A fairly large body of research which demonstrates this point is now available (see, for example, Blue 1991; Bosk 1979; Comaroff 1982; Eisenberg and Kleinman 1981; Gaines 1979, 1985a, 1987a; Gaines and Hahn 1982; Gilman 1988a; Good and Good 1981; Hahn 1985, 1987; Hahn and Gaines 1985; Hahn and Kleinman 1983; Kirmayer 1988; Lock 1980, 1985; Lock and Gordon 1988; Low 1988; Maretzki 1988; Maretzki and Seidler 1985; Mendelsohn and Elkana 1981; Norbeck and Lock 1987; Ohnuki-Tierney 1984; Pliskin 1987; Townsend 1978; Weisberg and Long 1984; Young 1978, 1988).

The distinctiveness emerging from the research on these biomedical traditions emphasizes the formative influence of local culture rather than the ideological or practical "hegemony" of a single, unitary biomedicine as argued by CMA writers (e.g., Baer, Singer and Johnson 1986; Singer, Baer and Lazarus 1990; Frankenberg 1980, 1988). Thus, medical knowledge, like all cultural knowledge, is problematic and necessarily equal in epistemological standing with other ethnomedicines (Hahn and Kleinman 1983; Young 1978, 1982). Critical medical views implicitly privilege professional medical views, blunting the very bases of constructivist interpretation and the deconstruction of medical realities.

It should be noted, however, that many medical anthropologists working in international health, in ecology and epidemiology of illness, and in physical/biological medical anthropology accept U.S. biomedical knowledge as unproblematic and apply it globally (see Greenwood et al. 1988; Young 1982). One also notes that not all (socioculturally oriented) ethnomedical researchers have seen biomedicine as a culturally constructed professional ethnomedicine. Rather, they see it as a more or less unchallengeable standard by which other medical systems or medical action is judged (e.g., Foster and Anderson 1978; Hughes 1968; Prince and Tcheng-Laroche 1987; Simons and Hughes 1985).

Neither the objects of medical and psychiatric research and therapeutic gaze are things of an independent, acultural "Nature," an entity that is itself a cultural construct (see Sahlins 1976; Gordon 1988). The development of a nosological entity in biomedicine should not be seen as independent of its isolation, description, and labeling. As Devereux (1980b) pointed out, diagnosis is a comparison of a presenting problem with known cultural *models* of pathology, not the assessment of the pathological nature of the presentation in its own terms (see Nuckolls, this volume).

Ethnomedicines, including ethnopsychiatries and ethnopsychologies, are to be seen as, to paraphrase Evans-Pritchard's postfunctionalist view of society, *moral, not natural, systems* (Evans-Pritchard 1962). They must be recognized as human creations ever in the process of recreation and alteration. The constructivist approach to psychiatric nosology for example, can make sense of and challenge not only the validity of specific nosological entities such as Post-Traumatic Stress Disorder (PTSD), (Young 1991), depression (Gaines and Farmer 1986; Kleinman 1986; Kleinman and Good 1985; Lutz 1985), or personality disorders (Nuckolls, this volume), but also the asserted acultural nature of the classificatory system itself (Gaines 1982b, 1991, 1992; Farmer 1980; Kleinman and Good 1985; Lock 1987; Marsella 1980; Nuckolls 1992).

Constructivist work reveals the nature and logic of medical practice and the marked differences among and within specialties in medicine and psychiatry (e.g., Bosk 1979; Hahn and Gaines 1985; Johnson 1985; Kleinman 1988a; Light 1980). Attempts to find and describe a homogeneous psychiatric establishment in the United States instead find a highly heterogeneous mix of ideologies and institutions that are largely autonomous but grounded in their local areas (e.g., Castel, Castel and Lovell 1982). Such highly significant internal differences are regularly effaced by deductive macrosystem or world system approaches (e.g., Baer, Singer and Johnson 1986; Frankenberg 1980; 1988; Navarro 1976; Morgan 1987). CMA approaches produce simplified pictures of reality and doubtful accounts of hegemony and power (Estroff 1988; Richters 1988; Rhodes, this volume; Morgan 1987; Sindzingre 1988).

2. ETHNOMEDICAL KNOWLEDGE IS CONSTITUTED
THROUGH EMBODIED AND DISEMBODIED DISCOURSE

Ethnomedical and ethnopsychiatric realities are created, recreated and altered through social interactions and communications. Communicative forms may be embodied (speech) or disembodied (texts, telecommunications). The realities of our own studies are largely constituted in discourse about "things" such as "physician competence" (DelVecchio Good 1985) or "Christian Psychiatry" (Gaines 1982c), not by that thing itself. This is analogous to the anthropological studies of witchcraft. Anthropologists and historians interested in witchcraft actually study witch discourse, i.e., the embodied or disembodied talk about witches (confessions, accusations, expressed beliefs, divination, archives, trial records), not witches themselves (e.g., Douglas 1970; Evans-Pritchard 1937; Larner 1981). Clinical realities are defined, clarified, transformed, and maintained through interactions (Kleinman 1980). Cultural realities germane to ethnopsychiatric transactions, particularly notions of the self, likewise are to be viewed as constructed, maintained, and transformed in and through social interaction and as incorporating aspects of the Other (Gaines 1992; Kirmayer 1989a; Kleinman and Kleinman 1990).

3. AN ETHNOMEDICAL SYSTEM IS AN UNFINISHED PRODUCT OF CULTURE HISTORY

The third central notion of cultural constructivism maintains that an ethnomedicine can not be understood without knowledge of its culture history. Medical systems are never-finished, historically derived products-under-construction. In this I suggest a processional view of medical systems in the stead of static, synchronic functionalist views. Constructivist research allows us to apprehend the central conceptual structures on which are based the productive and reproductive processes of medical knowledge/practice (Gaines 1991, Swartz, this volume; Young 1978, 1991). And, much is borrowed from other traditions and refashioned locally over time.

It is without merit to suggest that medical knowledge is grounded in some "need" of the or a world or national system. Systems cannot have neither needs nor requirements, for the systems are actually researchers' abstractions, not organic realities. Attributions of a system's "needs" simply anthropomorphize academic conceptions. As well, nothing human springs *de novo* into the world; all is historically conditioned. But political economists of health argue that medical knowledge, including nosologies, organizations, or practices, are the results of a contemporary world system's "needs" and requirements for order, control, and/or profit (Baer 1982; Frankenberg 1988; Navarro 1976; Waitzkin 1979, 1981).

4. ETHNOMEDICINES ARE CONSTITUENTS AND EXPRESSIONS OF THEIR RESPECTIVE CULTURES

The cultural constructivist position takes popular and professional ethnomedicines, including ethnopsychiatries, or any other identifiable human enterprise, as expressions of their respective cultures. Because critical approaches ignore the ideological commonalties of professional and lay groups in a society, physicians appear as acultural creatures as is biomedicine. In this view, biomedical practitioners are completely without sincerity or conviction and medical practice is merely an elite conspiracy against society (e.g., Frankenberg 1980, 1988; Ingleby 1983; Navarro 1976; Scheper-Hughes 1988; Waitzkin 1979). But, seen as products of cultural discourses, ethnopsychiatries are ever-incomplete cultural productions even when much of what is 'produced' is imposed or imported, as the selective process itself has cultural bases (Blue 1991).

Ohnuki-Tierney states this point quite clearly with respect to

Japanese biomedicine. She demonstrates that the categories of "thought operative in the medical domain are related to thought governing other domains of Japanese culture, and that these categories show historical continuity" (1984:3). While few would dispute that local culture generates and frames folk ethnopsychiatry, many deny its impact on professional biomedical and psychiatric knowledge, practice and organization. However, the impress of popular culture is clear on all studied professional medicines, whether in the U.S. (Gaines and Hahn 1982; Hahn and Gaines 1985; Lock and Gordon 1988), France (Baszanger 1985; Herzlich 1973), Germany (Maretzki 1988; Maretzki and Seidler 1985; Townsend 1978), Japan (Lock 1980; Norbeck and Lock 1987; Ohnuki-Tierney 1984), Latin America (Low 1988; Scheper-Hughes 1988), the Mediterranean (e.g., Pliskin 1987), or in Southeast Asia (Weisberg and Long 1984).

As aspects of cultures, professional ethnomedical thoughts and actions parallel, and are grounded in, lay cultural domains. Methodologically, then, the investigation of other domains can serve as a check on interpretations of the ethnomedical domains themselves. Key implicit ethnopsychological assumptions in a biomedicine would be those discernable in nonmedical domains in a culture. The assumptions of ethnomedicines must thus be seen as cultural assumptions whose form expresses and conceals popular ideas. The notion that medical and cultural ideas are separate is merely a replication of a particular Western cultural point of view.

5. ETHNOMEDICINES CONCERN HUMAN, EXPERIENCE-NEAR REALITIES

Analyses of lay and professional ethnomedical systems should see them in human experiential terms, e.g., pain, suffering, relief, frustration, loss, joy, anger, fear, sense of self, or worthiness or worthlessness, and the like. Analyses which seek explanations in experience- and culture-distant terms omit the crucial factors in health and illness, the phenomenal persons and groups wherein human experience and intersubjective (not subjective) realities are constructed (Gaines 1991; Kleinman and Kleinman 1990). (Western) scientific medicine is thought to be objective while social sciences are often said to be subjective. Cultural constructivism seeks to comprehend the intersubjective reality underlying both forms of human endeavor. Constructivist approaches seek the voices of patients, healers, and suffering. The voices of all three, in critical medical anthropologies, are obliterated, recast into structural terms (e.g., Navarro 1976; Scheper-Hughes and Lock 1986; Susser 1988), or "disembodied," as Kleinman and Good (1985) note occurs in the study of depression and dysphoric affect.

Biomedicine, on the other hand, sees itself, and has been seen by some anthropologists (e.g., Scotch 1963; Foster and Anderson 1978) as neutral and scientific and dealing in natural facts (Gordon 1988) and natural classes (Lock 1987), in deviations from measurable biophysiological norms which themselves are asserted to be universal and generic (Engel 1977; Mishler et al. 1981). Critical medical anthropologists see economic classes, world systems and the like in precisely the same ahistorical empiricist, universalist terms. They argue, with biomedicine, for a rationalist view of humans and a positivist view of disease, thus managing to eliminate the cultural (i.e., ethnic and general culture), the personal, and the unique, as well as the very experience, from illness realities, and healing interactions.

The focus of ethnomedical, including ethnopsychiatric, work must be a concern for the individual and his/her relationship to the local and wider culture. To concern ourselves with "wider issues" in the critical medical anthropological sense, a reference to a focus on economy, social structure, and disembodied systems of power, is simply to avoid human experience and to replace it with foci on anthropomorphized systems and structures. Such foci serve to divert our attention from, rather than to, human agency, responsibility, experience, and suffering.

The Future

As we look toward the future and the kinds of studies that will be importance to pursue, it must be said that any perspective worthy of the name of anthropology must have a concern for the experience of both healers and patients and with all others involved in ethnopsychiatric systems, i.e., families, friends, neighbors, villages, etc. Some of the areas of the new ethnopsychiatry which will be important are echoed in this collection of essays. These and others are discussed below.

Expanding Horizons

An important goal of future ethnopsychiatric studies should be that of expanding the horizons of inquiry. This expansion is suggested because most of the ethnopsychiatric care in complex, industrial societies is provided by people who are not psychiatrists. One would not suspect this from the antipsychiatry literature of the 1960s (e.g., Szasz 1961) or the critical medical literature of the 1980s (Ingleby 1980; Scheper-Hughes 1988).

It is known, however, that the great majority of mental problems (leaving aside the problem of the validity of disease entities) are commonly seen and cared for not in the context of professional ethnopsychiatry, but in the context of nonprofessional or alternative ethnopsychiatric circles, i.e., the family itself, family medicine and general practice, *curanderos*, shamans, various counselors and psychotherapists (Finkler 1985; Good 1977; Kleinman 1980; 1986, 1988a; Kleinman, Eisenberg and Good 1978; Low 1988). A physician- and institution-centered approach misses the majority of psychiatric events of sickness and caring occurring in large industrial societies. As a consequence, there will be a tendency to replicate implicit conventional professional definitions of the psychiatric.

In this regard, almost unexplored as ethnopsychiatrists are the huge numbers of alternative therapies, therapists-counselors (such as Hershel, Swartz, and Oths of the present volume) and social workers (Goleman 1985). Through these therapists and therapist scholars, ethnopsychiatric researchers and practitioners are clearly having an impact on diagnosis and therapy outside of professional ethnopsychiatry (Goleman 1989; Pedersen et al. 1989; Sue and Morishima 1982; Waxler-Morrison 1990; Westermeyer 1989).

Ethnopsychiatry's influence on professional psychiatry is likewise now more palpable. For example, a number of psychiatrist-anthropologist scholars come to mind, e.g., J. Hsu, Foulks, Mars, F. Raveau, Levy, Tseng, Lambo, Kirmayer, D. Young, Eisenberg, E. Brody, Kiev, T.-Y. Lin, Fábrega, Prince, Wintrob, Hartog, Littlewood, Weiss, Westermeyer, Beiser, F. Cheung, Shore and Kleinman, among others. In his oft-cited 1982 review of medical anthropology, Allan Young noted that Kleinman was then "the most influential and prolific writer" in the field (1982:264). Today, the same can be said of Kleinman with reference also to the field of ethnopsychiatry based on his work in the 1970s and 1980s. This includes his published research on problematic conceptions and organization of psychiatry from a "critical rational" perspective (Manschreck and Kleinman 1977), his studies of depression, anxiety, therapeutic efficacy, pain, and suffering in chronic illness experiences and politics in China, Chinese psychiatric illness and etiologies, treatment and management in, and the refiguring of, U.S. psychiatry (e.g., see Kleinman 1980, 1986, 1987, 1988a, b, c; Hahn and Kleinman 1983; Kleinman et al. 1975; Kleinman and Gale 1982; Kleinman and Good 1985; Katon and Kleinman 1981; Kleinman and Kleinman 1985; Manschreck and Kleinman 1977).

Other workers, while doubtless serving ethnopsychiatric functions, may do so in a variety of different local ideological contexts (e.g, Buddhist and "dream centers," astrology and "shamanic" and "goddess studies," all among the literati (and *gliterati*) of the San Francisco Bay Area). It might also be of interest to study the influence of anthropological ethnopsychiatric knowledge and methods on the practice of ethnopsychiatry and the character and nature of resistance thereto (see Brody 1987; Farmer, this volume; Kleinman 1988a). Such a consideration leads to an appropriate characterization of the very great diversity contained within popular and professional ethnopsychiatries (e.g., Devereux 1957; Gaines 1985a, 1987b; Lazare 1973; Light 1976).

In accounting for diversity, its range, causes and consequences, we might consider an illuminating comparative approach to professional medical specialties, that is, an ethnology of ethnopsychiatry. Such an approach would serve to highlight features of each unit chosen for study more so than ethnography (e.g., Gaines, this volume; Gilman 1988a; Hershel, this volume; Nuckolls, this volume). Geertz (1990) has recently made a comparable point with respect to social and cultural anthropology, calling for studies of the intellectual niches (ruts?) of modern science.

Physician-centeredness may also be seen as a reflection of a Western cultural emphasis on individuals as healers. By way of contrast, for example, we find that one of the sources of ethnopsychiatric healing in Morocco is not a person, but rather a religious brotherhood which the afflicted join and which, in turn, simultaneously provides the context for the healing of newcomers and continuous therapy for existing members (Crapanzano 1973). This is also found in the *Zar* cults in Africa (Boddy 1988).

Although it took some time for medical anthropologists to finally see Western physicians as appropriate objects of study (Hahn and Gaines 1985; Maretzki 1985), we need not become completely physician-centered (or fixated). This collection unhesitatingly combines studies of professional and folk medicine and considers them epistemologically analogous. Herein, I have included Oths's article on Chiropractic as "unintended (psycho)therapy" and Dwyer's historical study, drawn from her larger work on asylum attendants (1987), and Maretzki's study of Groddeck, in order to point in the direction of an expanded conception of ethnopsychiatry. In enlarging our explicit notion of ethnopsychiatry, it is important for researchers to recognize the fact of the ever ongoing cultural construction of ethnopsychiatric realities. This realization suggests a need to develop research that is diachronic and attends to the actual construction of disorders in lay or professional ethnopsychiatries.

Young has brought us close to this with his series of papers (several unpublished) on PTSD (1988, 1990, 1991). While needing prospective studies of disease and also of the construction of related health roles (e.g., for Sexually Transmitted Diseases (STDs), see Brandt [1986] and for Acquired Immune Deficiency Syndrome (AIDS) in the United States, see Gilman [1988a], and Farmer [1990] for AIDS in rural Haïti), we need also to attend to interpretive culture histories of other extant illnesses and roles. These would include such roles as those pressed on women physicians (Morantz-Sanchez 1985), and the "diseases" of schizophrenia (e.g, Gilman 1988b) and depression (Jackson 1985, 1986). More work is needed on dysphoric affect, its shaping and often *positive* experience and expression cross-culturally (Gaines, this volume, 1987a; Gaines and Farmer 1986; Kleinman and Good 1985; Marsella 1980; Obeyesekere 1985). Important in this interpretive enterprise are the "representations" (e.g., symbols, portraits, models) of the afflicted or the disease (Gilman 1988a, b) and their implications for care, treatment, and funding for constructed problems.

Several disorders are currently under construction in United States professional ethnopsychiatry, e.g., CFS (chronic fatigue syndrome)

(HMSHL 1989). Several, such as PMS (premenstrual syndrome) (Dalton 1980), self-defeating personality and late luteal phase dysphoric disorder (APA 1987) seem to be rather clear reflections/expressions of gender bias against women (Gaines 1992; Gilman 1988b). We also see a variety of new diseases being constructed in Japan (see Norbeck and Lock 1987), as is the case elsewhere. All suggest the dynamic nature of professional and popular ethnopsychiatries as systems of understanding, explanation, and critiques of self-experience and of the Other.

Suffering and Violence

While issues of change and of stress will continue to be addressed (Dressler 1985; Lock 1988; Young 1988, 1990, 1991), another area needing expanded attention was but briefly noted above. This is the area of illness in terms of the nature of suffering, its experience and expression, and the means by which such are constructed and communicated (see Csordas, this volume; DelVecchio Good 1988; Good 1988; Kleinman 1988a, b). In this domain, ethnopsychiatry becomes a part of the "anthropology of experience" (Turner and Bruner 1986). As such, this aspect of ethnopsychiatry will delve into reflexivity, narrativity, symbolism, self, performance and other constructions. In some sense, this work will involve the cultural and personal authoring of the self (Geertz 1986). Here ethnopsychiatry builds bridges to studies of cultural psychology (Shweder 1990).

Another area of study relating to suffering is that of the plight of many refugees, especially now from Latin America and earlier from Southeast Asia. Some of this work moves between the control of emotion discourse by the state to the "state's construction of affect" (Mary-Jo DelVecchio Good, in Jenkins 1991b) in terms the state sees as appropriate at particular historical moments (Good and Good 1988; Jenkins 1991b). This research is one of the avenues in ethnopsychiatry which leads out of it into ethnopsychology because of the intimate relationship of the medical/psychiatric with seemingly nonmedical notions of self, person, and gender, with social cynosures, affect and the cultural history from which all such notions derive (e.g., Csordas 1990, this volume; Gaines and Farmer 1986; Good and Good 1988; Jenkins, 1991a, this volume; Lutz 1985). At the same time, such work may lead back into ethnopsychiatry in that issues of war and refugees include the problems of torture, terror, and responses to unimaginable and unassimilable experiences (Jenkins 1991b; Kinzi et al. 1984; Kirmayer 1989b; Scarry 1985; Westermeyer 1989; Young 1990).

This enterprise will be difficult, for it will not only pose problems of research and analysis, but of expression and presentation as well. This need may be filled by studies focally concerned with suffering and its conceptual and linguistic constitution (DelVecchio Good 1988; Pandolfi 1988), as parts of fine-grained analyses of healing (e.g., Csordas 1983, 1990, this volume), of ethics and morality (Young 1990) or in the context of critiques of a biomedical practice (e.g., Scheper-Hughes 1988).

Such interests also lead us to a consideration of violence. This topic is but slightly opened in this collection in the chapters of Swartz, Hershel, Dwyer, and Katz, but promises to be an important topic of research. Violence within (Caudill 1958; Katz and Kirkland 1990) and outside of mental institutions, as well as state-supported violence, its construction, and consequences, are all topics needing further exploration. The problem of violence and the expression of emotion from "somatizing" cultures has recently been explored from the standpoint not of ethnopsychology or ethnopsychiatry, but from a focus on the situated discourse of emotion and healing (Good, Good and Fischer 1988; Watson-Gegeo and White 1990), i.e, on the discourse from which our objects of study are created, constituted, and maintained.

Chronic Illness

Also related to the issue of suffering is the consideration of chronic sicknesses and how these are endured and managed by self and others. We have tended in ethnopsychiatry to focus on acute problems except when dealing with institutions or deinstitutionalization (Estroff 1981; Scheper-Hughes 1981) or studies of help-seeking (Good 1977; Kleinman 1980). Management of chronic problems, and the means of their cultural/clinical construction and maintenance, is not the central focus of our research though increasingly this is found in other fields (e.g., Biegel, Sales and Schulz 1991). Recent studies emphasize more the nature of chronic afflictions (Kleinman 1986) but other topics remain to be explored. These include the study and deconstruction of such conceptions as substance abuse or "addictions" (e.g., Kennedy 1987; Marshall 1979; Westermeyer 1982) and the chronic, often tragic conditions, glossed (and reduced) as Alzheimer's or schizophrenia by biomedicine, in their social and cultural contexts (Gaines 1989; Jenkins, this volume, 1991a; Valle 1989).

While some work has appeared outside of ethnopsychiatry on chronic conditions (e.g., Alexander 1981; Kaufman 1988), we need more ethnopsychiatric work on problems analogous to Edgerton's exceptional study of individuals labeled "retarded" and the construction of that sociomedical identity and clinical reality (1967; see also Langness and Levine 1986). We have Reynolds and Farborow's study of life in psychiatric aftercare facilities (1977) and Estroff's sensitive account of the deinstitutionalized individual's life on the streets (1981), but much more is needed concerning living with mental disorders in a wide variety of cultural settings. Current relevant work is largely in the public health, psychiatric, and social work domains (e.g., Biegel, Sales and Schulz 1991; Goldman and Luchins 1984; Goldman and Manderscheid 1987; Goldstein 1987). In the present volume, Jenkins's evocative study suggests some directions in this area for future research.

GENDER. It should be important to focus attention on gender differences not only in the construction of illness and idioms of distress (Nichter 1981), but also, and especially with respect to, suffering (Finkler 1985; Kleinman 1986; Pandolfi 1988) and medical treatment (Ehrenreich and English 1989; Russett 1988) because illness, experience, resort, gender, and treatment all are cultural constructions. Relating gender to healing and caring should attract our attention (e.g., McClain 1989). Also important in relation to gender are the classification systems of illness, especially in professional ethnopsychiatries (e.g., Diagnostic and Statistical Manuals-I to III-R) and their inhering gender biases or "cultural thought models" (Devereux 1978) which in the U.S., simultaneously express and conceal (see Gaines 1992; Nuckolls, this volume, 1992). This is precisely the sort of cultural deconstruction that *is* critical and should encompass our own culture-bound or culture-specific disorders, as suggested by Thomas Johnson (1987) and Devereux. The same caution may be expressed about models proposed in feminist circles about the afflictions of women of other cultures (see Morsy [1978] for an excellent critique). Insuring the presentation of multiple cultural voices, rather than one, is clearly an important direction in which to move and to which this volume makes only a small contribution.

More on the Self

The role of self and person constructions were introduced just a decade ago in the context of the study of illness manifestations of interest to professional ethnopsychiatry (Marsella 1980) and as they relate to Western professional biomedical theory and practice (Gaines 1979, 1982b). Conceptions of person continue to attract attention (e.g., Gordon 1988; Kirmayer 1988) now even in the popular press (Goleman 1989). Of potential importance in this area of research is an internal cultural division which can be drawn in the seemingly unitary "West." The recognition of a cultural division "in the West" grew out of fieldwork in France among Alsatian Catholics and Protestants and study of and talk with ethnographers of the Mediterranean (with inspiration from Geertz [1976] and Hallowell's early work [1955]) (Gaines n.d., 1982b, 1985a, b, c; Gaines and Farmer 1986). This distinction reflects the fact that the "West," usually seen as unitary, and contrasted with a seemingly homogeneous "East," is actually composed of at least two distinct cultural traditions which manifest themselves at all cultural psychological levels including notions of person. I have distinguished the *indexical* and the *referential* person conceptions (Mediterranean and Northern European, respectively) (Gaines 1982b, 1985a, c).

The distinction, which emphasizes the self defined and presented in social interaction, appears to have had some utility for authors in ethnopsychiatry and ethnomedicine (e.g., Gordon 1988; Van Moffaert and Vereecken 1989; White and Kirkpatrick 1985; White and Marsella 1982) and history (e.g., Lawrence 1988). It is worth developing further to avoid a kind of implicit homogenizing Occidentalism or Orientalism. In this light, the distinctions in person conceptions drawn by Shweder and Bourne (1982), the *sociocentric* and the *egocentric* (East vs. West) may be seen as too broad (White and Marsella 1982). They emphasize a patterned cognitive focus in their portrayal of the egocentric self, i. e., the referential self in my scheme. I would suggest this refers only to the Northern European person conception, not to that of the Mediterranean (i.e., the indexical). The result of the notion of the West as egocentric is an attribution of uniformity of culture to the people of Europe and by extension, Asia.[4]

Related to the question of self is the nature of suffering and the issue of efficacy, or lack thereof. In reality, we refer here to the cultural construction of efficacy (Finkler 1985; Good, Herrera, Good and Cooper 1985; Kleinman 1980, 1988a, b, c). Efficacy is necessarily culturally constructed because criteria of evaluation are clearly relative (e.g., Pattison et al. 1973; Westermeyer and Wintrob 1979; Young 1977a).

Aging and Ethnopsychiatry

It seems reasonable to suggest here that another area of interest of future ethnopsychiatric research is aging. Such interests may relate to chronic illness, as a response, or to the problems of aging as conceptualized locally. Already an important area of research outside of ethnopsychiatry in medical anthropology (e.g., Biegel, Sales and Schulz 1991; Ikels 1983, 1991; Kayser-Jones 1981), it would seem to be an area of future interest and amenable to ethnopsychiatric illumination. That is, we need to establish some sort of *geriatric ethnopsychiatry* that pays attention to the cultural construction of aging, aged, elders and their needs, and culturally constructed age-specific problems. In addition, (psychiatric) burdens of care-givers should be considered as a topic of research.

One topic might be the emergence of a geriatric psychiatry, one of the more recent forms or specialties in U.S. psychiatry. And, because elder status in Chinese culture is respected (Ikels 1983), even elevated to the status of a social cynosure (LaBarre 1946), one might presume that elder status would have different psychological consequences in different societies; what is a problem in one, may have its blessings in another.

Ethics

Finally, we will need to begin to engage ourselves in the field of ethnopsychiatric ethics (e.g., Post 1992; Young 1990), as a branch of medical ethics (for which see, for example, Veatch 1989; Weisz 1990). We will need to consider "ethnoethics" (e.g., Farmer 1988) as well as the ethics of cross-cultural ethnopsychiatric practice, including diagnosis, treatment, management, and disease classification (Gaines 1991,1992; Post 1992). Ethical analyses also should consider the culturally constructed locus of distress (i.e., gender, "racial" group, class, or occupational groups) and the ethics of such social categories. This must be part of the analysis of the appropriateness, efficacy, or conflictual nature of diagnosis, therapy and/or management.

A consideration of issues of authority and power is also related but as noted by Rhodes (this volume), power cannot be considered an external, invariant force (Young 1982). Rather, power must be seen as a cultural construct, here based on expertise, there on knowledge; here on gender, there on strength or kin ties. The study of power should not merely replicate the conventional wisdom of nineteenth-century empiricist social (and popular) science. Rather, we need to break new ground in seeing our own distorting lenses *and* those of others. Interpretive approaches provide us with the appropriate orienting assumption; there are other valid ways for understanding and acting in one's constructed world. This allows us to go beyond explanations which are sensible only in our own cultural context (e.g., economics, interests, strategies, etc.) (see also Morsy 1978).

New studies should not include just the narrow and distorting (and blame-pinning) treatment of non-Western patients by Westerners, but the opposite as well, a flavor of which we see in Katz's article in this volume (see also Basker and Domínguez 1984). While decrying Orientalism, we do not improve matters with rank Occidentalism, even that curiously mixed with Euro- or "Americocentrism" (Gaines 1991).

Summary

In the future of the new ethnopsychiatry, there appears to be room for both the expansion of current areas of research and the development of new areas of investigation. As we move more toward a recognition that our world and our ethnopsychiatries, and those of others, are likewise constructed, we expand the nature and breadth of our research endeavor. At the same time, we demonstrate the cultural construction of the disciplinary and conceptual boundaries as research leads us into nonpsychiatric and nonmedical fields and back again. It is appropriate, then, to use constructivist approaches which do not falsify our own and other cultural worlds and which do not deny or ignore local realities. Rather, we need to improve upon our ability to recognize and deconstruct cultural constructions, including the notions and activities called science and medicine, as well as notions of sickness, person and the Other so that we can find better ways to understand, rather than deny them.

Notes

1. This formulation, that the body is an object and an objectification of culture, originates in Csordas's 1988 Stirling Award Paper published in *Ethos* (Csordas 1990). See Douglas (1966), Foucault (1979), Ots (1988), O'Neill (1985), and Turner (1984), among others, for related perspectives in the anthropology of the body.

2. The contributors were unaware of my editorial mission of encompassing and representing diversity of lived experiences in the discourse of the new ethnopsychiatry. Unfortunately, still other vantage points could not be accommodated due to time and space constraints, e.g., V. Garrison on Afro-American popular ethnopsychiatry, A. Lovell on Bioenergetics in France and Qi Hu on Chinese professional ethnopsychiatry. Previous volumes in the field have tended to be a bit androcentric, e.g., Kleinman and Good 1985; Gaines and Hahn 1982; Hahn and Gaines 1985; Marsella and White 1982.

The contributors to this volume include veritable novices in their first publishing ventures (Nomura, Oths and Blue), junior scholars (Farmer, Nuckolls, Hershel), scholars in or near mid-career (Csordas, Dwyer, Katz, Gaines, Jenkins, Rhodes, Swartz), and a senior scholar, recently retired (Maretzki). The authors are from a variety of national, religious and cultural backgrounds, South African, German, Japanese, Eastern and Western European-American and Cosmopolitan. Faiths represented include Buddhism, Protestantism, Catholicism, and Judaism. Cosmopolitan is a term from Hawai'i used to describe the many individuals there with ancestry in three or more distinct ethnic or cultural groups. The colloquial term, as I learned while there, is either "chop suey" or "mixed plate," the latter referring to a local dish which includes aspects of the cuisines of Japan, Hawaii, China, Portugal and, often, *Ha'ole* (any European (American) ethnic except for Portuguese).

3. The author had the pleasure of meeting the congenial Dr. Mars, our field's name-giver, in Paris (1974) while visiting Professor Devereux's ethnopsychiatry seminar at the École Pratique des Hautes Études en Science Sociales.

4. For person conceptions in Oceania, see White and Kirkpatrick (1985), for South Asia, China, and Japan, see Carithers, et al. (1985), Daniel (1984); Kapferer (1979), Lebra (1976), Marsella, DeVos and Hsu (1985), and Weidman (1969); for the United States, the Mediterranean, and Europe see Blue (1991), Gaines (1979, 1982b, 1985a,b), Geertz (1976), Hahn (1985), and Lee (1959a); for Native North America, see Hallowell (1955) and Lee (1959b); for Morocco and Indonesia see Geertz (1976) and also Conner (1982) for Indonesia, among others considering the self.

References

Alexander, Linda
1981 The Double-Bind Between Dialysis Patients and Their Health Practitioners. In The Relevance of Social Science for Medicine. Leon Eisenberg and Arthur Kleinman (eds.). Dordrecht: D. Reidel.

American Psychiatric Association (APA)
1952 Diagnostic and Statistical Manual I (DSM-I). Washington, D.C.: American Psychiatric Association.

1968 Diagnostic and Statistical Manual II (DSM-II). Washington, D.C.: American Psychiatric Association.

1980 Diagnostic and Statistical Manual III (DSM-III). Washington, D.C.: American Psychiatric Association.

1987 Diagnostic and Statistical Manual III-Revised (DSM-III-R). Washington, D.C.: American Psychiatric Association.

Baer, Hans

1982 On the Political Economy of Health. Medical Anthropology Newsletter 14(1):1–17.

1986 Sociological Contributions to the Political Economy of Health. Medical Anthropology Quarterly 17:129–131.

Baer, Hans, Merrill Singer and John Johnson, eds.

1986 Toward a Critical Medical Anthropology. Social Science and Medicine Special Issue 23.

Basker, Eileen and Virginia Domínguez

1984 Limits to Cultural Awareness: the Immigrant as Therapist. Human Relations 37(9):693–719.

Baszanger, Isabelle

1985 Professional Socialization and Social Control: From Medical Students to General Practitioners. Noal Mellott, trans. Social Science and Medicine 20:133–143.

Biegel, David, Esther Sales and Richard Schulz

1991 Family Caregiving in Chronic Illness. Newbury Park, CA: Sage.

Blue, Amy V.

1991 Culture, *Nevra*, and Institution: the Making of Greek Professional Ethnopsychiatry. Unpublished Dissertation in Anthropology. Case Western Reserve University. Cleveland, Ohio.

Bosk, Charles

1979 Forgive and Remember. Chicago: University of Chicago Press.

Boddy, Janice

1988 Spirits and Selves in Northern Sudan. American Ethnologist 15(1):1039–1046.

Brandt, Alan

1986 No Magic Bullet. Oxford: Oxford University Press.

Brody, Howard

1987 Stories of Sickness. New Haven: Yale University Press.

Carithers, M., S. Collins and S. Lukes, eds.

1985 The Category of the Person: Anthropology, Philosophy, History. Cambridge: Cambridge University Press.

Castel, Robert, Françoise Castel and Anne Lovell

1982 The Psychiatric Society. New York: Columbia University Press.

Caudill, William

1958 The Psychiatric Hospital as a Small Society. Cambridge, MA: Harvard University Press.

Caudill, W. and Tsung-Yi Lin, eds.
1969 Mental Health Research in Asia and the Pacific. Honolulu: East-West Center Press.

Comaroff, Jean
1982 Medicine: Symbol and Ideology. In The Problem of Medical Knowledge. Peter Wright and Andrew Teacher (eds.). Edinburgh: University of Edinburgh Press.

Conner, Linda
1982 The Unbounded Self. In Cultural Conceptions of Mental Health and Therapy. Anthony Marsella and Geoffrey White (eds.). Dordrecht: D. Reidel.

Crapanzano, Vincent
1973 The Hamadsha. Berkeley: University of California Press.

Csordas, Thomas
1983 The Rhetoric of Transformation in Ritual Healing. Culture, Medicine and Psychiatry 7(4):333–375.
1990 Embodiment as a Paradigm for Anthropology (Stirling Prize Essay). Ethos 18(1):5–47.

Dalton, Katherine
1980 Cyclical Criminal Acts in Premenstrual Syndrome. The Lancet, November:1070–71.

Daniel, Valentine
1984 Fluid Signs. Berkeley: University of California Press.

Devereux, George
1944 The Social Structure of a Schizophrenic Ward and Its Therapeutic Fitness. Journal of Clinical Psychotherapy 6(2):231–265.
1949 The Social Structure of the Hospital as a Factor in Total Therapy. American Journal of Orthopsychiatry 19(3):492–500.
1957 Dream Learning and Individual Ritual Difference in Mohave Shamanism. American Anthropologist 63(5):1088–90.
1969 Mohave Ethnopsychiatry. Washington, D.C.: Smithsonian Institution Press.
1978 Cultural Thought Models in Primitive and Modern Psychiatric Theories. In Ethnopsychoanalysis: Psychoanalysis and Anthropology as Complementary Frames of Reference. Berkeley: University of California Press.
1980a Schizophrenia: An Ethnic Psychosis. In Basic Problems of Ethnopsychiatry. George Devereux. Chicago: University of Chicago Press.
1980b Basic Problems of Ethnopsychiatry. Chicago: University of Chicago Press.

Douglas, Mary
1966 Purity and Danger. London: Routledge and Kegan Paul.
1970 Witchcraft, Confessions and Accusations. A.S.A. Mgr. #9. London: Tavistock.

Dressler, William
1985 Psychosomatic Symptoms, Stress and Modernization. Culture, Medicine and Psychiatry 9(3):257–294.

Dwyer, Ellen
1987 Homes for the Mad. New Brunswick, NJ: Rutgers University Press.

Edgerton, Robert
1967   The Cloak of Competence. Berkeley: University of California Press.

Ehrenreich, Barbara and Deirdre English
1989 [1979]   For Her Own Good. New York: Anchor Doubleday.

Eisenberg, Leon
1977   Disease and Illness: Distinctions Between Professional and Popular Ideas of Sickness. Culture, Medicine and Psychiatry 1(1):9–24.

Eisenberg, Leon and Arthur Kleinman, eds.
1981   The Relevance of Social Science for Medicine. Dordrecht: D. Reidel.

Elkana, Yehuda
1981   A Programmatic Attempt at an Anthropology of Knowledge. In Science and Cultures. E. Mendelsohn and Yehuda Elkana (eds.). Dordrecht: D. Reidel.

Engel, George
1977   The Need for a New Medical Model: A Challenge for Biomedicine. Science 1965:129–135.

Estroff, Sue E.
1981   Making it Crazy: An Ethnography of Psychiatric Clients in an American Community. Berkeley: University of California Press.
1988   Whose Hegemony? A Critical Commentary on Critical Medical Anthropology. Medical Anthropology Quarterly 2(4):421–426.

Evans-Pritchard, E. E.
1937   Witchcraft, Oracles and Magic Among the Azande. Oxford: Clarendon Press.
1962   Social Anthropology and Other Essays. Glencoe: The Free Press.

Farmer, Paul
1980   New Approach to Psychiatric Diagnosis: Acultural or Anglicized? First Contact 6(2):11–14.
1988   Bad Blood, Spoiled Milk: Bodily Fluids as Moral Barometers in Rural Haïti. American Ethnologist 15(1):62–83.
1990   Sending Sickness: Sorcery, Politics and Changing Concepts of AIDS in Rural Haïti. Medical Anthropology Quarterly *(n.s.)* 4(1): 6–27.

Finkler, Kaja
1985   Spiritualist Healers in Mexico. New York. Bergin and Garvey.

Foster, George and Barbara Anderson
1978   Medical Anthropology. New York: John Wiley.

Foucault, Michel
1973 [1965]   Madness and Civilization. Richard Howard, trans. New York: Vintage Books.
1975 [1963]   The Birth of the Clinic. A. M. Sheridan, trans. New York: Vintage Books.
1978 [1975]   Discipline and Punish. A. M. Sheridan, trans. New York: Pantheon.
1979   A History of Sexuality, Vol. 1. R. Hurley, trans. London: Allen Lane.

Frankenberg, Ronald
1980   Medical Anthropology and Development. Social Science and Medicine. 14B (4):197–207.
1988   Gramsci, Culture and Medical Anthropology: Kundry and Parsifal? or Rat's

Tail to Sea Serpent? Medical Anthropology Quarterly (*n.s.*) 2(4):324–337.

Gaines, Atwood D.

1979 Definitions and Diagnoses. Culture, Medicine and Psychiatry 3(4):381–418.

1982a Knowledge and Practice: Anthropological Ideas and Psychiatric Practice. In Clinically Applied Anthropology. N. Chrisman and T. Maretzki (eds.). Dordrecht: D. Reidel.

1982b Cultural Definitions, Behavior and the Person in American Psychiatry. In Cultural Conceptions of Mental Health and Therapy. Anthony Marsella and Geoffrey White (eds.). Dordrecht: D. Reidel.

1982c The Twice-Born: 'Christian Psychiatry' and Christian Psychiatrists. Culture, Medicine and Psychiatry 6(3):305–324.

1985a The Once- and the Twice-Born: Self and Practice Among Psychiatrists and Christian Psychiatrists. In Physicians of Western Medicine. R. Hahn and A. Gaines (eds.). Dordrecht: D. Reidel.

1985b Alcohol: Cultural Conceptions and Social Behavior Among Urban 'Blacks.' In The American Experience with Alcohol. Linda Bennett and Genevieve Ames (eds.). New York: Plenum.

1985c Faith, Fashion and Family: Religion, Aesthetics, Identity and Social Organization in Strasbourg. Anthropological Quarterly 58(2):47–62.

1987a Cultures, Biologies and Dysphorias. Transcultural Psychiatric Research Review 24(1):31–57.

1987b Shamanism and the Shaman: A Plea for the Person-Centered Approach. Anthropology and Humanism Quarterly 12(3 & 4):62–68.

1988 Delusions: Culture, Psychosis and the Problem of Meaning. In Delusions: Interdisciplinary Perspectives. Thomas Oltmanns and Brenden Maher (eds.). New York: John Wiley.

1989 Alzheimer's Disease in the Context of Black (Southern) Culture. Health Matrix 6(4):33–38.

1991 Cultural Constructivism: Sickness Histories and the Understanding Ethnomedicines Beyond Critical Medical Anthropologies. In Anthropologies of Medicine. B. Pfleiderer and G. Bibeau (eds.). Wiesbaden: Vieweg Verlag.

1992 From DSM-I to III-R; Voices of Self, Mastery and the Other: A Cultural Constructivist Reading of United States Psychiatric Classification. In The Cultural Construction of Psychiatric Classification. Charles Nuckolls (ed.). Social Science and Medicine Special Issue/Section. (In press).

n.d. The Word and the Cross: Identity and Paradox in Alsace. m.s.

Gaines, Atwood and Paul Farmer

1986 Visible Saints: Social Cynosures and Dysphoria in the Mediterranean Tradition. Culture, Medicine and Psychiatry 10(4):295–330.

Gaines, Atwood and Robert Hahn

1985 Among the Physicians: Encounter, Exchange and Transformation. In Physicians of Western Medicine: Anthropological Approaches to Theory and Practice. R. Hahn and A. Gaines (eds.). Dordrecht: D. Reidel.

Gaines, Atwood and Robert Hahn, eds.

1982 Physicians of Western Medicine: Five Cultural Studies. Culture, Medicine and Psychiatry Special Issue 6(3).

Geertz, Clifford
1973 The Interpretation of Cultures. New York: Basic Books.
1976 "From the Native's Point of View." In Meaning in Anthropology. K. Basso
      and H. Selby (eds.). Albuquerque: University of New Mexico Press.
1983 The Way We Think Now: Toward an Ethnography of Modern Thought. In
      Local Knowledge. C. Geertz. New York: Basic Books.
1984 Anti-Anti-Relativism. American Anthropologist 86(2):263–278.
1986 Making Experiences, Authoring Selves. In The Anthropology of Experience. Vic-
      tor Turner and Edward Bruner (eds.). Urbana, IL: University of Illinois Press.
1990 Towns. Countries. Cultures. The Hitchcock Lectures. University of Califor-
      nia at Berkeley. April 1990.

Gilman, Sander
1988a Disease and Representation: Images of Illness from Madness to AIDS. Ithaca,
      NY: Cornell University Press.
1988b Constructing the Image of the Appropriate Therapist: The Struggle of Psychi-
      atry and Psychoanalysis. In Disease and Representation: Images of Illness
      from Madness to AIDS. Sander Gilman. Ithaca, NY: Cornell University Press.

Goffman, Erving
1961 Asylums. New York: Anchor Books.

Goldman, H. H. and R. W. Manderscheid
1987 Chronic Mental Disorders in the United States. In Mental Health, United
      States. R. W. Manderscheid and S. A. Barrett (eds.). Washington, DC: U.S.
      Government Printing Office.

Goldman, L. S. and D. J. Luchins
1984 Depression in the Spouses of Demented Patients. American Journal of Psy-
      chiatry 141:1467–1468.

Goldstein, E. G.
1987 Mental Health and Illness. Encyclopedia of Social Work (18th edition). Silver
      Spring, MD: National Association of Social Workers.

Goleman, D.
1985 Social Workers Vault Into a Leading Role in Psychotherapy. Washington
      Post, April 30.
1989 From Tokyo to Tampa, Different Ideas of Self. New York Times. March 7.

Good, Byron
1977 The Heart of What's the Matter. Culture, Medicine and Psychiatry (1):25–58.
1988 A Body in Pain. Paper presented at the Conference, Anthropologies of
      Medicine: Western European and North American Perspectives. University
      of Hamburg. Hamburg, Germany. December 4–8.

Good, B., H. Herrera, M.-J. DelVecchio Good, and J. Cooper
1985 Reflexivity, Countertransference and Clinical Ethnography: A Case from a
      Psychiatric Cultural Consultation Clinic. In Physicians of Western Medicine:
      Anthropological Approaches to Theory and Practice. R. Hahn and A. Gaines
      (eds.). Dordrecht: D. Reidel.

Good, Byron and Mary-Jo DelVecchio Good
1981 The Semantics of Medical Discourse. In Science and Cultures. E. Mendelsohn
      and Y. Elkana (eds.). Dordrecht: D. Reidel.

1982 Toward a Meaning-Centered Analysis of Popular Illness Categories. In Cultural Conceptions of Mental Health and Therapy. Anthony Marsella and Geoffrey White (eds.). Dordrecht: D. Reidel.
1988 Ritual, the State, and the Transformation of Emotional Discourse in Iranian Society. Culture, Medicine and Psychiatry 12(1):43–63.

Good, Mary-Jo DelVecchio
1985 Discourses on Physician Competence. In Physicians of Western Medicine. Robert Hahn and Atwood Gaines (eds.). Dordrecht: D. Reidel.
1988 The Practice of Biomedicine and the Discourse on Hope: A Preliminary Investigation into the Culture of American Oncology. Paper presented at the Conference, Anthropologies of Medicine: Western European and North American Perspectives. University of Hamburg. Hamburg, Germany. December 4–8.

Good, Mary-Jo DelVecchio, Byron Good and Michael Fischer, eds.
1988 Emotion, Illness and Healing in Middle Eastern Societies. Culture, Medicine and Psychiatry Special Issue 12(1).

Good, Mary-Jo DelVecchio, Deborah Gordon and Mariella Pandolfi, eds.
1990 Traversing Boundaries: European and North American Perspectives on Medical and Psychiatric Anthropology. Culture, Medicine and Psychiatry Special Issue 14(2).

Gordon, Deborah
1988 Tenacious Assumptions in Western Medicine. In Biomedicine Examined. Margaret Lock and Deborah Gordon (eds.). Dordrecht: Kluwer Academic Publishers.

Gordon, Daniel
1991 Female Circumcision and Genital Operations in Egypt and the Sudan. Medical Anthropology Quarterly (n.s.) 5(1):3–14.

Greenwood, Davydd, Shirley Lindenbaum, Margaret Lock and Allan Young, eds.
1988 Medical Anthropology Theme Issue. American Ethnologist 15(1).

Grim, John A.
1983 The Shaman. Norman, OK: University of Oklahoma Press.

Hahn, Robert
1985 A World of Internal Medicine: Portrait of an Internist. In Physicians of Western Medicine: Anthropological Approaches to Theory and Practice. R. Hahn and A. Gaines (eds.). Dordrecht: D. Reidel.

Hahn, Robert, ed.
1987 Obstetrics in the United States. Medical Anthropology Quarterly (n.s.) Special Issue 1(3).

Hahn, Robert and Atwood Gaines, eds.
1985 Physicians of Western Medicine: Anthropological Approaches to Theory and Practice. Dordrecht: D. Reidel.

Hahn, Robert and Arthur Kleinman
1983 Biomedical Practice and Anthropological Theory: Frameworks and Directions. In Annual Review of Anthropology. Palo Alto, CA: Annual Review Press.

Hallowell, A. I.
1955 The Self and Its Behavioral Environment. In Culture and Experience. A.I.
      Hallowell. Philadelphia: University of Pennsylvania Press.

Harvard Medical School Health Letter (HMSHL)
1989 Chronic Fatigue. Harvard Medical School Health Letter. 14(5):1–3.

Herzlich, Claudine
1973 Health and Illness. New York: Academic Press.

Hughes, Charles
1968 Ethnomedicine. In International Encyclopedia of the Social Sciences. New
      York: The Free Press.
1990 Ethnopsychiatry. In Medical Anthropology. Contemporary Theory and
      Method. Thomas Johnson and Carolyn Sargent (eds.). Westport, CT: Green-
      wood Press.

Hunt, Lynn, ed.
1989 The New Culture History. Englewood Cliffs, New Jersey: Prentice-Hall.

Ikels, Charlotte
1983 Aging and Adaptation: Chinese in Hong Kong and the United States. Ham-
      den, CT: Archon Books.
1991 Aging and Disability in China: Cultural Issues in Measurement and Interpre-
      tation. Social Science and Medicine 32(6):649–665.

Ingleby, David, ed.
1980 Critical Psychiatry. New York: Pantheon Books.

Ingleby, David
1983 Mental Health and Social Order. In Social Control and the State: Historical
      and Comparative Essays. S. Cohen and A. Scull (eds.). Oxford: Martin.

Jackson, Stanley, Jr.
1985 *Acedia* the Sin and Its Relationship to Sorrow and Melancholia. In: Culture
      and Depression. A. Kleinman and B. Good (eds.). Berkeley: University of
      California Press.
1986 Melancholia and Depression. New Haven: Yale University Press.

Jenkins, Janis Hunter
1988 Conceptions of Schizophrenia as a Problem of Nerves. Social Science and
      Medicine 26(12):303–331.
1991a Anthropology, Expressed Emotion and Schizophrenia. Ethos 19:387–431.
1991b The State Construction of Affect: Political Ethos and Mental Health Among
      Salvadoran Refugees. Culture, Medicine and Psychiatry 15(2):139–165.

Johnson, Mark
1987 The Body in the Mind. Chicago: University of Chicago Press.

Johnson, Thomas
1985 Consultation-Liaison Psychiatry: Medicine as Patient, Marginality as Prac-
      tice. In Physicians of Western Medicine. R. Hahn and A. Gaines (eds.). Dor-
      drecht: D. Reidel.
1987 Premenstrual Syndrome as a Western Culture-Specific Disorder. Culture,
      Medicine and Psychiatry 11(3):337–356.

Kapferer, Bruce
1979 Mind, Self, and Other in Demonic Illness. American Ethnologist 6(1):110– 133.

Katon, Wayne and Arthur Kleinman
1981 Doctor-Patient Negotiation. In The Relevance of Social Science for Medicine. L. Eisenberg and A. Kleinman (eds.). Dordrecht: D. Reidel.

Katz, Pearl
1979 Rituals in the Operating Room. Ethnology 20(4):335–350.

Katz, Pearl and Faris Kirkland
1990 Violence and Social Structure on Mental Hospital Wards. Psychiatry 53:262–277.

Kaufman, Sharon
1988 Toward a Phenomenology of Boundaries in Medicine: Chronic Illness Experience in the Case of Stroke. Medical Anthropology Quarterly *(n.s.)* 2(4):338– 345.

Kayser-Jones, Jeanie Schmit
1981 Old, Alone, and Neglected: Care of the Aged in Scotland and the United States. Berkeley: University of California Press.

Kennedy, John
1987 The Flower of Paradise: Institutionalized Use of *Qat* in North Yemen. Dordrecht: D. Reidel.

Kinzi, J, et al.
1984 Posttraumatic Stress Disorder Among Survivors of Cambodian Concentration Camps. American Journal of Psychiatry 141:645–650.

Kirmayer, Laurence J.
1988 Mind and Body as Metaphors: Hidden Values in Biomedicine. In Biomedicine Examined. Margaret Lock and Deborah Gordon (eds.). Dordrecht: Kluwer Academic Publishers.
1989a Psychotherapy and the Cultural Concept of the Person. Santé, Culture, Health 6(3):241–270.
1989b Cultural Variations in the Response to Psychiatric Disorders and Emotional Distress. Social Science and Medicine 29:327–339.

Kleinman, Arthur
1977 Problems and Prospects in Comparative Cross-Cultural Medical and Psychiatric Studies. In Renewal in Psychiatry. Theo Manschreck and Arthur Kleinman (eds.). Washington, D.C.: Hemisphere Publishing.
1980 Patients and Healers in the Context of Culture. Berkeley: University of California Press.
1986 Social Origins of Distress and Disease: Depression, Neurasthenia, and Pain in Modern China. New Haven: Yale University Press.
1987 Anthropology and Psychiatry. British Journal of Psychiatry 151:447–454.
1988a Rethinking Psychiatry. New York: Free Press.
1988b The Experience of Suffering and its Professional Transformation. Paper presented at the Conference, Anthropologies of Medicine: Western European and North American Perspectives. University of Hamburg, Hamburg, Germany. December 4–8.
1988c The Illness Narratives. New York: Basic Books.

Kleinman, A. L. Eisenberg and B. Good
1977 Culture, Illness and Care. Annals of Internal Medicine 88:251–258.

Kleinman, Arthur and J. Gale
1982 Patients Treated by Physicians and Folk Healers: A Comparative Outcome Study in Taiwan. Culture, Medicine and Psychiatry 6(4):405–423.

Kleinman, Arthur and Byron Good, eds.
1985 Culture and Depression: Studies in the Anthropology and Cross-Cultural Psychiatry of Affect and Disorder. Berkeley: University of California Press.

Kleinman, Arthur and Joan Kleinman
1985 Somatization. In Culture and Depression. Arthur Kleinman and Byron Good (eds.). Berkeley: University of California Press.
1990 Suffering and Its Professional Transformation: Toward an Ethnography of Experience. November. ms.

Kleinman, Arthur, Peter Kunstadter, E. Russell Alexander,

and James L. Gale, eds.
1975 Medicine in Chinese Cultures: Comparative Studies of Health Care in Chinese and Other Societies. Washington D.C.: USDHEW for the Fogerty Center.

LaBarre, Weston
1946 Social Cynosure and Social Structure. Journal of Personality 14(3):169–183.

Langness, L. L. and Harold Levine
1986 Culture and Retardation. Dordrecht: D. Reidel.

Larner, Christine
1981 Enemies of God. Baltimore: the Johns Hopkins University Press.

Latour, Bruno and Steven Wolgar
1979 Laboratory Life. Beverly Hills, CA: Sage.

Lawrence, Bruce B.
1988 Defenders of God. New York: Harpers.

Lazare, Aaron
1973 Hidden Conceptual Models in Clinical Psychiatry. New England Journal of Medicine 288:345–351.

Lazarus, Ellen
1988 Theoretical Considerations for the Study of the Doctor-Patient Relationship: Implications of a Perinatal Study. Medical Anthropology Quarterly *(n.s.)* 2(1):34–58.

Lebra, Takie
1976 Japanese Patterns of Behavior. Honolulu: The University Press of Hawaii.

Lebra, William, ed.
1972 Transcultural Research in Mental Health. Honolulu: University Press of Hawaii.
1976 Culture-Bound Syndromes, Ethnopsychiatry, and Alternate Therapies. Honolulu: University Press of Hawaii.

Lee, Dorothy
1959a View of the Self in Greek Culture. In Freedom and Culture. D. Lee. Englewood Cliffs, New Jersey: Prentice-Hall.

1959b The Wintu Self. In Freedom and Culture. D. Lee. Englewood Cliffs, New Jersey: Prentice-Hall.

Le Goff, Jacques
1980 Time, Work and Culture in the Middle Ages. A. Goldhammer, trans. Chicago: University of Chicago Press.

Light, Donald
1976 Work Styles Among American Psychiatric Residents. In Anthropology and Mental Health. Joseph Westermeyer (ed.). The Hague: Mouton.
1980 Becoming Psychiatrists. New York: W.W. Norton.

Littlewood, Roland
1990 From Categories to Contexts: A Decade of the New Cross-Cultural Psychiatry. British Journal of Psychatry 156:308–327.

Lock, Margaret
1980 East Asian Medicine in Urban Japan. Berkeley: University of California Press.
1985 Models and Practice in Medicine: Menopause as Syndrome or Life Transition? In Physicians of Western Medicine: Anthropological Approaches to Theory and Practice. R. Hahn and A. Gaines (eds.). Dordrecht: D. Reidel.
1987 DSM-III as a Culture-Bound Construct. Culture, Medicine and Psychiatry 11(1):35–42.
1988 A Nation at Risk. In Biomedicine Examined. M. Lock and D. Gordon (eds.). Dordrecht: Kluwer Academic Publishers.

Lock, Margaret and Deborah Gordon, eds.
1988 Biomedicine Examined. Dordrecht: Kluwer Academic Publishers.

Low, Setha
1988 The Diagnosis and Treatment of *Nervios* in Costa Rica. In Biomedicine Examined. Margaret Lock, and Deborah Gordon (eds.). Dordrecht: Kluwer Academic Publishers.

Lutz, Catherine
1985 Depression and the Translation of Emotional Worlds. In Culture and Depression. A. Kleinman and B. Good (eds.). Berkeley: University of California Press.

Manschreck, Theo and Arthur Kleinman
1977 Renewal in Psychiatry. Washington, D.C.: Hemisphere/Halsted Books.

Marcus, George and Michael Fischer
1986 Anthropology as Cultural Critique: An Experimental Moment in the Human Sciences. Chicago: University of Chicago Press.

Maretzki, Thomas
1985 Including the Physician in Healer-Centered Research: Retrospect and Prospect. In Physicians of Western Medicine. R. Hahn and A. Gaines (eds.). Dordrecht: D. Reidel.
1988 Cultural Studies of Medical Institutions, Hierarchies and Training Practice: Therapy Spectrum and Cultural Traditions: Choices for Cures. A Reflexive Report. Paper Presented at the Conference, The Anthropologies Medicine: Western Europe and North American Perspectives. University of Hamburg. Hamburg, Germany. December 4–8.

Maretzki, Thomas and Eduard Seidler
1985 Biomedicine and Naturopathic Healing in West Germany: A History of a
      Stormy Relationship. Culture, Medicine and Psychiatry 9(4):383–427.

Marsella, Anthony
1980 Depressive Experience and Disorder Across Cultures. In Handbook of Cross-
      Cultural Psychology. Vol. 5. Culture and Psychopathology. H. Triandis and
      J. Draguns (eds.). Boston: Allyn and Bacon.

Marsella, Anthony and Geoffrey White, eds.
1982 Cultural Conceptions of Mental Health and Therapy. Dordrecht: D. Reidel.

Marsella, Anthony, George DeVos and F. L. K. Hsu, eds.
1985 Culture and Self. New York: Tavistock.

Marshall, Mac, ed.
1979 Beliefs, Behaviors and Alcoholic Beverages. Ann Arbor: University of Michi-
      gan Press.

McClain, Carol Shepard
1989 Women as Healers. New Brunswick: Rutgers University Press.

Mendelsohn, Everett and Yehuda Elkana, eds.
1981 Science and Cultures. Dordrecht: D. Reidel.

Menninger, Karl with M. Mayman and P. Pruyser
1963 The Vital Balance. New York: Viking.

Mishler, Elliot, S. Osher and L. Amarasingham, et al.
1981 Social Contexts of Health, Illness and Patient Care. Cambridge: Cambridge
      University Press.

Morantz-Sanchez, Regina Markell
1985 Sympathy and Science. New York: Oxford University Press.

Morgan, Lynn
1987 Dependency Theory in the Political Economy of Health: An Anthropological
      Critique. Medical Anthropology Quarterly *(n.s.)* 1(2):131–154.

Morsy, Soheir
1978 Sex Roles, Power, and Illness in an Egyptian Village. American Ethnologist
      5(1):137–150.
1991 Safeguarding Women's Bodies: The White Man's Burden Medicalized. Medi-
      cal Anthropology Quarterly *(n.s.)* 5(1):19–23.

Murphy, Jane
1976 Psychiatric Labeling in Cross-Cultural Perspective. Science 191:1019–1028.

Navarro, Vincente
1976 Medicine Under Capitalism. New York: Prodist.

Nichter, Mark
1981 Idioms of Distress. Culture, Medicine and Psychiatry 5(4):379–408.

Norbeck, Edward and Margaret Lock, eds.
1987 Health, Illness and Medical Care in Japan. Honolulu: University of Hawaii
      Press.

Nuckolls, Charles, ed.
1992 The Cultural Construction of Psychiatric Classification. Social Science and
      Medicine Special Issue/ Section. (In press)

Obeyesekere, Gananath
1985 Depression, Buddhism and the Work of Culture in Sri Lanka. In Culture and Depression. Kleinman, Arthur and Byron Good (eds.). Berkeley: University of California Press.

Ohnuki-Tierney, Emiko
1984 Health and Illness in Contemporary Japan. Cambridge: Cambridge University Press.

O'Neill, J.
1985 Five Bodies: The Human Shape of Modern Society. Ithaca: Cornell University Press.

Ortner, Sherry
1984 Theory in Anthropology Since the Sixties. Comparative Studies in Society and History 26(1):126–166.

Ots, Thomas
1988 Phenomenology of the Body. Paper presented at the Conference, Anthropologies of Medicine: Western European and North American Perspectives. University of Hamburg. Hamburg. Germany. December 4–8.

Pandolfi, Mariella
1988 Refusing Knowledge: Embodying Emotion: Women in a Southern Italian Village. Paper presented at Conference, Anthropologies of Medicine: Western European and North American Perspectives. University of Hamburg. Hamburg, Germany. December 4–8.

Parsons, Talcott
1951 The Social System. Glencoe, IL: Free Press.

Pattison, E., N. Lapins and H. Doerr
1973 Faith Healing: A Study of Personality and Function. Journal of Nervous and Mental Disease 157(6):397–409.

Pedersen, Paul, J. Draguns, W. Lonner and J. Trimble, eds.
1989 [1976] Counseling Across Cultures. 3rd edition. Honolulu: University of Hawaii Press.

Pliskin, Karen
1987 Silent Boundaries. New Haven: Yale University Press.

Post, Stephen
1992 DSM-III-R: Psychiatry, Religion and Bias. In The Cultural Construction of Psychiatric Classification. Charles Nuckolls, ed. Social Science and Medicine Special Issue/Section. (in press)

Prince, Raymond and Françoise Tcheng-Laroche
1987 Culture-Bound Syndromes and International Disease Classifications. Culture, Medicine, and Psychiatry 11(1):3–20.

Press, Irwin
1990 Levels of Explanation and Cautions for a Critical Clinical Anthropology. Social Science and Medicine 30(9):1001–1009.

Rabinow, Paul and William M. Sullivan, eds.
1979 Interpretive Social Science. Berkeley: University of California Press.
1987 Interpretive Social Science: A Second Look. Berkeley: University of California Press.

Reynolds, David and Norman Farbarow
1977   Endangered Hope: Experiences in Psychiatric Aftercare Facilities. Berkeley:
       University of California Press.

Rhodes, Lorna Amarasingham
1986   The Anthropologist as Institutional Analyst. Ethos 14(2):204–217.
1991   Emptying Beds. Berkeley: University of California Press.

Richters, Annemiek
1988   Fighting the *Peists* of Our Times: Medical Anthropology and Cultural Hege-
       mony. Medical Anthropology Quarterly *(n.s.)* 2(4):438–446.

Russett, Cynthia Eagle
1988   Sexual Science: The Victorian Construction of Womanhood. Cambridge, MA:
       Harvard University Press.

Sahlins, Marshall
1976   Culture and Practical Reason. Chicago: University of Chicago Press.

Scarry, Elaine
1985   The Body in Pain: the Making and Unmaking of the World. New York:
       Oxford University Press.

Scheder, Jo C.
1988   A Sickly-Sweet Harvest: Farmworker Diabetes and Social Equality. Medical
       Anthropology Quarterly *(n.s.)* 2(3):251–277.

Scheper-Hughes, Nancy
1981   Dilemmas in Deinstitutionalization: A View from Inner City Boston. Journal
       of Operational Psychiatry 12(2):90–99.
1988   The Madness of Hunger. Culture, Medicine and Psychiatry 12(4):429–458.

Scheper-Hughes, Nancy and Margaret Lock
1986   Speaking Truth to Illness: Metaphors, Reification and a Pedagogy for
       Patients. Medical Anthropology Quarterly 18(1):6–41.
1988   The Mindful Body: A Prolegomenon to Future Work in Medical Anthropolo-
       gy. Medical Anthropology Quarterly *(n.s.)* 1(1):6–41.

Scotch, Norman
1963   Medial Anthropology. In Biennial Review of Anthropology: 1963. B. Siegal et
       al. (eds.). Stanford, CA: Stanford University Press.

Shweder, Richard
1990   Cultural Psychology—What Is It? In Cultural Psychology. J. Stigler, R.
       Shweder and G. Herdt (eds.). Cambridge: Cambridge University Press.

Shweder, Richard and Edmund Bourne
1982   Do Conceptions of Person Vary Cross-Culturally? In Cultural Conceptions of
       Mental Health and Therapy. Anthony Marsella and Geoffrey White (eds.).
       Dordrecht: D. Reidel.

Simon, B.
1978   Mind and Madness in Ancient Greece: The Classical Roots of Modern Psychi-
       atry. Ithaca: Cornell University Press.

Simons, Ronald C. and Charles Hughes, eds.
1985   Culture-Bound Syndromes. Dordrecht: D. Reidel.

Sindzingre, Nicole
1988 Comments on Five Manuscripts. Medical Anthropology Quarterly *(n.s.)* 2(4):447–453.

Singer, Merrill
1986 Developing a Critical Perspective in Medical Anthropology. Medical Anthropological Quarterly 17(5):128–129.

Singer, Merrill, Hans Baer and Ellen Lazarus
1990 Critical Medical Anthropology in Question. Social Science and Medicine 30(2):v–viii.

Skultans, Vieda
1979 English Madness. London: Routledge and Kegan Paul.

Sue, Stanley and James Morishima
1982 The Mental Health of Asian Americans. San Francisco: Josey Bass.

Susser, Ida, ed.
1988 Health and Industry. Medical Anthropology Quarterly *(n.s.)* Special Issue 2(1).

Szasz, Thomas
1961 The Myth of Mental Illness. New York: Hoeber-Harper.

Tomm, Winnifred and Gordon Hamilton, eds.
1988 Gender Bias in Scholarship: The Persuasive Prejudice. Waterloo, Ontario: Wilfrid Laurier University Press.

Townsend, J. M.
1978 Cultural Conceptions and Mental Illness. Chicago: University of Chicago Press.
1979 Stereotypes and Mental Illness: A Comparison with Ethnic Stereotypes. Culture, Medicine and Psychiatry 3(3):205–230.

Turkle, Sherry
1978 Psychoanalytic Politics: Freud's French Revolution. New York: Basic Books.

Turner, Bryan
1984 The Body and Society. New York: Basil Blackwell.

Turner, Victor
1964 An Ndembu Doctor in Practice. In Magic, Faith and Healing. Ari Kiev (ed.). New York: Basic Books.

Turner, Victor and Edward Bruner. eds.
1986 The Anthropology of Experience. Urbana, IL: University of Illinois Press.

Valle, Ramón
1989 Outreach to Ethnic Minorities with Alzheimer's Disease: The Challenge to the Community. Health Matrix 6(4):13–27.

Van Moffaert, Myriam and André Vereecken
1989 Somatization of Psychiatric Illness in Mediterranean Immigrants in Belgium. Culture, Medicine and Psychiatry 13(3):297–313.

Veatch, Robert, ed.
1989 Cross-Cultural Perspectives in Medical Ethics: Readings: Boston: Jones and Bartlett.

Waitzkin, Howard
1979 Medicine: Superstructure and Micropolitics. Social Science and Medicine
      13A:601–609.
1981 A Marxist Analysis of the Health Care Systems of Advanced Capitalist Soci-
      eties. In The Relevance of Social Science for Medicine. Leon Eisenberg and
      Arthur Kleinman (eds.). Dordrecht: D. Reidel.

Watson-Gegeo, Karen and Geoffrey White, eds.
1990 Disentangling. Stanford: Stanford University Press.

Waxler-Morrison, Nancy et al.
1990 Cross-Cultural Caring: A Handbook for Health Professionals in Western
      Canada. Vancouver, B.C.: University of British Columbia Press.

Weidman, Hazel H.
1969 Cultural Values, Concept of Self and Projection: The Burmese Case. In Men-
      tal Health Research in the Pacific. W. Caudill and T. -Y. Lin (eds.). Honolu-
      lu: East West Center Press.

Weisberg, D. and S. O. Long, eds.
1984 Biomedicine in Asia: Transformations and Variations. Culture, Medicine and
      Psychiatry Special Issue 8(2).

Weisz, George, ed.
1990 Social Science Perspectives on Medical Ethics. Dordrecht: Kluwer Academic
      Publishers.

Westermeyer, Joseph
1982 Poppies, Pipes and People. Berkeley: University of California Press.
1989 Mental Health for Refugees and Other Migrants. Springfield, IL: C. C. Thomas.

Westermeyer, Joseph and Ronald Wintrob
1979 Folk Criteria for the Diagnosis of Mental Illness in Rural Laos. American
      Journal of Psychiatry 136:755–761.

White, Geoffrey and Anthony Marsella
1982 Introduction: Cultural Conceptions in Mental Health Research and Practice.
      In Cultural Conceptions of Mental Health and Therapy. A. Marsella and G.
      White (eds.). Dordrecht: D. Reidel.

White, Geoffrey and John Kirkpatrick, eds.
1985 Person, Self and Experience: Exploring Pacific Ethnopsychologies. Berkeley:
      University of California Press.

Wright, Peter and Andrew Treacher, eds.
1982a The Problem of Medical Knowledge: Examining the Social Construction of
      Medicine. Edinburgh: University of Edinburgh Press.

Wright, Peter and Andrew Treacher
1982b Introduction. In The Problem of Medical Knowledge: Examining the Social
      Construction of Medicine. Peter Wright and Andrew Treacher (eds.). Edin-
      burgh: University of Edinburgh Press.

Yap, P. M.
1974 Comparative Psychiatry: A Theoretical Framework. J. Lau and A. Stokes
      (eds.). Toronto: University of Toronto Press.

Young, Allan

1976   Some Implications of Medical Beliefs and Practices for Social Anthropology. American Anthropologist 78(1):5–24.

1977a Order, Analogy and Efficacy in Amhara Medical Divination. Culture, Medicine and Psychiatry 1(1):183–199.

1977b Internalizing and Externalizing Medical Belief Systems. Social Science and Medicine 10(1):141–156.

1978   Mode of Production of Medical Knowledge. Medical Anthropology 2(1):97–122.

1981   The Creation of Medical Knowledge: Some Problems of Interpretation. Social Science and Medicine 15B:379–386.

1982   The Anthropologies of Illness and Sickness. In Annual Review of Anthropology. Palo Alto: Annual Review Press.

1988   A Case Study Describing How An Institutional Ideology Shapes Knowledge of a Mental Disorder (Posttraumatic Stress Disorder). ms.

1990   Moral Conflicts in a Psychiatric Hospital Treating Combat-Related Posttraumatic Stress Disorder (PTSD). In Social Science Perspectives on Medical Ethics. George Weisz (ed.). Dordrecht: Kluwer Academic Publishers.

1991   Emil Kraepelin and the History of American Psychiatric Classification. In Anthropologies of Medicine. B. Pfleiderer and G. Bibeau (eds.). Wiesbaden, Germany: Vieweg Verlag.

2

The Subject of Power
in Medical/Psychiatric Anthropology[*]

Lorna Amarasingham Rhodes

TO TURF: definition; To get rid of...
(Shem 1978:428)

Introduction: Power and Clinical Practice

Power has become a subject of explicit interest in medical anthropology. In a recent article, for example, Singer, Davison, and Gerdes (1988) distinguish between the "webs of significance" that many of us, following Geertz, have been entangled in for years, and the "webs of mystification" they feel are overdue for unraveling. Some, however, wonder whether this concern is, itself, a new form of mystification that sees "homogeneous hegemony" everywhere (Estroff 1988; see also Gaines, this volume) and that reframes but does not really change the focus of our perennial concern with suffering.

At issue in this debate are questions about the relationship between domination and understanding, and about the nature and purpose of anthropological interpretation. We find ourselves asking not only *what* is the subject of power in medical anthropology, but also *who* is the subject of power. "Critical" medical anthropologists share with their (perhaps) less critical colleagues the anthropologist's fascination for the speaking subject: the voice, or the multiplicity of voices, explaining, describing, perhaps haranguing, that are, for many of us, the foundation of our work.[1]

One task of this moment in the history of medical anthropology seems to be a more self-conscious working through of the dilemmas and contradic-

---

[*]This chapter is drawn from my book, *Emptying Beds: The Work of an Emergency Psychiatric Unit*; copyright © 1991, The Regents of the University of California. The material is used with the kind permission of University of California Press.

tions provoked by a double awareness. We are listeners, entangled willy-nilly in the web of micro-level research, where we experience directly the significance of what is spoken by those we study. At the same time we are participants in the demystifying, deconstructing discourses of our time, discourses that seem to give us a foothold outside, looking on with anger, or despair (depending on our temperament), at the entanglements and multiple oppressions of our subjects.

This paper centers on a story that has been, for me, evocative of the possibility of a productive, though perhaps awkward, intersecting of these perspectives. This story comes out of two years of research I conducted in the emergency psychiatry unit of a large community mental health center. My focus was the staff of this unit and their relationship to work that was regarded (by others and by them) as difficult and problematic.[2] In choosing this particular story to represent questions about the "subject" I have chosen a case in which the patient could not speak. I see this, in part, as a way of highlighting the fact that all clinical situations are polyphonous; though the voices of patients are, of course, of great importance, sometimes our privileging of the "patient's perspective" threatens to become a sophisticated form of objectification (cf. Arney and Bergen 1984). In this account the staff are the speaking subjects, and they speak, in part, of the temptations and dangers that emerge from their patient's silence.

Before turning to the emergency unit, I want to make two points about issues that emerge in writing about psychiatric institutions. First, in considering the situation of patients in institutions it is useful to recognize that the current controversy between applied and critical approaches in medical anthropology is replicated in the dispute between clinical and critical psychiatry. On the one hand, much of the literature in psychiatry is concerned with the treatment of patients—interpretation and intervention based on more or less close scrutiny of symptoms, feelings, relationships—and, sometimes, with examining the relationship between practitioner and patient. Though this literature is vastly diverse and contradictory, in the main it is based on the assumption that agency (excepting countertransference issues) is relatively straightforward. Those who treat are helping, or trying to.

On the other hand, critical or antipsychiatric literature construes practitioners as agents of social control whose primary role is to contain deviance. In a typical statement David Ingleby says:

> [The] "critical view" argues that "mental illness" is to a large extent
> socially caused, or even socially constructed; that the goal of treatment
> has to do with the maintenance of social order; and that the domination
> of the medical profession is neither warranted nor desirable. (1983:143)

Views on the nature of and reasons for this social construction and control of mental illness vary widely; but there is general agreement that psychiatric professionals are agents of forces that are not, at bottom, in the interests of the patient. Therapy is mystification, concealing (and masking in ideology) a variety of forms of oppression. Andrew Scull, for example, sees the community psychiatry movement as a direct consequence of the government's intention to provide cheaper, not better, accommodation for those "qualified" to drop out of the surplus labor pool (1979, 1984). Its rationale is as delusional as (or maybe more delusional than) the patients it claims to help. (For general discussions of these issues see also Cohen and Scull [1983].)

While the clinical perspective reveals the richness and sometimes the subtlety of individual relationships, and the critical perspective opens up a macro-level vista often invisible to individuals, neither seems sufficient when one is immersed in the daily of life of a psychiatric institution. Goffman discovered long ago that at close quarters the institution reveals itself to be constituted of endless self-perpetuating "binds"—ambiguous relationships between form and content, constraint and opportunity—to which practitioners and patients respond in pragmatic and strategic ways (1961). From the perspective of those who work or live in institutions, the tension between context and agency is ongoing and unresolvable. To use the words of Jean Comaroff: resistance and acquiescence are perpetually in balance (1985). Power is always present, but the question of precisely who has it evades one at every turn.

This brings me to my second point: the usefulness of Michel Foucault's work on power for an understanding of institutions. Foucault writes about institutions not merely as places that reflect or contain societal problems, but as sites for the construction of the relationship between the individual and society. In his studies of the asylum, the hospital, and the prison, Foucault shows that in the late eighteenth and early nineteenth centuries the inner space of these institutions developed a configuration that provided for the development of the peculiarly modern relationship between subject and object; through the manipulation and management of the body, the inmate became an object of knowledge and a subject of discipline (1973, 1975, 1978).

I do not have space here for a detailed consideration of Foucault's notions of disciplinary space, power/knowledge, and subjectivity. I want to point out, however, that I found striking similarities between the talk of the staff of the emergency unit and the writing of Foucault (especially 1973, 1979, 1980). Surely these similarities are not accidental; they reflect the fact that the staff of the unit spoke from the center of the kind of disciplinary space Foucault describes, a space in which confinement of "others" contributes to an objectification of self.

In Foucault's view, power does not "rest" in the hands of individuals or groups; rather it is fluid, and diffuse, operating in a net-like grid of relationships. This analogy to a net or web corresponds to my observation of the way the unit worked. The staff members described their power as paradoxical and contradictory; they were both discipliners and disciplined. They did not employ a single kind of power (as, for example, the power to label patients as mentally ill, or, conversely, the power to make them well) in a clear, unidirectional way, nor were patients passive in the face of such power. Rather, administrators, staff and patients were engaged in a situation of shifting, reciprocal, and multidirectional power relations. I do not mean by this that the unit's staff did not exercise more power than the patients; they did. But in order to understand the nature of clinical practice on the unit, we cannot depend for explanation on an arrow of "power over" that points only from the staff to the patients (or, for that matter, from the state or the economy to the staff). Rather, staff, patients, administrators, and other institutions have to be seen as bound together in the same disciplinary space, one in which all, to varying degrees, exercise and are subjects of power.

The staff of the Acute Psychiatry Unit (APU) did not accede passively to an enmeshment in a system of power. "Where there is power there is resistance" (Foucault 1978); and they found ways to resist, through strategy, humor, and subversion of discipline. The resistance of the staff was covert, ephemeral, and oblique; it served to throw into relief, at every turn, ways in which the work constantly threatened to become absurd. Many of the "techniques for making useful individuals" that pervaded the hospital—from the patient interview to the writing of charts—had the potential to be subverted or mocked.

This subversion is not, it seems to me, peripheral to the "real" work of clinical practice, something that would end were the institution to be retooled to more perfectly meet the needs of its constituents. It was clearly part and parcel of the work itself and to the extent that the work had meaning to the staff, it was because they made something tangible out of their experience of disjunction, contradiction, and absurdity. Novels and popular accounts of clinical work sometimes make this point indirectly, as when, in *The House of God*, the intern/antihero is asked by those outside the hospital how he can laugh about what he is doing (Shem 1978).

I am concerned, then, with the way in which the micro-settings of institutions offer us a play of power and resistance, of visibility and invisibility, of objectivity and subjectivity. On the one hand, the staff are enmeshed in strategic action, exerting and acquiescing to power in a complex and nonlinear fashion. On the other hand, they resist. In this paper I want to make the point that one aspect of this resistance is interpretation. The staff try to maintain, in the chinks of invisibility between the threads of capillary power, a subjective capacity to redefine and give subversive meaning to their actions. Seen in this way, the interpretation of events does not result in meanings that lend themselves to the construction of models of clinical practice; rather the meanings themselves are recognized by their creators to be contingent, partial, and prone to dissolution in the face of the ongoing contradictions of the work.

The Acute Psychiatry Unit

The Acute Psychiatry Unit[3] was an acute treatment facility in the inner city area of a large midwestern city. The unit was part of a 100-bed public psychiatric hospital called a "community mental health center" because of its location, orientation to short-term therapy, and ideology of community treatment. The unit had nine beds, and 25–30 patients passed through these beds in a month. The unit's staff consisted of thirty psychiatrists, psychiatric residents, nurses, social workers, and mental health aides.

The patients who passed through the Acute Psychiatry Unit were poor, acutely ill or distressed, and often completely without resources of any kind. Because of the deinstitutionalization of psychiatric patients begun in the late 1960s, few long-term care facilities were available for these patients, who often returned repeatedly to the unit.[4] Thus the task of the unit was to treat patients quickly, moving them on to other facilities, out to their families or, in some cases, to "the street" (see Mizrahi 1986).

The APU was a locked ward on which patients occupied single rooms. The unit, which occupied the first floor of the community mental health center, was extremely simple in design, consisting of a locked area that included a day room, and a nurses' station facing onto the patients' hallway. The staff prided themselves on the stark, bare-bones nature of this environment which was intended, in their view, to discourage the return of patients. Patients were generally on the unit too briefly to become well known to the staff.[5]

Four staff members play important roles in the account that follows. A psychiatrist, Sam Wishinski, was the unit's clinical director; his immediate supervisor, Ben Caldwell, was the psychiatrist who directed the hospital's emergency wing. Lillian Morgan was the unit's head social worker, and Walter Boyd was the addictions counselor. Residents, nurses, and aides were also involved, but I have not named them here.

Sam Wishinski kept a sharp eye out for metaphors and stories that expressed aspects of the unit's work. One was a play, *Terra Nova*, about Admiral Scott's ill-fated expedition to the South Pole (Tally 1981). Scott and all of his men died on the way back from the pole, having been beaten to it by a few days by the Norwegian explorer Amundsen. In the play, Amundsen is a pragmatic man who taunts Scott with his unwillingness to bend to the practical exigencies of his situation. Scott, an Englishman, maintains to the end the strictest rules of gentlemanly decency. He refuses to use his dogs for food or to leave injured men behind. But there is one moment when he looks out on the frozen wastes stretching away from his tent and says suddenly, as though seeing the place for the first time, "Good God, this is an *awful* place!"

Sam felt that this scene provided a useful image for understanding the APU.

1. The unit was an "awful place" because of its position as what the staff called the unconscious of psychiatry, a place where the patients were acutely ill and socially marginal. About 30 percent of the patients had been sent to the unit by the police or the court system. The staff could count few "successes" and felt that they were expected to accomplish an impossible task in a field of ever-dwindling resources.

2. The staff concentrated on that aspect of the work that was most immediately compelling: getting patients out. Their emphasis was on disposing of, turfing, discharging; they were obliged to keep beds open for emergencies, and in order to do so, they had to move patients already on the unit. Patients might be moved to other facilities, or back onto the streets, to families or to homeless shelters; regardless, the staff had to produce empty beds. Thus, they had to be like Amundsen. Amundsen taunts Scott with being "the most dangerous kind of decent man" (Tally 1981), someone not willing to look at what is really in front of him. The APU staff felt that the rules of the outside world—"decency"—had to give way on a daily basis to choices among painful and unavoidable alternatives.

3. The staff of the unit considered their position unusual and not easy for outsiders to understand. One of the psychiatrists told this story:

    > A man sees a sign in a shop window that says: 'We press pants.' The next day he takes in a pair of pants to be pressed. 'Oh no,' said the shopkeeper, 'We don't press pants, we make signs.'

The unit advertised itself as offering treatment but in fact it offered movement; it served as a brief way station in a complex landscape of hospitals, shelters, and streets, a place that "patched them up and sent them out" until the next time. The staff felt that their acceptance of the need to "eat their dogs," to do many things that might be unacceptable in what they imagined was the neater, better-lighted world of "regular" psychiatry, was hidden by a many-faceted collusion among the hospital administration, the state, and perhaps even the patients, a collusion in which they were full participants.

The Game of "Hot Shit"

One day in June a man named Charles Judge was brought into the unit by the director of a local nursing home. Judge had become unmanageable at the nursing home, and the unit was considered a placement of last resort for difficult patients who had nowhere else to go.

Charles Judge was in his early fifties, but he looked at least sixty-five. An alcoholic all his life, he suffered from brain damage; he was unable to care for himself and could not speak more than a few words. He had episodes in which he fell down, he wandered uncontrollably, and he was sometimes incontinent. The nursing home had used restraints to keep him from wandering around.

Judge stayed on the APU for more than five months. He was an anomaly and, for this reason, he came to represent to the staff many aspects of their situation. He was a patient they couldn't get rid of, thereby highlighting the nature of their strategies and the essence of their relation to the outside world. At the same time, they developed a relationship with him that became paradigmatic of their ability to resist, when they had to, the unit's definition as an emergency facility. Through their redefinition of Judge as a "child" and a "pet" they created an alternative image of the unit.

The APU had already had two experiences of having patients from the nursing home "dumped" on them. This time Ben Caldwell wanted to prove once and for all that these were inappropriate referrals. He wrote an eight-page evaluation documenting that Charles Judge was not a psychiatric patient, and admitted him on "holding status," which meant that he had no chart but was to be "held." Usually, this category was only used for a few hours for patients about to be transferred to other facilities.

Ben liked the fact that he had such an obvious and well-witnessed case, and hoped to "nail" the nursing home director and the Department of Mental Health on it. Talking later about his reaction to Charles Judge, Ben said, "When he came in I had two separate and contradictory feelings. One was, he should be in a state hospital, preferably in the old days when they had farms. And the other was, too bad, that's not what I'm the agent for, I'm the agent for a different set of values." One of these values was the protection of his unit from an influx of "inappropriate" admissions. "I wanted Sam *not* to solve [Judge's case] or we would have more of these problems to solve."

Judge was an inappropriate admission because he didn't have what staff considered a psychiatric disorder. They felt that he had a medical illness, dementia secondary to alcoholism. This illness was incurable and rendered him completely helpless. Sam said:

> When Judge came in he was defined as the offal—the piece of shit in the game of hot potato, or hot shit, among parts of the system. Whoever got stuck with him would be the person who takes care of the shit. What do you call those people in Japan? The *Eta*. Are psychiatrists the *Eta*? Or nursing homes? The chronic wards? The community?

The initial reaction of the staff to Charles's admission was one of resentment:

> Sam: I tried to avoid him. I said to the resident, 'this case has too many administrative complexities.' I let him manage it.
> Walter [who was assigned to take care of Judge on a daily basis]: Initially when he came in he was a headache. He was a square peg trying to fit into a round hole. Not much we could do for him, and not much he could do for himself, either.

For the first month or more, Judge was an invisible patient. He had no official chart (though the staff kept an unofficial one). He was not even discussed in the biweekly staff meeting (called "staffing") at which decisions were made about the unit's patients. When he was finally mentioned in staffing, it was with a certain defiance.

> Sam: On Judge, there's nothing new. We're still awaiting word from the Department of Mental Health [on how to resolve the dispute with the nursing home]. Well, we won't do a thing, just see how long we can keep him here before anyone *does* anything.

At this point, Charles Judge represented for the staff their position as the unconscious of psychiatry. They could not get the attention of those with the power to resolve the situation. During the fall, the APU staff tried to exercise their competence at what they did best. They tried every possible option for disposition. Charles could not be accepted by home-care programs because he needed too much care, even if his niece, who lived in the city, had been willing to have him. For a while it looked as though a diagnosis of mental retardation might get him into a home for the retarded.

> Lillian: I'm going to try to get through to the Mental Retardation program; I'll call Dr. D. first to find out how to present it to them.
> Sam: (hopefully): We could have [the psychologist] test him. I'm sure he'd score retarded now.

But this plan fell through. The program only accepted retarded people who had been wrongly diagnosed as mentally ill, not those with organic brain damage. Sam joked in staffing, "…we could interview his niece, she's not too swift. Maybe we could establish some genetic [tendency]…" But, as Walter remarked later,

> [There was] a painful side [to Judge's case]. We made light of it, but we were very aggressive in trying to get him out. It was a blow to my ego dealing with him because we're used to getting people out at a rapid pace.

In the meantime, Charles Judge was becoming a fixture on the unit; people were getting used to him.

> Sam [in staffing]: I think everyone's getting comfortable with him here.
> I think if he gets very ill, Ben and Giuliani will get scared he'll die here
> and do something about him.
> Walter: He sleeps late, he's been hoarding stuff under his bed, ice
> cream, soda. So we have to watch it. But he's been up.

As this conversation indicates, there was concern, for a while, about
his health, as he seemed to be going into a decline.

> Walter: I took him to the ER [emergency room] Friday. They said he
> was dehydrated. His teeth are bad.
> Sam: Maybe we should try a softer diet, milkshakes.
> Lillian: That [his teeth] is not making him feel good.
> Sam: There used to be a time when they pulled the teeth of chronic
> inmates.
> Walter: He was angry at me for taking him to the ER. [Walter imitates
> Charles trying to say, "You bastard."]
> Sam: Does he look depressed?
> Walter: He's down, stays in his room a lot.

By calling up the image of the old hospital/prison and its toothless inmates,
Sam throws into relief the care the staff are giving Mr. Judge. They want
him to be "up," walking around in the safety of the APU environment, in
contrast to the nursing home where he was kept in restraints.

As this last conversation suggests, Walter, who was most involved in
Judge's daily care, had by this time become the interpreter of his moods.
The staff had ceased to remain aloof from the patient's humanity. Sam
said:

> Eventually I felt uncomfortable about this man lying on the floor. It
> was hard to pretend he wasn't there. One of the great moments was
> when we finally got his niece in with her baby and Judge's eyes lit up
> and he talked to the baby—"dadada"! Judge was like a child.

The staff began to talk as though they had a special understanding of
Judge's needs.

> Walter: We're checking out the VA [Veteran's Administration]. They
> said to document that he's not a behavior problem. He has "seizures"
> and slides to the floor, but if he's ignored he goes to his room.
> Nurse: We walk right over him!
> Walter: If you say, "want a drink" he'll get up. Going to an old folks
> home is not good for him, no one would joke around with him.
> Sam: So you're recommending nursery school?
> Nurse: Remember the baby? They got along perfectly—"da-da-da!"

Walter talked about the way his attitude toward Judge shifted as he
accepted the hopelessness of the situation:

Things didn't lessen and there was no end in sight. [Judge] became a continual headache. Then I got empathetic, though still annoyed. I was beyond the point of being angry at being imposed on; it became a routine, knowing we didn't have *any* alternatives.

At this point, the implications of Judge's name began to be felt. Sam said, "Then we lose, we've got him. But then he becomes a human being, we realize he's not a piece of shit. He's *The Judge*."

Judge's health improved, and staff were proud of their success. As Walter put it, "We're doing good work; the Judge is getting better." When Thanksgiving came around Judge's family wanted him to come home for the day. But Ben and Sam decided against it. Ben was worried that Judge might overeat and get sick. And, on principle, he felt that, "They can't just take him when they feel like it, we will not provide an interim rest home for the family." Here again Ben was interested in defining the limits of the unit's role. But there was also a sense in which Judge had become like a child to the staff; they defended him against the competing, but erratic, attentions of his family.

Increasingly, the Judge was accepted as he was. He was always the last to be brought up in staffing, a recurring addendum to the normal business of moving people along, often greeted with the (by now) timeworn joke: "Here come de Judge!" Staff still felt their failure to place him as a challenge to their competence, but they also found that treating Judge as a guest had its own rewards. Enjoyment of his personality began to change into feelings of self-respect for the appreciation and care they were giving him. Sam recalled later: "Judge would play in the bathtub, which endeared him to us. At first it was seen as a behavior problem because he didn't want to get out, but we redefined it that he enjoyed it and started putting him in there to play and sing." The staff were proud that Judge's "wandering," "fits," and babbling were not problematic for them.

By late November the Judge was a fixture on the unit. All attempts to place him had failed. Sometimes now he was referred to as a "pet." In the day room, Judge, who has been sitting at the table, suddenly starts to lean to one side with his eyes closed. Another patient tries to stop him. One of the mental health workers says, "One thing about the Judge, he never falls." The other patient asks, "Is he sick?" "Yeah," she says, "we have real sick people in here. This is a mental hospital." She says to me, "The Judge, he's the head nurse's pet, that's why he's still here."

At this point the hospital's administrator became concerned about the use of "holding status" to keep a patient indefinitely. He consulted legal authorities at the state level, who said that this practice was probably illegal. To make the situation look better, Ben abolished "holding status," replacing it with a new category called "awaiting disposition." The only way out of holding the Judge seemed to be the one that was rejected at the beginning to make the point, that is, to give him a legal status and transfer him to a long-term unit.

A hearing was scheduled for the Judge. In the hearing room he sat straight and seemed to listen as Ben presented the problem, describing how he was admitted as a "guest" and could not be placed; Ben emphasized his complete inability to care for himself. The public defender asked Judge: "Do you want to stay here?" nodding as he said it, and Judge said "Yes," nodding back (he nodded "yes" to anything). Ben presented his doubts about voluntary admission since Judge would not understand what he was signing. But the hearing officer thought that it was the only solution. He recommended that Judge be signed into the unit as a "voluntary" patient.

When they get back to the unit from the hearing Lillian asks Judge, "Do you want to stay?" Judge's head seems to clear and he says: "I want to get out of here." "Where would you go?" "I've got a place to go...I've got four...," says Judge, but then he falters. He can't remember the names of his children.

When this incident was described to Ben—it suggested that Judge did not want to stay—he said, "I don't care, I'm keeping him." Judge's human needs had won out over the administrative agenda; it seemed pointless to make an issue of the involuntary quality of Judge's "voluntary" admission. Sam outlined the larger picture:

> He became human to us. Clearly the Judge belongs on a decent chronic care unit. But the history of the mental health movement has distorted our faculties so we can't reach those elementary decisions. Instead, the medical establishment says he's psychiatric, psychiatry says it's medical. The Department of Mental Health says it doesn't matter what you say because we are implementing deinstitutionalization as a policy.

Judge did "sign" a "voluntary" and, because there were no beds available at the state hospital, he was transferred to another, longer-term unit at the mental health center. For Ben, whose mind was on administrative consequences, Judge represented the fact that, ultimately, anyone could be placed. For him, the unit's power rested in the confidence of the staff that all patients had a "niche."

> I don't believe anything different about the Judge now...just another guy, no different from others who tramp through here, they all have a niche to which we can send them.

But for most of the staff he became paradigmatic of their capacity to be flexible; they developed their own local, situated understanding of this patient for whom they had struggled so long to find a place. By the time the Judge left he had become a source of self congratulation for the staff and a category had been generated to describe him. He was no longer someone "awful" who "doesn't belong here" but a "pet," "someone we give good care to." Sam said,

Gradually the fact that no other place can deal with him becomes the system's fault. We perceive the awfulness of the system instead of his awfulness. So he becomes a test case, a Judge.

A few months after Judge's departure from the unit, Lillian reported with delight that he had finally been accepted into a long-term ward at the state hospital. In the meantime his story had become part of the unit's incorporation of new students. One day in staffing a patient was referred to as a "young Charles Judge." The new resident said, wistfully, "I wish I could meet the Judge."

Conclusion

We can point to many "macro-level" forces that might be seen to underlay (or perhaps overlay) this drama—perhaps DNA costarring with alienation in the guise of Judge's alcoholism, the capitalist health care system in the role of the nursing home, and class interests as players in Judge's poverty and the staff's paternalism. But to see these as "forces" somehow separate from the events themselves, with arrows, perhaps, pointing from one "level" to another, is to miss the way they are embedded and enacted in practice and to miss, as well, the richness to be discovered in the disorder of their mutual interaction. Thus, I come back to Foucault's point: power does indeed manifest itself in institutions, but we can understand it best if we see it as diffuse and multiple, as spread out rather than imposed from above.

(The) Judge was one point of articulation in a field of intersecting interests, strategies, and definitions. Each point in this field had its strength, its ability to exert force, and its weakness. The hospital could admit and yet "not admit" Judge; Ben could strategically refuse to solve the problem yet solve it after all (or was it a solution?); Sam could hold still, defiantly, forcing action from above, yet he could not *not* act; the staff could 'strategize' through diagnostic manipulations while pretending the Judge did not exist And it would demean the Judge not to accord him his mite of power as well, for he eluded restraints and, by sheer force of silent personality, found a temporary lodging.

"Clinical reality" cannot be understood separately from such ambiguous relationships. The task of the staff was to exert their strength (for example, their power to change a diagnosis) to try to influence and shift the balance of power in their own interests; other forces counteracted and counterbalanced them. For example, one aspect of their work, only slightly apparent in this account, was a constant shifting between visibility and invisibility. On one hand, their work was highly visible, manifest in charts, schedules, supervision, and the openness of their workplace to inspection.

On the other hand, they operated also through invisibility, through what was not written, or what was written to deceive, through the hidden character of their workplace and the darkness implicit in their patients' silence. Thus the staff were "supervisors perpetually supervised" (Foucault 1979), always open to inspection, and yet they also resisted and hid themselves.

The Judge presented the staff with an anomaly and, in so doing, with a space for commentary. The staff used their powers of irony and whimsy and outrageous expression of feeling to create him as a pet and a child, inverting conventional categories and making of him someone "good to think with." As "hot shit," he represented their position in the hospital; as "pet," their provision of a safe, if stark, haven, and as "child," their ability to nurture. As "The Judge," he was a silent witness both to the "awfulness" of "the system" itself and to the impossible task they were required to carry out.

Commentary filled many such spaces on the unit, areas hidden from various kinds of authoritative gaze, where the voices of the staff were subversive and irreverent. In *Discipline and Punish*, it seems that Foucault presents us with a subjectivity entirely shaped, imprinted, and normalized by the discipline of institutions (1979). Historical and subjective agency is a delusion, the mechanisms that give institutions their distinctive character as loci of power relations shape the "inner" life of individuals, who find themselves in an "iron cage worse than any Weber ever dreamed of" (Berman 1982). But in other places Foucault also suggests that disciplinary space has chinks and crannies in which we can, if we will, recover the possibility of agency. In a later interview he says that his intent is to show "the arbitrariness of institutions" and "which space of freedom we can still enjoy." One such space of freedom is suggested by the margins in which "subjugated knowledges" are created—knowledge that is local, ephemeral, and emergent, knowledge that is rarely written, organized, or even orderly (1980).

The commentary of the APU staff around their care of the Judge seems to me such a "subjugated knowledge." Formed in the chinks of power, it made meanings (more than one, and not consistently) out of the contradictions of situated action. To return now to the question with which I started: what is, who is, the subject of power? Perhaps the story of the Judge can best be taken as a cautionary tale. It seems we cannot decide in advance who is the subject of power; the notion of diffuse power helps us see clinical practice as ambiguous and contradictory in ways that belie representation in terms of one or two global, but narrow, kinds of oppression. Nor can we see those on whom power acts as merely mystified. We have to listen and, in listening, discover the many ways in which subjugated knowledges are formed, dissolve and form again. I suspect that the tension between the speaking subject and the object of power is an irreducible given in clinical, and other, settings, and that we must try to make the most of it.

Notes

1. This emphasis on the everyday lives and speech of their subjects is evident in the work of many critical medical anthropologies (e.g., Taussig 1980; Frankenberg 1988) and suggests that a working out of the relationship between micro and macro contexts is a necessity for anthropologists trained to an appreciation of the importance of the details of social life.

2. The research on which this paper is based was carried out over a two-year period in which I was a participant observer on the emergency unit described here. My research centered on the work of the unit's staff and, specifically, on the way a particular orientation to practice emerged from the context in which that work took place. I would like to thank the staff of the unit and the director of the mental health center for supporting my work. See Rhodes (1986) for a discussion of fieldwork in this institution.

3. All names and identifying features have been changed. Some of the individuals named are composite figures, and some details of the account that follows have been changed to conceal participants' identities. Quotes are taken from notes and tapes made during meetings and interviews.

4. See Estroff (1981a, b), Klerman (1977), Scheper-Hughes (1981), Jones (1979), and Scull (1984) for discussion of deinstitutionalization and its effect on patients.

5. Involuntary patients could not be held for more than three days without going through a hearing to determine whether they could be legally retained against their will. Hearings were held in the hospital on a weekly basis; the patient was represented by a public defender who argued his or her case before the hearing officer.

References

Arney, William Ray and Bernard J. Bergen
1984 Medicine and the Management of Living: Taming the Last Beast. Chicago: University of Chicago Press.

Berman, Marshall
1982 All That Is Solid Melts Into Air: The Experience of Modernity. New York: Simon and Schuster.

Cohen, S. and A. Scull
1983 Social Control and the State: Historical and Comparative Essays. Oxford: Martin Robertson.

Comaroff, Jean
1985 Body of Power, Spirit of Resistance: The Culture and History of a South African People. Chicago: University of Chicago Press.

Estroff, Sue E.
1981a Psychiatric Deinstitutionalization: A Sociocultural Analysis. Journal of Social Issues 37(3):116–132.
1981b Making it Crazy: An Ethnography of Psychiatric Clients in an American Community. Berkeley: University of California Press.
1988 Whose Hegemony? A Critical Commentary on Critical Medical Anthropology. Medical Anthropology Quarterly 2(4):421–426.

Foucault, Michel
1973 Madness and Civilization: A History of Insanity in the Age of Reason. Richard Howard, trans. New York: Vintage Books.
1975 The Birth of the Clinic: An Archeology of Medical Perception. A. M. Sheridan, trans. New York.
1978 The History of Sexuality: Vol. 1, An Introduction. Robert Hurley, trans. New York: Pantheon.
1979 Discipline and Punish: The Birth of the Prison. Alan Sheridan, trans. New York: Vintage Books.
1980 Power/Knowledge: Selected Interviews and Other Writings. Colin Gordon (ed.). New York: Pantheon.

Frankenberg, Ronald
1988 Gramsci, Culture and Medical Anthropology: Kundry and Parsifal? or Rat's Tail to Sea Serpent? Medical Anthropology Quarterly (*n.s.*) 2(4):324–337.

Goffman, Erving
1961 Asylums, Essays on the Social Situations of Mental Patients and Other Inmates. New York: Doubleday.

Ingleby, David
1983 Mental Health and Social Order. In Social Control and the State: Historical and Comparative Essays. S. Cohen and A. Scull (eds.). Oxford: Martin.

Jones, Kathleen
1979 Deinstitutionalization in Context. Health and Society: Milbank Memorial Fund Quarterly 57(4):552–569.

Kaufman, Sharon R.
1988 Toward a Phenomenology of Boundaries in Medicine: Chronic Illness Experience in the Case of Stroke. Medical Anthropology Quarterly (*n.s.*) 2(4):338–345.

Klerman, Gerald L.
1977 Better But Not Well: Social and Ethical Issues in the De-Institutionalization of the Mentally Ill. Schizophrenia Bulletin 3(4):617–631.

Mizrahi, Terry
1986 Getting Rid of Patients: Contradictions in the Socialization of Physicians. New Brunswick, N.J.: Rutgers University.

Rhodes, Lorna Amarasingham
1986 The Anthropologist as Institutional Analyst. Ethos 14(2):204–217.

Scheper-Hughes, Nancy
1981 Dilemmas in Deinstitutionalization: A View from Inner City Boston. Journal of Operational Psychiatry 12(2):90–99.

Scull, Andrew
1979 Museums of Madness: The Social Organization of Insanity in Nineteenth Century England. London: A. Lane.
1984 Decarceration: Community Treatment and the Deviant: A Radical View. (2nd ed.). Cambridge: Polity Press.

Shem, Samuel
1978 The House of God. New York: Dell.

Singer, Merrill, Lani Davison and Gina Gerdes
1988   Culture, Critical Theory, and Reproductive Illness Behavior in Haïti. Medical Anthropology Quarterly (*n.s.*) 2(4):370–385.

Tally, Ted
1981   Terra Nova. New York: Doubleday.

Taussig, Michael
1980   Reification and the Consciousness of the Patient. Social Science and Medicine 14B:3–13.

Illness, Experience, and the Problems of Ethnopsychiatric Knowledge

3

Notes on a Defrocked Priest: Comparing South Indian Shamanic and American Psychiatric Diagnosis[1]

Charles W. Nuckolls

Introduction

When I was doing fieldwork in India, in a single-caste fishing village on the southeastern coast, I noticed that villagers showed no deference to the village headman, to the elders, or to the village priest. I reasoned that, in this society, authority was not communicated in idioms familiar to an American—at least not to an American who, just out from Chicago, was accustomed to rather open displays of what the natives call "clout." On the one hand, I could explain what I saw by relating authority to two features of village life: kinship and consensus. Authority exists within a network of kinship relations and is exercised by kinship groups according to their statuses. There is nothing surprising in this, given what we know about South Asian kinship and social organization. On the other hand, even though I could account for the positions of the headman, the elders, and the priest, I could not account for the position of one man, Teddi Naidu, who did seem to have "authority" in my crude Chicagoan's sense of the word. In a village so thoroughly structured by kinship relations and so given to establishing consensus, how was this to be explained?

Various ideas suggested themselves. Naidu was comparatively wealthy. He operated the village's only subsidized rice store. He had been a district representative in the municipal council. Naidu had also been the village priest, an office he held for twenty years before being succeeded by his nephew. Among all these possibilities, financial, political, religious, I was at a loss. Other men in the village have more money. And others now hold the offices (district representative and village priest) which Naidu once held. I listened for references in villagers' conversations for clues to Naidu's authority and what I found surprised me: "Naidu," they said, "has goddesses." He sends his goddesses to attack people he doesn't like. People know this and avoid situations likely to make Naidu mad. His authority therefore seemed to depend largely on fear.

What I want to do in the first part of this paper is to use Devereux's idea of "social mass" to explain both what Naidu and what the community derive from Naidu's anomalous authority. I will suggest that Naidu's authority resolves, for him, deep-seated personality conflicts which result from being the former village priest. I will suggest that Naidu's authority establishes, for the villagers, a benchmark against which to gauge themselves. Specifically, I show that in Jalari diagnosis the measurement of "intentionality" is crucial and that Naidu helps to calibrate the scale according to which measurements of intentionality are made. In the second part, I compare the uses of personality attributions in Jalari and American psychiatric diagnosis.

"Social mass" was defined by Devereux as follows:

> It is the essence of psychiatric symptoms that they are more or less conspicuously at variance with the mores and, indeed, must be provocatively at variance with them if they are to gratify the idiosyncratic and socially negativistic needs of the patient. In other words, the psychiatric patient is a 'social trouble unit' and, precisely for that reason, possesses a great deal of what I have called 'social mass.' (1980b:256)

Naidu's authority, his ability to threaten, frighten, coerce, and cajole, is an indicator, in this society, of his social mass. He offends basic societal mores, mores which stress that authority resides in no one individual and cannot be exercised on any individual's behalf. Naidu's authority therefore may spring from his conspicuously variant and socially negativistic needs. What are these needs and where do they come from? Two details are pertinent here, first, the role of the priest in Jalari culture and, second, the effect of dismissal from that office on Naidu.

In Jalari culture the village priest (*pujari*) is said to "carry" the village goddesses. The priest is supposed to use this special relationship for the good of the village, by controlling the goddesses which the Jalaris otherwise regard as extremely dangerous. In his role as goddess carrier and goddess controller, the priest becomes a little like a goddess himself, peripheral and powerful simultaneously. On festival occasions, the identities of priest and goddess are fused as the goddess possesses the priest and speaks through him. But something happens when the priest loses his priesthood. There is no overtly defined role for the "ex-village priest." It is as if the roles of "goddess" and "goddess-carrier," normally linked or fused in ritual performances, become delinked, leaving, in Naidu's case, only the role of "goddess." For a goddess, or here, for one who is "like" a goddess, to be loose in the village without the paired presence of a controlling "carrier" is a very dangerous thing. This is what makes Naidu's present position as former village priest necessarily anonymous. But it is not enough to explain how or why he takes advantage of it, or why the villagers permit him to.

Naidu's story is an interesting one. His patriline holds the village priesthood, which is passed down through primogeniture. However, if a priest's eldest son is too young to succeed, the position passes to the father's younger brother until the rightful heir is old enough. Naidu, who held the priesthood after the former priest, his elder brother, died, was forced to relinquish it to this elder brother's son when the son reached maturity. I say "forced" because, from all accounts, Naidu did not give up his office voluntarily. In conversations with Naidu, I learned that he deeply resents his dismissal as priest. For years, he tried to recover his lost status by seeking elected office and by struggling in a business career. He succeeded only temporarily in both. He is now obsessed with asserting authority through the only other idiom at his disposal, i.e., the role of "defrocked priest."

An analogy may help to characterize this role. The former priest in Jalari culture is a little like the former president in our own. The afterglow of office accompanies both, surrounding them with a protective aura and imbuing them with a power not easily defined or delimited. For the Jalaris, to have once been village priest is to retain at least potential control over the goddesses, just as, for Americans, to have once been president is to retain at least potential influence over national affairs. A former president, for instance, can "speak out" on matters of public concern and attract considerable media attention when he does so. But because the "office" of the presidency no longer constrains him, he is uncontrollable and potentially disruptive. Much depends on his own self-control and self-maintained distance from involvement in political affairs. Perhaps the same may be said of Jalari priesthood. Without the constraint of office, the former Jalari priest can, if he wishes, wield considerable power, and use that power for good or ill purposes. He risks little since the afterglow of office protects him from dismissal at the same time it assures him of a receptive and susceptible audience.

Teddi Naidu achieves social mass by doing what a former priest should not do, by abusing the status which attaches to him by virtue of his past office. People assume that he still has the power to communicate with and control the goddesses he once "carried." But ungoverned by the duties of goddess controller, he now uses that influence selfishly and directs the goddesses to his own ends. He thus offends basic Jalari norms by taking on the attributes of the ultimate negative persona, the "witch" (*cillingi vadu*). Naidu's ex-priesthood *is* witchcraft, and Naidu is, significantly, the only person identified as a witch in the village.

Naidu represents himself as a witch in several ways. First, he identifies himself publicly, to all who will listen, as the most important man, not only in the village, but in the whole of India. Second, he asserts that he, not the current priest (his nephew), is more knowledgeable in spiritual matters. Third, he claims he has control of all village goddesses. Finally, he threatens anyone who opposes him with unpleasant consequences. Behavior of this kind would be grounds for excommunication from the caste for any ordinary Jalari. Naidu is not only tolerated, but permitted to flourish. The result is the anomaly that originally caught my attention: Naidu's open and effective display of personal authority.

What all this achieves for Naidu is clear: integration of the roles (goddess carrier and goddess controller) originally sundered by his dismissal from priestly office. Of course the meaning of this integration is different, because it is based on the category of "witch" and not "priest." But for Naidu, the role of despised "witch" comes closest, by direct opposition, to duplicating the authority and power he enjoyed in the office of "priest." What Naidu's position achieves for the village is clear from its role in diagnosis and in the larger context of group psychodynamics. These both will be examined below.

Jalari Diagnosis

Illness or poor fishing will lead, depending on their magnitude and duration, to an examination of causes though an elaborate diagnostic system (Nuckolls 1987). Jalari shamans, called *dasudu-s*, perform or participate in four distinct modes of diagnosis, matching patient conditions (physical, emotional, and moral) to stereotypic event sequences. These sequences constitute well-organized knowledge structures best described, using cognitive terminology, as "scripts" (see Hutchins 1980). Causal scripts exist at two levels of abstraction. Primary scripts describe goddesses' reactions to human transgression and account for the simple or "efficient" causes of typically diagnosed events (illness and poor fishing). Secondary scripts describe disruptions in social relations and account for the more complex, "precipitating" causes. In a case referred to in more detail below, a primary script explained a child's fever. The child's family had committed an offense against another family, causing the goddesses of the second family to attack. A readily available secondary script explained the offense: a structurally predictable dispute, stemming from allegiance to conflicting kinship values, make it impossible for the first family to honor its affinal obligations to the second family. That explained the precipitating cause.

The efficient causes of events are goddesses. The precipitating causes are social disputes. But what links efficient to precipitating causes or, to put it differently, how do social disputes trigger attacks by family goddesses? Jalaris answer these questions in diagnosis by examining the "intentionality" or personal willfulness of the individual whose goddesses attacked.

When a Jalari gets sick, s/he goes to a *dasudu* who examines his/her pulse in order to identify the attacking goddesses. Offerings to this goddess are then promised, but not actually made until the patient recovers and a second diagnosis establishes the social or precipitating causes of the goddess's attack.

The goal of secondary diagnosis is not to cure the patient, since that, presumably, has been achieved already. The purpose of secondary diagnosis is to determine why someone's goddess attacked to make sure that it doesn't attack again. The case referred to above is an example. After the child recovered, his father went to a *kaniki*, a kind of secondary diagnostic encounter. In the *kaniki*, the *dasudu* asks a long series of questions and, after each question, the *kaniki* performer (a woman of the washerman caste) drops a handful of rice into a vessel filled with water. If the rice sinks, the answer is "no." If the rice floats, the answer is "yes." The setting resembles a court: the patient is the claimant, the *dasudu* his attorney, and the goddesses are the chief witnesses as well as the jury. The purpose of both, court and *kaniki*, is similar: to construct an argument structure convincing enough to win the case and motivate resolution of the precipitating dispute. There is insufficient space here to consider the mechanics of this process (see Nuckolls 1987), but suffice to say that building an argument structure is a complicated interactive process, as the participants make inferences and test their conclusions.

The *kaniki* diagnosis resulted in an argument structure that linked the goddess's attack on the child to disturbed social relations between the child's father and his sister. In Jalari culture, brothers and sisters have certain very important obligations to each other, e.g., to arrange the marriages between their children and to participate in simple material exchanges. In the present case, the brother had been selling fish to his sister, but the sister had not paid him. When the brother asked for the money, the sister was insulted because demands for money are offensive by social standards which value extreme indirectness. Her household goddess responded by attacking the brother's child. The purpose of the argument structure assembled in the *kaniki* was this: first, to show that the sister had felt badly toward her brother; second, to show that her goddess had attacked a valued member of the brother's family (his son); and third, to show that business transactions between her and her brother should cease, lest the same thing happen again. The goal, in other words, was to sever economic relations between the brother and sister. Why should the brother want to do that? Apparently he felt that his sister provided an uncertain market for his fish and so preferred to take his business elsewhere.

It is a relatively easy thing to show that the sister's goddess attacked and to show that relations between the sister and brother were disturbed. Both, as far as the Jalaris are concerned, are observable. It is relatively difficult, however, to prove that the sister felt badly, since her feelings were not open to scrutiny. Yet demonstrating this is essential for the argument structure to work; without it, the case would falter and the brother's effort to sway public opinion would fail. The diagnosis therefore paid special attention to establishing the sister's feelings, or more precisely, to the level of "intentionality" with which these feelings corresponded.

Intentionality, as I use the term, means this: the sister *could have* responded to her brother's insulting request for money: a) by feeling angry, but not consciously knowing that she felt angry; b) by feeling angry, knowing that she felt angry, but not knowing that her angry feelings caused her goddess to attack; or c) by feeling angry, knowing that she felt angry, and deliberately praying to her goddess to make it attack her brother's child. The first option describes intentionality at its lowest level, i.e., anger which is realized but which represents no conscious intention to do harm. The third describes intentionally at the highest level, i.e., anger which is realized and which represents both the intention and the act of causing harm.

The consequences of intentionality at these three levels are what we must consider with respect to the case at hand. A secondary diagnosis which demonstrates intentionality at the first level cannot justify severing social relations between the attacking and the attacked families. After all, relations between the brother and sister could not be too bad if the sister's anger toward her brother had not been consciously realized. Public opinion would respond cautiously: let the brother and sister resume trading and try to work things out. A secondary diagnosis which results in proof of intentionality at the second level is different. If the sister felt angry and knew it, then relations between her and her brother may already be so strained that no effort to "work things out" can succeed. Village opinion might support separation. But how to prove that the sister's intentions were of this magnitude?

Demonstrating intentionality at the second level is the objective when the *dasudu* explicitly invokes a comparison to the third level. Level three is the level of ultimate intentionality, the level at which the feeling of anger, its conscious realization, and the attempt to harm accompany each other. Prototypically, level three is the domain of witchcraft and as we know, only one man in the village is categorized as a witch, the former priest, Teddi Naidu. In diagnosis, references to Naidu are common in the form of a question: "Did the *cillingi vadu* ('the witchcraft man') get mad and pray to his goddesses?" The answer may be (and usually is) "no," except when there is reason to expect Naidu's involvement. So what purposes do such references usually serve? Very possibly, they frame the attribution of intentionality in the case at hand, to indicate the logical extreme toward which the intention of the agent tends.

To return to the brother-sister case: it is in the brother's interest to demonstrate that his sister felt badly toward him and that she knew it. This represents a level of intentionality (level two) high enough to suggest that the two can never be reconciled, hence freeing the brother of an obligation to trade with his sister. To do this, the brother, or rather the *dasudu* who, like a lawyer, acts on his behalf, compares those feelings implicitly to Naidu's. It is like saying that the only thing which distinguishes the two is Naidu's deliberate wish to harm and his ability to act on it; otherwise, the sister and Naidu are the same.

The brother's argument structure successfully convinced his fellow kinsmen and the villagers at large that his sister, with whom he had been trading fish, consciously felt angry toward him. What clinched the argument, however, was not just the reference to Naidu. That established a framework for comparison, but by itself proved nothing. Rather, it was the fact, attested to in the diagnosis and validated by public opinion, that the sister and Naidu also possessed the same *kind* of goddess. Naidu, it will be recalled, claims to control many goddesses, including the village goddesses and various other goddesses he has "acquired." It is the second category, acquired goddesses, that is relevant here. In a social controversy a disputant may, as the Jalaris say, "strike the earth" and promise, "If I have not been truthful, let me be attacked by Sati Polamma (the promise goddess)." If he lied, Sati Polamma, the goddess of promises, attacks him or one of his family members. He thereby "acquires" Sati Polamma and must make offerings to her as one of his own household goddesses. The significance of this fact to the attribution of intentionality is crucial. To be subject to passions so strong that one "strikes the earth" and "makes promises," even at the risk of personal attack, is to be a highly "intentional" or willful person, the kind of person who, quick to anger, does not repress inner promptings but consciously acts on them. Relations with such an individual entail risk, lest at some little provocation that individual grow angry and let his goddess attack. It is better, in the Jalari view, to limit social relations and thus reduce the risk of attack.

This is precisely what the brother hopes to achieve; and it is by comparing his sister to Naidu and linking them by virtue of their mutual possession of the *promise goddess* that he succeeds. His sister is "too hot to handle" and public opinion, therefore, supports dissolution of their economic relationship.

Group Processes and the Role of the Despised Other

The question posed at the beginning of this discussion was, what does Naidu's "social mass" achieve for the village? One answer is clear from the case presented above. Naidu "calibrates" the scale of intentionality by setting its upper limit at the extreme intentionality of the "witch." Any "agent" whose actions, possessions, or personality attributes make him comparable to Naidu therefore tends to be classed near the upper end of this scale. This suggests that before Naidu, there was no such scale or, if there was, that it had a much lower upper limit. In fact, there is evidence to the contrary. The position of "defrocked priest" is reproduced structurally every time a village priest dies and is succeeded by his younger brother, who then must relinquish the office when the dead priest's son reaches maturity. This has happened at least twice in living memory. What this means is that there is always, at least potentially, one individual who "has goddesses" and who, like a witch, can send them to attack people. For Jalari diagnosis, it means that there has always been an upper limit for judgments of intentionality and that this limit has always been more or less the same.

Beyond causal explanation and shamanic diagnosis, can we say that Naidu's social mass achieves anything? That is, does the community's identification of Naidu as their only witch and their complete toleration of him in that role speak of any interesting psychodynamic processes at work? In a study of social deviancy, Devereux wrote,

> ...society accords an explicit recognition to every deviant—even to the most extreme ones—and sometimes in very surprising ways. The 'glamor' of the deviant presupposes, within limits, the imperfect acceptance of norms, even by very well-adjusted individuals, who can therefore identify with the 'hero,' the 'great criminal,' or the 'eccentric' or dares defy the norm. (1980b:101)

Community acceptance of Naidu signifies displacement of socially negativistic desires and the projection of such desires onto a convenient other. The "other" is openly despised but secretly admired for being the embodiment both of what people hate and love most about Jalari identity: high valuation of sociocentric attributes expressed in symbols which strongly emphasize the primacy of the group, not the individual. These manifest themselves in the Jalari emphasis on concealing strong feelings which could be interpreted as hostile. They are reflected, also, in the Jalari presumption that when hostile feelings are experienced, the experiencer does not (or should not) consciously realize them or deliberately act on them (unless, of course, he is a witch.)

All nonsociocentric, ego-centered feelings are displaced onto two available targets: the goddesses and the goddess surrogate, Teddi Naidu. Consider the first. A Jalari person experiences anger toward someone, but culturally is prohibited from consciously knowing or acting on that experience. He "does" nothing and "knows" nothing himself. Instead, his goddess knows and acts for him, excusing him of egocentric responsibility. That is how displacement works on the human-goddess level. Now consider the second category, Teddi Naidu. He is a human being who is "like a goddess," that is, a being who possesses great *ahankaramu* ("ego-ness") and is able to know and to act directly. Like the goddesses, he is free from many forms of social constraint which bind ordinary human beings. He is therefore despised for behaving in contravention of the rules "normal" humans obey, but admired for his ability to get away with it. Naidu is a classic example, then, of a "pattern of misconduct" (Linton 1936), an expression of "social negativism" (Devereux 1980b), and a "social cynosure" (LaBarre 1956).

American Psychiatric Diagnosis

American psychiatric diagnosis, by comparison, seems very remote. The use of increasingly sophisticated diagnostic criteria in evaluative techniques, *à la* the perpetually revised DSM, makes the Jalari reliance on specific cases and contexts seem subjective and impressionistic. While American psychiatrists employ a checklist to determine, say, a patient's conformity to the prototypical "borderline" personality disorder, Jalari shamans refer to a well-known, named individual and ask, in essence, "Is the case under consideration like him or not?" The two systems would seem to have little in common.

However, introspective reports from a nonscientific sample of American psychiatrists do not confirm this contrast. In fact, several psychiatrists remarked that the complex diagnostic criteria of the DSM play almost no role in diagnosis except secondarily as terms for justifying medical insurance reimbursements. Other psychiatrists were more generous. According to one, objective criteria actively enter diagnostic decision making in evaluations of the major ("Axis I") disorders, like the psychoses. Visual and auditory hallucinations, formal thought disorders, looseness of associations, and so forth, are easy to identify and therefore easy to attribute. As one psychiatrist put it, "If somebody's hallucinating—that is, perceiving internal stimuli which aren't really there—it's quite obvious what they're doing." Applying well-defined criteria is thus possible and practicable for some conditions.

There is, however, a continuum along which disorders vary in the ease with which diagnostic criteria can be applied. The further away from the "psychoses" and the more toward the "affective" and "personality" disorders one moves, the less usable formal diagnostic criteria become. Particular cases and well-remembered contexts play increasingly important roles, replacing cut-and-dried criteria as the psychiatrist's chief instruments of diagnostic interpretation. This is nowhere more evident than in two sets of cases: those labeled "manic" and those labeled "borderline" and "narcissistic."

Well-remembered episodes seem to cluster in great numbers around conditions so labeled. If, in fact, this part of the psychiatrist's interpretive repertoire is the analogue of the Jalari shaman's standard reference to Teddi Naidu, then it may display characteristics similar to those already described for Jalari diagnosis. To test this hypothesis, it is necessary first to examine what such psychiatric diagnoses look like. A psychiatrist described a well-remembered "manic" case this way:

> The individual was very irritable, non-compliant, was refusing treatment. Interestingly, he was a very wealthy person. A wealthy and powerful person. It was hard for people to distinguish what was legitimate from what was irrational. But, for instance, he had bought his eight-year-old grandson a three or four thousand dollar toy car for Christmas. And done other things which were eccentric. In the process of interviewing, he plainly was manic. And in the course of the next three days of treatment he was able slowly to perceive himself coming down to baseline. He is one that sticks in my mind.

And in a second case, also very well-remembered, the psychiatrist reported:

> He was a biochemist. He was not irritable. He was quite amusing, actually. Very amicable. He had become increasingly involved in his own delusional system, to a point at which he realized that he was hearing the voices of his co-workers spreading rumors about him. Although he was ready to believe that these voices were hallucinations, he couldn't accept that the rumors were untrue. He became increasingly involved in his delusional system, to the point that he thought his house was being bugged, he was being followed, etc. One weekend he stayed up all night writing notes on brilliant new ideas. He had recently gone out and priced a BMW. He had bought a whole bunch of imported prints and had them framed. He had evidence of hypersexuality. He had episodes of irritability. Atypical irritability at home. This case will be remembered as an acute manic episode.

What these cases seem to share, at first glance, are descriptions of individuals whose behavior is variously eccentric, compulsive, and delusional. These, anyway, are the labels attached to cases diagnosed as "manic." But such terms and the behaviors associated with them have culturally meaningful correlates which, in any discussion of their applicability in diagnosis, must be construed. Certainly one clue to this is the psychiatrist's own reaction to the cases reported above: Manic cases are considered "interesting," even "amusing." Personality disorders, on the other hand, and particularly the borderline and narcissistic personalities, are "unappealing," "disagreeable," and "difficult to deal with." Most psychiatrists, he continued, have an "instinctive aversion" to them. Clearly, when we face disorders that the psychiatrists diagnose using past case examples, and not formal criteria, we enter a new domain hedged around by new meanings and feelings.

Consider first the "manics" represented in the first two accounts and identified by the psychiatrist as basic to his diagnostic repertoire. They spend money extravagantly on expensive presents for others and on luxuries for themselves. They are up at odd hours or for prolonged periods, involved in the projects they consider vitally important. They are wary and suspicious of others. There is something, said one psychiatrist, strangely engaging about such people. That something, I think, is this: removed from the context of the hospital and professional psychiatry and placed, let us say, in the context of popular American mythology, they differ very little from the typical stage and screen personas of the actors Charles Bronson and Clint Eastwood or the rock star Jim Morrison. They are, in a word, "heroic," but in that special sense Americans reserve for figures who are ruggedly individual, unconventional, self-involved and often self-destructive: the loners, misfits, and drunks incarnated on the screen as cowboys, gunslingers, and urban vigilantes.

Of course it is different offscreen. "It was hard," said the psychiatrist, referring to difficulty in diagnosing the first case, "for people to distinguish what was legitimate from what was irrational." The manic represents in extreme form values and attitudes associated with American culture's "positive identity" (Erikson 1963). But by virtue of their expression in extreme form such features must be constrained, either through the mechanism of controlled fantasization (in films, for example) or through controlled displacement onto obliging individuals (people in "manic episodes") who are then subjected to "cure" and brought "back to baseline." Confusion in evaluating such cases results partly from ambivalence: are we to admire such people or fear them?

Before we consider in more detail the problem of manics and the group's positive identity, let us turn to the personality disorders for what, I will suggest, is the other side of the coin. Particular cases of borderline and narcissistic personalities are well-remembered and used by the psychiatrists in making subsequent diagnoses. Borderlines are "infinitely needy" and "demanding." They refuse to accept "appropriate distances," particularly in relation to their therapists. One case recalled by a psychiatrist was notorious for having broken into her therapist's house and lived there while he was out of town. Another parked his car in front of the therapist's house and slept there at night. Narcissistic persons, on the other hand, feel themselves to extremely "entitled," to be justified, that is, in requiring of others more than social convention normally allows. Both the borderline and narcissistic cases are described as extremely unpleasant.

The personality disorders discussed here, like the manics, correspond closely with personality types and character attributes linked to an American stereotype: the compulsive patient, usually associated with the displaced New York neurotics of Woody Allen movies. These characters serve as a framework for the group's "negative identity," typifying the very un-Rambo-like (and therefore, potentially, un-American) characteristics of illness, psychological trauma, and (worst of all) the eagerness to tell anyone, from the analyst to the casual acquaintance to the movie viewer, the excruciatingly personal details of these conditions.

When not obsessed with these himself, the character insists that his interactants or viewers be equally obsessed; worse, he demands that they reciprocate, either directly (among his fellow characters) or indirectly (in the minds of moviegoers who perhaps cannot help wondering if they, too, behave and suffer as he does). Like the narcissistic personality, the Woody Allen characters (and the apparently "negative" identity they represent) are needy, dependent, self-obsessed, and refuse to acknowledge appropriate boundaries between themselves and others.

It is important to remember that the two sets of identities, the manic and the disordered personality types, Rambo and Woody Allen, inhabit the same world. It is hypothesized here that they represent opposite sides of the same coin, for which the Eriksonian terms "positive" and "negative" identity do not really suffice. One or the other may be positive or negative, depending on the context. I suggest that the manic and his larger-than-life correspondents in popular mythology (the cowboys, etc.) represent in extreme form an egocentric ideal in American culture. The disordered personalities (borderline and narcissistic, especially), on the other hand, represent a sociocentric ideal.

The egocentric ideal is simply the self-contained and self-protecting individual, who needs no one but makes others dependent on his eccentric power for relief from problems which they, as people who *are* enmeshed in social relations, cannot address directly. The sociocentric ideal is the opposite: the person who needs and clings, who reduces boundaries and coercively establishes relations, and who compels others' concern for him by forcing them out of their own egocentric involvements.

We variously admire and disparage the embodiments of egocentric and sociocentric ideals in popular mythology. In "real life," we do the same thing, but with one important difference. Mythic embodiments are "good to think with" only for as long as they remain "mythic," and thus conveniently distanced targets for displacement. "Real life" embodiments, the manics and personality-disordered people, are too close to serve as effective displacement objects. In our society, psychiatric treatment or psychiatric confinement is needed to keep the boundary between mythic and real worlds intact, either by returning (through treatment) temporarily lost individuals to "normalcy" or by locating them (through confinement in asylums) in places outside society. In Jalari society, proximity to the displacement object is possible only because Teddi Naidu is given the status of witch, thus distancing him and assuring society of his continued availability as a displacement object, to be both admired and hated, envied and feared.

Conclusions

The chief objective of this paper has been to suggest that in Jalari culture, and in our own, particular categories of people are cynosures and, in that role, serve as calibrators, setting the limits according to which departures from normalcy are measured.[2] In the Jalari diagnosis of spirit-related events, references to the calibrator, Teddi Naidu, are explicit. Any persons whose intentions compare closely to Naidu's, that is, any person whose background, conscious enmity, and suspected hostile actions make him like a witch, may be attributed with causing a goddess to attack. In American psychiatric diagnosis, references to specific calibrators are implicit and confined, apparently, to cases for which there are poor diagnostic criteria. These cases include primarily the manics and the two personality disorders, borderline and narcissistic. The psychiatrist's memory of highly illustrative past cases is his diagnostic repertoire, used whenever he confronts cases in these categories.

The second purpose of the paper has been to examine whether, and to what extent, similarities in Jalari and American diagnostic technique reveal similarities in Jalari and American constructions of normalcy. I have suggested that the scales defining the limits of normalcy are established, for both societies, by their contradictory ideal typifications of themselves. For Jalari society, strongly sociocentric ideals, ideas which deny authority to individuals except as acknowledged group representatives, find their opposite expression in Teddi Naidu, defrocked priest and witch, who wields strong personal authority and who represents no one but himself. Naidu is a social cynosure and is tolerated mainly because he functions as an embodiment of the group's opposite (not necessarily negative) identity, successfully concentrating in human form the egocentric authority and capacity for direct action otherwise reserved for the goddesses alone. Every Jalari person at some point becomes the focus of diagnostic reference (i.e., suspected of causing a goddess to attack someone) and therefore, in the eyes of other villagers, a little like Naidu. Every person, that is, is suspected from time to time of disobeying Jalari cultural ideals and of acting directly and selfishly. But the diagnostic process itself reveals that, just as everyone approaches being a "Naidu" (and therefore a witch), everyone stops short of actually becoming one.

For U.S. society, on the other hand, strongly egocentric ideals, ideals which stress rugged individualism and limited reliance on "society," find their opposite expression in the typical Woody Allen persona. He is feared and admired for what he represents: the failure (or fulfillment) or American personhood in the vulnerable, clinging, and dependent self. In myth there is a place for such a figure; in society there is not. Consequently, people who typify in extreme form the sociocentric ideal may be attributed with personality disorders and, in the most severe cases, classified as "border-lines." Such people receive treatment, not Academy Awards.

The egocentric ideal is no less problematic, as public concern over former President Reagan's "Ramboesque" foreign interventions makes plain. As much as Americans admire decisiveness and independence, they fear them lest they seem to justify acting "outside the law," "selfishly," or without "bipartisan consensus." Again, for their caricatures in popular mythology (the Bronsons and Stallones) such values have a place, though not an uncontroversial one; in everyday life, their realizations in equally extreme form have a much harder time. The "manic" is often intelligent, witty, quick to act and quick to respond, independent, decisive, and hyper-sexual: all qualities that, on film, would inspire interest if not admiration. But he is simply too hard to live with, and society accords him only one role: the psychiatric patient who needs treatment and rehabilitation.

Finally, it should be noted that these conclusions, though tentative, do not lend complete support to the thesis that Americans and Indians sub-scribe to radically different "world premises." Shweder and Bourne (1982) and others (Miller 1982; Ramanujan 1988) argue that United States culture is predominantly egocentric and individualistic and that Indian culture is predominantly sociocentric and relational.[3] The authors mentioned have compiled a valuable corpus of confirming data, produced from extensive interviews, and surveys of a vast literature, and it is not my purpose to quibble with them. Rather, the point is this: while such ideals (United States egocentrism, Indian sociocentrism) may be elicited in certain con-texts, they are not unequivocal, and different studies in other contexts easi-ly reveal their opposites. Americans, the egocentrics, are as much troubled by egocentrism as they are fascinated and appalled by sociocentric behav-ior. Indians, the sociocentrics, may or may not be troubled by sociocen-trism (the data are not available on this point), but they are certainly both-ered and tantalized by its egocentric opposite. The fact that such ideals exist as alternatives to each other is in many ways more interesting than the fact that one or the other (egocentrism or sociocentrism) may, in certain circumstances, be upheld as the ideal. The usefulness of such constructs analytically will be enhanced to the extent we stop trying to make them watertight, mapping them onto cultures whose dynamics are in fact much more complex.

Acknowledgments

Gratitude is expressed to Richard Shweder, Howard Stein, Atwood Gaines, Janis Nuckolls, and several anonymous psychiatrists for sugges-tions. The usual disclaimers apply.

Notes

1. The comparative research on which this paper is based was made possible by grants from the National Science Foundation, the American Institute of Indian Studies, the Charlotte W. Newcombe Foundation, the National Endowment for the Humanities, and the American Council of Learned Societies.

2. Devereux (1980b:273) notes, "...in primitive psychiatry explicitly and in modern psychiatry implicitly diagnosis is made in terms of the patient's conforming to a marginal model of 'singularities of behavior' and not in terms of his deviation from (a) norm."

3. See Gaines (1982) and chapter 1, this volume, for a view of the West as comprising two distinct cultural traditions.

References

American Psychiatric Association
1987 Diagnostic and Statistical Manual of Mental Disorders-III-Revised. (DSM-lll-R). Washington, D.C.: American Psychiatric Association.

Devereux, George
1980a Basic Problems of Ethnopsychiatry. George Devereux. Chicago: University of Chicago Press.
1980b Primitive Psychiatric Diagnosis: A General Theory of the Diagnostic Process. In Basic Problems of Ethnopsychiatry. George Devereux. Chicago: University of Chicago Press.

Erickson, Erik
1963 Childhood and Society (2nd ed). New York: W. W. Norton.

Gaines, Atwood D.
1982 Cultural Definitions, Behavior and the Person in American Psychiatry. In Cultural Conceptions of Mental Health and Therapy. Anthony Marsella and Geoffrey White (eds.). Dordrecht: D. Reidel.

Hutchins, E.
1980 Culture and Inference. Cambridge, MA: Harvard University Press.

LaBarre, Weston
1956 Social Cynosure and Social Structure. In Personal Character and Cultural Milieu. Douglas Haring, (ed.). New York: Syracuse University Press.

Linton, Ralph
1936 The Study of Man. New York: Appleton-Century-Crofts.

Miller, J.
1982 Culture and the Development of Social Explanation. Unpublished dissertation. Department of Anthropology, University of Chicago.

Nuckolls, Charles
1987 Culture and Causal Thinking: Diagnosis and Prediction in Jalari Culture. Unpublished dissertation in Anthropology. University of Chicago.

Ramanujan, A.
1988 Is There an Indian Way of Thinking? Nuclear Policy, Culture and History. Chicago: Center for International Studies.

Shweder, R. and E. Bourne
1982   Does the Concept of the Person Vary Cross-Culturally? In Cultural Concep-
       tions of Mental Health and Therapy. A. Marsella and G. White (eds.). Dor-
       drecht: D. Reidel.

4

Unintended Therapy:
Psychotherapeutic Aspects of Chiropractic

Kathryn S. Oths

Introduction

The utilization of alternative medical therapies is currently on the rise in the United States, continuing a trend that began in the late 1800s and gained momentum during the 1960s. This conversion to alternative forms of treatment, which include chiropractic, homeopathy, naturopathy, massotherapy, and many more, is often attributed to a growing dissatisfaction of consumers with the quality and efficacy of biomedicine.

Evidence suggests that alternative therapists pay more attention to the psychosocial aspects of sickness because they primarily treat chronic disorders which are known to contain a large psychosomatic element. Here, I wish to elucidate the characteristics of one alternative therapy, chiropractic, which has inherent in its structure and delivery the capacity to effectively employ psychotherapeutic techniques with which to enhance patient satisfaction and recovery. Consequently, by design or default, chiropractors often employ such techniques to a greater extent than their biomedical counterparts, with resulting therapeutic benefits for patient healing.

Some providers of mental health services in urban U.S. clinics have expressed interest in discovering what alternative resources are used in their communities, but little is known about the patterns of resort among people with problems of living and minor psychological and psychosomatic complaints[1] (Fábrega 1990). Landy (1983:243), in a comprehensive review of the field of medical anthropology, calls for more field studies which deal with healing alternatives to mainstream biomedicine. My clinical fieldwork in the office of a Doctor of Chiropractic (D.C.) has allowed me to draw some tentative conclusions in support of the proposition that chiropractors make use of psychotherapeutic techniques (Oths 1985). I believe my findings regarding chiropractic will be applicable to other alternative paradigms as well. I will outline what indications exist in order to suggest sufficient cause for further investigation.

It is our quest as anthropologists to understand humans as simultaneously organic and cultural beings. Traditional healers everywhere—whether rural or urban, in the West or the Third World—manipulate cultural experience, knowledge, and beliefs, intentionally or unintentionally, to influence the mental and or physical status of patients (Oths 1991). It is accepted that though they are not scientific, they know and understand their people's problems, and that in so far as most diseases have some psychosomatic aspects, these healers are usually helpful (Murphy 1964). Similarities between shamanism and psychotherapy have been noted by Kiev (1964), Lévi-Strauss (1963), Torrey (1972), and many others.

While United States-based Puerto Rican spiritists and Christian faith healers have also been compared to psychotherapists in their ability to address psychic disturbances in their patients and heal through belief and practice (e.g., Garrison 1977; Harwood 1987; Koss 1975; Rogler and Hollingshead 1961), anthropology has neglected to examine the mechanisms and appeal of the less exotic, unorthodox U.S. healers, much less what nonmedical elements of therapy they might use.

Alternative health-care therapists such as chiropractic, like traditional and spiritist healers, tend to specialize in treating chronic and somatized complaints and focus on the personal and social aspects of illness. It might be assumed on the surface that the same principles which demonstrate the spiritists' effective use of psychotherapy can be applied wholesale to explain that of chiropractic. However, many differences in the structure and content of their practices distinguish the two cases. As the following account will detail, chiropractic is a psychotherapeutically oriented healthcare resource, heretofore unidentified and undocumented, which operates in the midst of mainstream United States society and culture.

Here, psychotherapeutic techniques will be simply defined as any method employed to relieve distress by facilitating attitude change through personal insight, communication, support, and empathy. "Psychotherapist" will be be used broadly to include any trained professionals whose primary form of treatment is talk therapy (i.e., psychoanalysts, behavioral psychiatrists, psychologists, social workers).

The ensuing discussion will be limited to sanctioned healer-patient encounters, although psychotherapeutic means may be globally viewed as any effect of personal influence on another's state of health and well-being. Given the diversity of United States society, it is natural to conclude that there are many viable routes to achieving increased personal integration and social adjustment. One should keep in mind that cultural values and beliefs determine the existence and definition of mental illness and the nature of its treatment as well.

Methods and Sample

This work is based on observational research that I conducted in the clinic of a suburban Cleveland chiropractor in 1985. My methods consisted of tape recording and observing all clinical interaction for a two-week period. The sample consisted of fifty-seven patients of all ages, mixed ethnicity (70 percent Anglo, 9 percent Black, 19 percent Italian, 2 percent Hispanic), and slightly more females (53 percent) than males. Their occupations were reported as 42 percent white collar and 33 percent blue collar. The remainder were unemployed and included children, students, retirees, and house-wives, many of the latter two groups being widowed or divorced. Evidently, the chiropractor has a broad appeal and does not simply attract those of a particular socioeconomic or cultural group.

Differences Between M.D.s and Chiropractors

The Cartesian dualism, though widely employed, has long been an untenable assumption. It disregards the impact of emotion on somatic states (Moerman 1983; Kleinman, Eisenberg and Good 1978). Purely psychic and purely bodily disorders exist only as logical extremes of a continuum (Frank 1961:217). Using the distinction early made in medical anthropology between disease (physiological dysfunction) and illness (one's perception or experience of the disease state) (for further discussion see Kleinman 1980:72), nearly 50 percent of biomedical patients come for care of illness problems, not for problems immediately relatable to disease conditions (Stoeckle, Zola and Davidson 1964). Also, studies estimate that as many as 88 percent of medical patients exhibit noticeable emotional or psychological disorder (Houpt et al. 1980; Shapiro 1964; Stoeckle et al. 1964). The incorporation of the biopsychosocial approach to sickness into medical clinical practice has been limited, at best (Engel 1977). There are numerous examples in the literature that show physicians' failure to recognize and/or deal with the psycho-social-emotional component of their patients' problems, with resultant poor treatment outcomes (Thompson et al. 1983; Duffy, Hamerman and Cohen 1980). For example, Stoeckle et al. (1964) found that 84 percent of patients in a medical clinic were suffering from psychological distress. In most cases, patients had a history of chronic problems.

Aware of the psychosocial component or not, M.D.s are trained to systematically ignore illness (Kleinman and Sung 1979) and few are therapeutically oriented or willing to deal with such considerations. With few exceptions, biomedicine does not aim to treat organic problems psychotherapeutically (but see Maretzki [this volume] for an historical account from Germany).

To be unaware of patients' psychosocial problems is not simply unfortunate but can lead to misdiagnosis of cases as medical or surgical ones. In short, the M.D. cures disease but fails to address illness. This results in patient dissatisfaction and often to a change to alternative treatment agencies (see Kleinman 1979; Kleinman and Sung 1979).

Chronic pain may be caused or aggravated by psychological problems or physical habits that patients can change if the problems are attended to. Persons with chronic pain often unsuccessfully try multiple conventional approaches to treatment of their pain, frequently leading to resort to alternative therapy after biomedical options have been exhausted (Marquis, Davies, and Ware 1983; Ben-Sira 1976; Oths 1985). That at least half of spiritist, chiropractic, and psychotherapy patients have received previous nonpsychiatric M.D. care for their chief complaint attests to this (Garrison 1977; Kadushin 1969; Oths 1985). I will return to this point later.

Unorthodox therapies may be unscientific, but they meet unscientific needs in patients. A patient is concerned with feeling better, not proving the theoretical soundness of a practice. Chiropractors are in demand because they supply what is often absent from overly logical and rational modern medicine—more social, psychological, and physical interaction, more listening, empathy, support, reassurance, and touching (Anderson 1980).

In contrast to biomedicine's narrow healing concept, a holistic paradigm has long been the forte of alternative therapists, including chiropractic. While the various alternative therapists and healers share no uniform set of theories or therapies, they do share a fundamental orientation which views the individual as an indivisible integration of body, mind, and spirit. Social, cultural, psychological, and physical dimensions of the person are recognized as shaping the disease and illness experiences (Sirott and Waitzkin 1984; Cmich 1984; Kotarba 1983; Leonard 1976).

Words, acts, and rituals become even more important when no pharmacological substances are used in treatment. Given their drug-free, noninvasive orientation, alternative practitioners such as chiropractic do not and cannot ignore the root of the patient's chronic problem by anesthetizing or removing it. Rather, they search for the underlying dysfunction in addition to treating the symptoms, which forces them to direct more attention to the emotional elements creating or aggravating the problem.

Evidence from my observations leads me to contend that chiropractic, as practiced by this D.C., can be considered a 'nonanalytic psychotherapy' (Kiernau 1974), as neither the therapist's main focus, nor at times his intention, is to engage in patient psychological assessment. He deals with the body as a physical problem. However, as he addresses minor psychological and life problems, his can be considered—to borrow the term—"a culturally disguised form of psychotherapy" (Kleinman et al. 1979).

Chronic pain such as backache may contain a large psychosomatic element (Cornacchia 1982:65). Given that chiropractic and others specialize in the treatment of chronic conditions, in contrast to biomedicine's attention to infectious and acute problems, it is understandable why non-medical therapists frequently and effectively employ more psychotherapeutic techniques than do their biomedical counterparts.

Similarities and Differences Among
Three Psychotherapeutically Oriented Practices:
Psychotherapy, Spiritism, and Chiropractic

Shared Features

In the following, I compare psychotherapy in general with one well-studied supernatural healing modality, namely Puerto Rican spiritism, and the one alternative therapy that is the focus of this research—chiropractic. Contrasts will be drawn with the predominantly medically oriented practice of biomedicine.

To begin, the basic features that Frank (1961:2–3) has postulated as shared by all psychotherapies are clearly evident in psychotherapy, spiritism and chiropractic. These are: 1) a trained, socially sanctioned healer acceptable to the patient and at least a portion of the patient's social network, 2) a suffering person seeking relief, and, 3) systematic contacts between the healer and client in which the healer attempts to reduce distress by changing the sufferer's behavior, attitudes, and emotional state.

Although chiropractic, like biomedicine, purports to treat only somatic complaints—in their case musculoskeletal and functional problems—there are many parallels and similarities between the elaborations of psychotherapy and spiritism, which both treat psychic problems, and chiropractic. To begin with, the aim of psychotherapy, spiritism and chiropractic is the better functioning of a person at all levels: emotional, social, and physical. All view themselves mainly as facilitators of patient change, realizing that the patient ultimately controls his or her improvement. These practices share a respect for the absolute power of the mind to heal or to destroy itself and the soma; agreeing as Hahn and Kleinman (1981) point out, that "belief kills; belief heals" (also see Fishman 1979:13). Self-healing is made evident by the placebo effect, as self-destruction is apparent in the case of chronic pain.

Placebo Effect

The effects of psychotherapeutic techniques and placebos are similar (Frank 1974). The efficacy of both relies on the same principle: that the mental state of an individual *in* and *of* itself can bring about recovery when a patient's expectation of help is aroused (Frank 1961). The mechanism of the mind's power to heal with psychotherapeutic methods is this: A positive attitude (like a placebo) combats anxiety, depression, and other negative emotions which aggravate and prolong painful symptoms, possibly by causing a release of mood-elevating hormones, endorphins, in the brain (Prince 1980). Temporary relief can eventually lead to permanent recovery through positive reinforcement. Furthermore, the mind can help to speed recovery by enhancing the effectiveness of mechanical or chemical treatment combined with it. In fact, the best treatment for psychosomatic conditions has been found to be a combination of psychotherapeutic and medical treatment (Luborsky, Singer and Luborsky 1975).

That the mind also has the ability to destroy its own and the body's health is shown clearly in the case of chronic disease. Chronic medical problems have been found to have an emotional-psychological basis as much as a degenerative-physical one (Swanson 1984; Szasz 1957; Engel 1961). Studies have shown that perhaps as many as 98 percent of chronically ill patients have mental illness, usually depression (Blumer and Heilbronn 1981; Reich, Tupin and Abramowitz 1983).

It is not often apparent whether the physical begets the psychological degeneration or vice versa. Nor is the sequence that important, as either condition exacerbates the other. What is important is that mental and physical impairment exist in unison.

Also, emotional distress can manifest itself in somatic disorders, leading to heightened psychological distress and so on. Such a reaction is self-perpetuating and self-defeating. The goal of therapy is to break the vicious cycle and reverse the process. Table 1 shows some of the more salient therapeutic components common to psychotherapy, spiritism, and chiropractic (also see Frank 1961).

A. Primary Focus of Treatment

PSYCHOLOGICAL VERSUS PHYSICAL EMPHASIS

Psychotherapists (often) and spiritists are nonmedical practitioners. Their explicit domain of treatment is problems of living, psychosocial distress, and mild to moderate personality disorders and neuroses. Neither customarily handle serious and severe psychiatric disorders such as schizophrenia and psychoses. Both psychotherapy and spiritism tend to encourage resort to biomedicine for physical disorders present (Harwood 1987:83; also see Fishman 1979:5, 18).

In Garrison's study, 48 percent and 58 percent of spiritist and physician patients, respectively, reported somatic and paramedical complaints of a chronic nature, compared to only 35 percent of persons in the general Puerto Rican population (1977:187, 190). Those going to spiritists, however, usually did not go for treatment of these complaints. If these problems were attended to by the spiritist, it was secondarily to "spiritual," or psychological problems. But it is noteworthy that 28 percent reported one reason for going to spiritists was:

Table 1. Similarities and Differences in Therapeutic Techniques
of Psychotherapy, Spiritism, and Chiropractic

	Generalized Characteristics		
	Psy	Spir	Chir
1. Primary focus on psychological problems	*	*	◊
2. Treatment consonant with sociocultural aspects	*	*	*
3. Oriented to particular social or cultural group	*	*	◊
4. Patient somatizes	◊	*	*
5. Extended family involved	◊	*	* ◊
6. Meaningful cognitive framework	*	*	*
7. Treatment criteria provided	◊	*	*
8. Physical contact	◊	*	*
9. Trance induction	◊	*	* ◊
10. Strong patient-practitioner relationship	*	*	*
11. Long-term relationship	*	*	*
12. Ritual object use	◊	*	*
13. Brings about behavior and attitude change	*	*	*
14. Locus of responsibility on patient	*	◊	◊
15. Transition to new status/role	◊	*	◊
16. Use of group psychology	* ◊	*	◊

* Characteristic present
◊ Characteristic absent

somatic complaints about which they had seen a doctor and the doctor had purportedly, "said there was nothing wrong," or "couldn't find anything," or "didn't cure" them. The complaints were most frequently headaches, backaches, stomachaches, or a variety of vague nonspecific pains or "not feeling well." All but four of these clients also reported a variety of psychological and interpersonal complaints and some were explicit that their somatic complaints were related to their mood and feeling state rather than to physical disorder. (Garrison 1977:142)

Eight percent of Garrison's sample reported only somatic complaints, with no accompanying psychosocial problems. Fishman, in his study of Christian prayer healing, also mentions that patients sometimes suffer from headaches, backaches, and stomachaches which, they are told, are caused by spirit possession (1979:10; also see Csordas, this volume) .

Seldom do spiritists diagnose a patient's problem as purely "material," or physical in origin. Usually problems are considered spiritual or a combination of spiritual and physical. Although they generally refer somatic problems to a physician, the spiritist mediums feel competent to treat most psychological disorders. They explicitly treat emotional-psychological-psychiatric complaints, though they are often not presented as such by the

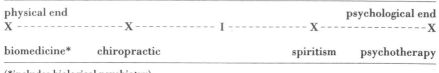

Figure 1. Continuum of Treatment Foci

patients themselves. However, spiritist patients report alleviation of physical symptoms concurrent with spiritual ministrations (Garrison 1977:149).

The exact opposite situation tends to occur with chiropractic patients.
Whereas the other two therapies advocate consulting a physician when medical problems persist, chiropractic functions to treat both psyche and soma,
that is, illness and disease. Clients of the chiropractor seek help for somatic
complaints which are often disguising problems of a psychological nature.
The chiropractor explicitly treats the patient's physical complaints with no
overt mention of his attention to patients problems of living, yet patients frequently report doing better with job, family, and friends after being under
the chiropractor's care for some time. The types of emotional-psychological
and living problems that patients were observed to discuss with the D.C.
include mainly difficulties with job, relations with spouse and children, and
adjustment to some form of physical incapacity. Life events, such as marriage, divorce, deaths in the family, and aging, and consumer purchases of
costly items such as houses, major appliances, and cars, were the topic of
many conversations. Patients also complained quite frequently about unsat-
isfactory medical care they had received from physicians and hospitals.

Chiropractic manifestly treats acute and chronic musculoskeletal disorders (especially back, neck, joint, and limb pain) and functional problems. However, given the emotional-psychological component so prevalent
in chronic pain which can cause or compound it, once a patient enters into
the chiropractor's care, the psychotherapeutic techniques the D.C.
employs are effective in hastening recovery. Thus, on the continuum of
treatment focus, with biomedicine falling on the physical extreme and psychotherapy falling on the mental end, spiritism lies more towards the mental than physical, while chiropractic tends to position itself closer to the
center, but in the direction of the physical.

Although chiropractors readily refer patients to a physician (e.g., sur-
geon, neurologist) when the problem is beyond their capability, they insist
they are fully trained and capable of dealing with most mild to serious physical problems, especially musculoskeletal and functional ones. They
attempt to help a patient with nonpharmacological, noninvasive procedures
before having the patient resort to more radical, potentially iatrogenic and
expensive methods. This philosophy is summed up in a popular chiroprac-

tic maxim, which hangs on the wall in this D.C.'s office: "Chiropractic First, Drugs Second, Surgery Last."

The psychosomatic nature of certain complaints helps to explain why chiropractors and patients alike also claim spinal manipulation effective for a host of problems that do not bear any apparent physiological relationship to nerve compression and vertebral misalignment, such as bed wetting, high blood pressure, constipation, acne, appendicitis, stomach trouble, shingles, asthma, and ulcers (from educational pamphlets in D.C.'s office; also, see Consumer Reports 1980:176).

The comparison presented above which shows the incidental treatment of somatic complaints by spiritists and the incidental treatment of psychic problems by chiropractic, clearly further support the contention of the strong interrelationship between chronic physical and chronic mental problems.

Although musculoskeletal complaints did occur, they were not among those chronic complaints most prevalent in the Puerto Rican community. Conditions such as asthma, *ataques* (attacks), headaches, stomach problems, insomnia, and poor appetite, ulcers, diabetes, and arthritis were salient. Back, joint, neck, and limb pain were rarely cited (also, see Anderson [1984] for a similar lack of medicalization of musculoskeletal pain in a rural nonindustrial population). In contrast, this latter class of complaints becomes a dominant idiom of distress when one looks at more acculturated U.S. populations, regardless of their ethnic origin. In the United States, back pain is one of the most frequent reasons for visiting a doctor, followed by physicals, coughs, and sore throat (McLemore 1979).

UNINTENDED CONSEQUENCES

In general, it could not be said that people seeking help from a chiropractor are explicitly/consciously seeking psychotherapy. Some go because they have tried the biomedical options available only to receive vague explanations and limited relief. Often they have heard about chiropractic as being "different." A friend of the patient is usually responsible for having suggested the chiropractor (Cowie and Roebuck 1975; Kelner, Hall and Coulter 1980), recounting stories—tantamount to testimonials—of their own success with this "unorthodox" therapy. (See Frank [1961], who has also noted the power of testimonials for psychotherapeutic efficacy.) This satisfied new patient recounts the successful episode to another friend and the cycle is repeated. Because chiropractors were for many decades barred from official means of advertising and still today suffer public censure, they have had to rely on building a clientele by reputation and word of mouth, much like any traditional healer.

The chiropractor disclaims his psychotherapeutic ministrations and, indeed, they may be unconscious or unintended to some extent. When the

D.C. rejects outright my suggestions that he is providing psychological support and therapy, he does so for the following reasons. First, the assertion diminishes his claims to the real therapeutic value of spinal manipulation and other treatment techniques, which are valid and restorative of structure and function. One of the major criticisms against chiropractic is that any benefit it might confer is "all psychological" (Consumer Reports 1980:182; Wardwell 1972:262.) Speaking of M.D. claims, "if they can't help you they think it's all in your head."

Second, he rightfully fears censure for overstepping the boundaries of licensure. Chiropractic professionals face endless persecution in the form of bad press, scientific criticism, and court battles which challenge the legitimacy of what they do and how effectively they do it. Therefore, chiropractors are hesitant to lay claim to the psychotherapeutic efficacy of their clinical art. Instead, they deny such efficacy in order to maintain their professional appearance.

Finally, it is not inconceivable that the chiropractor does not realize the tremendous psychological impact his "talk therapy" and his "laying on of hands" has on patients, being blinded to it by such a strong faith in the theory and practice of his manipulative techniques. My informant insists he was given no special training in psychology or counseling during his four years of chiropractic college. However, the curriculum in accredited chiropractic schools, such as the one he attended, includes a three-year sequence in both clinical art and chiropractic philosophy. These courses heavily emphasize patient care, the doctor-patient relationship, effective communication and developing professional attitudes (Palmer College 1983).

In most schools, during the third- and fourth-year chiropractic students have a thorough apprenticeship in the clinical art with a faculty chiropractor. The occupational description published by the American Chiropractic Association includes the point that "professional counsel is often given in such areas as...physical and mental attitudes affecting health...and the many other activities of daily living that would enhance the effects of chiropractic health care" (ACA 1978:3).

According to chiropractic theory, structural realignment will improve attitude and chemical balance through progressive positive feedback. If chemical or structural treatments are carried out with no corresponding improvement in health, a blockage of the mental health is searched for and rooted out. Thus, even if chiropractic training specializes in a mechanical treatment with less or no emphasis on counseling or psychological skills, the training at the same time teaches D.C.s to be on guard constantly for emotional imbalances in the person which, without amelioration, will render their own treatments worthless.

All in all, I found the D.C. quite ambivalent about admitting his use of "psychology," as he puts it. On the one hand, he muses: "Do I use psychology on my patients? I don't know if I do or not." And, "I've treated thousands of patients, but so far I've only run across one case where it was more psychological than anything else."

On the other hand, he also confesses that patients tell him "there's no one else that they'll talk to" and "people use me as a shrink." He confided to me, "They let it down, I'm telling you...I'm amazed at what people tell me sometimes. I mean I'm absolutely amazed." But he was quick to point out that he recommends his patients see a psychologist if he detects a serious problem. And indeed, on one occasion I did observe him suggest this to a young male patient in the case his "sensory kinds of things" continued. He also sometimes has patients fill out a symptom survey of psycho-emotional functioning.

B. Treatment Consonant with Sociocultural Characteristics

PSYCHOLOGIZATION VERSUS SOMATIZATION

The degree to which a patient articulates underlying emotional problems may follow socioeconomic and cultural lines. As Harwood pointed out (1987:2), some trained in psychotherapy have concluded that methods which stress insight and verbal skills are inappropriate for lower-class patients (Kaplan and Roman 1973:218–19; Prince 1969:22–29). Response to symptoms and pain varies among ethnic groups and social class (Zola 1966; Zborowski 1952; Elder and Acheson 1970). Some tend to localize symptoms in the physical body rather than in the mind, as do some Westerners (see Kleinman 1980; Ohnuki-Tierney 1984).

Working-class people are more prone to physical stress related to their job activities. Thus, the lower and working classes and certain ethnic groups are better represented among those with chronic and somatized complaints, due to occupation-related causes, the tendency to somatize, and culturally defined ways of reacting to stressors, thereby making alternative therapies which are receptive to these expressions much more attractive. The college-educated, on the other hand, are much more likely to seek psychotherapy (Kadushin 1969).

EXTENDED FAMILY

Another difference which highlights cultural differences between the three healing practices is the degree to which the extended family and friends, i.e., the social support network, is involved in therapy choice and the clinical process. A decisive factor in the treatment decision process is the degree of faith family members have in various practitioners, formed from previous experience, knowledge, and expectations (Shapiro 1964).

Individual psychotherapy is, as a general rule, private, although family or relationship counseling are exceptions. This reflects the strong emphasis on individualism in the dominant U.S. culture, especially in upper-class strata. In chiropractic, members of the immediate family are urged to participate, and when they do, are incorporated fully into the treatment and consultation sessions. However, this does not happen in the majority of cases. This approach emphasizes chiropractic's focus on emotional support of the sick person and is consistent with cultural norms of assistance expected from the nuclear family. Contrasting sharply with the other two therapies, Puerto Rican spiritism mirrors the strong familism characteristic of that culture (see Jenkins, this volume). The immediate and extended family are encouraged and often required to be involved in the healing sessions. Family and ritual kin (e.g., godparents) are typically in attendance.

SOCIAL REALITY

The more congruent the social reality between patient and therapist, the greater the chance for a positive therapeutic outcome. Lesser sociocultural differences between therapist and patient potentially reduce barriers to effective communication. These differences are often manifested by sociolinguistic differences, as patients tend to ask fewer questions the more perceived distance they feel from a doctor (Waitzkin and Stoeckle 1972), and, as doctors, who perceive patients to be of lower class, ethnic or educational background, tend to avoid giving explanations and information (Pratt, Seligmann and Reader 1957).

Whereas psychotherapists are generally from the same upper socioeconomic strata as their clientele, spiritist mediums and their clients are from the lowest income strata. (Forty-six percent of households in Harwood's study received public assistance [1987:26]). Chiropractic therapists and their patients come from a range of backgrounds centering around the middle strata, with the working class being well-represented (White and Skipper 1971; James, Fox and Guity 1983; National Analysts 1972).

Given that a practitioner has more success the less social and cultural distance separates him/her from the patient, how is it then that the chiropractor ostensibly appeals to both middle and upper socioeconomic groups? Chiropractors, including this D.C. are mainly drawn from the middle class in contrast to the predominance of upper-middle class M.D.s (White et al. 1971). The D.C. I observed is himself a professional now, but he retains a working-class demeanor and language; he thus straddles the fence between the status groups. Communication is greatly enhanced when they understand each other's meanings and expressions. Even if the D.C. does not share all the basic values, beliefs, and problems of all his clients, at least he understands and can relate to a wider range of people from the various socioeconomic strata.

Many have concluded that the low-income, less educated, and/or working class prefer the concrete over the abstract, are nonintrospective, desire immediate gratification, are not verbal but rather given to expressing psychological complaints in physical terms (Kaplan and Roman 1973; Prince 1969), and for these reasons they avoid entering psychotherapy (Brill and Storrow 1960; Bernstein 1964; Prince 1969) and tend to go to chiropractors (Cowie et al. 1975; James et al. 1983; McCorkle 1961; Wardwell 1972).

One could argue that this type of research by upper socioeconomic status social scientists regarding the lower classes has certain unexamined biases. Regarding the second premise, an equally probable assertion is that members of minority ethnic and low-income groups avoid utilizing psychotherapists because mental health professionals are often not willing or able to understand their values or problems (Gursslin, Hunt and Rosch 1964). But, however true the first and second arguments may be, the third statement, that these people make up the bulk of chiropractor's patients, is highly questionable.

First of all, there were few lower-class patients in my study (most manual laborers were lower-middle to upper-middle class). Moreover, many of the blue collar patients were very verbal and took the opportunity to unload problems on the chiropractor. And a few, of course, were noncommunicative, the most notable of my sample being a dentist, whose entire conversation with the D.C. consisted of salutations and a few instrumental questions.

Ethnicity combines with socioeconomic position as factors upon which the choice of therapist is based. While psychotherapy tends to draw patients more from the white, upper and upper-middle classes, spiritism is a uniquely Puerto Rican phenomenon attracting mostly low-income members of that ethnic group, particularly those on the margins of mainstream United States culture and society. Of the household heads in Harwood's study, 94 percent were born in Puerto Rico (1987:27).

Immigrants and the first generation of Hispanic origin may have a preference for religious or spiritual forms of treatment, which spiritism provides. Belief in spirits is more acceptable than institutional care. And, of course, spiritists and their clients speak the same language. On the other hand, chiropractors have a more broad-based appeal, treating patients of the middle to upper socioeconomic status from various ethnic groups who share a relatively mainstream sociocultural existence. There were few identifiable first generation or immigrant people among the chiropractor's patients.

The chiropractor uses cultural knowledge to positively influence the course of treatment. Two examples of this are his playing on the popular disenchantment with biomedicine and his use of mechanistic analogies to explain himself. Dissatisfaction with biomedicine was a frequent topic of conversation between the doctor and the patient: (patient) "M.D.s don't know anything about backs." (D.C.): "They'd be the last to admit that. They think they know everything about everything!"

A middle-aged female patient recalled the shooting pains in her head and neck that she has alleviated with chiropractic care:

> For 18 years, at least 18 years I went to doctors. Oh, my God, I went to the (x) clinic, (y) hospital, (z) hospital. And that doesn't include all the doctors...and I used to have to go to (y) hospital before I went to work of a morning and they would put me in that machine there (traction)...all different types of medication...anywhere from...20 to 25 pills a day. There were days when I would have 9 before I even went to work. They told me that it was part hereditary because every day of my mother's life that I can remember, she had a headache and they said it was passed on from mother to daughter, not mothers to sons; that was the only thing that they ever told me.

The D.C. uses analogy to help patients conceptualize their problems (see Oths 1985). Etiological explanations draw on mechanical examples from the everyday world, which can be easily understood regardless of one's socioeconomic or cultural background. He might say, for example:

> You've got to understand we're moving bones here. It's like moving teeth. You just don't put teeth into position in a day, just like that...they put braces on the teeth, right?...and it hurts like hell for awhile. You walk into the dentists office with no pain, you walk out and you're in tremendous pain...Sometimes you move the bones and it does create what seems like a negative reaction, but it's just the nature of moving bones.

Or, he compares misaligned vertebrae and disc compression to a brick and mortar wall:

> If the brick was sitting like this (demonstrates unparallel bricks with his hands) what would happen? Just the pressure alone would eventually wear out that side of the mortar. Well, just imagine, if that building had the ability to move, it would wear out even quicker.

C. Cognitive Framework

As Harwood notes, the importance of placing the client's behavior into a cognitive framework that provides a label or meaning for the behavior is characteristic of all who use psychotherapy (1987:194). A shared cognitive system helps bring about the placebo effect (Adler and Hammett 1973). Any therapeutic treatment includes as a distinct element the belief it elicits in both practitioner and patient, in addition to the more observable physiological effect of the treatment itself (Weil 1983). In other words, it is not simply the objective effect of therapeutic measures that are of interest, but also the ideas forming the basis of the therapeutic acts as well (Ackerknecht 1946).

Cowie and Roebuck have noted the importance to patient recovery of "buying into" the practitioner's approach and worldview (1975). Psychotherapists, spiritist mediums, and chiropractors—as opposed to biomedical physicians—operate on the basis of unique, cohesive ideologies, each a systematic comprehensive worldview of disease, illness, and health, which gives a rational understanding of any patient's problem, a coherent explanation of it, and a method of treating it. With a unified theory, patients' previously ill-defined problems are recognized and legitimated, a necessary condition for successful psychotherapeutic interaction.

The psychotherapist sees patient insight and awareness of inner needs and conflicts as the key to knowing and improving one's life. Patients who seek their help usually partake of similar etiological and theoretical constructs, even if the formal theory of psychotherapy is not understood. Spiritism is evaluated on the ability to connect the patient with the spiritual world, to eventually receive the protection of one or more protective spirits (Harwood 1987:189). This culturally acceptable framework is already familiar to new clients, and at *reuniones* one develops a personal understanding of the basic conceptual system of spiritism. Finally, chiropractic views the structural integrity of the body to be the main factor in health, and the instrumental cause of disease as vertebral misalignment, or "subluxation," and nerve impingement. Stress, especially occupational, can be a precipitating factor in subluxation (Palmer College 1983). This conceptual framework is not generally known to new patients but is inculcated promptly through an educational immersion process, as follows.

Chiropractors spend much office time educating patients about their own etiological belief system (Oths 1985). Given the unorthodox nature of the chiropractic system, the chiropractor goes to great lengths to educate new patients to a new way of thinking about their often longstanding problems. Initial educational explanations are given and films shown to the new patient, with frequent indoctrination to chiropractic theory during subsequent treatment sessions. Heavy emphasis is placed on leading patients to realize they can understand and influence their own condition. The D.C. sees this education process as essential because patient expectations for cure are unreasonable unless and until they understand the nature of the internal damage, why the healing process will take time, how he "moves" bones, the necessity of frequent office visits, etc. Their ability to describe and discuss an ailment is important because once it is made comprehensible it becomes tangible, thus easier to manage, with a resultant reduction in anxiety about it (Maslow 1963; Barsky 1981).

In essence, the chiropractor first manipulates a patient's belief structure before setting about to manipulate his or her physical structure, providing an analogous structural realignment in both the mind and body. A congruity between patient beliefs and behaviors gives a certain unity to the chiropractic experience, securing patient's faith in and adherence to the system of therapy (see Lévi-Strauss 1963:196). Thus, all those who use psychotherapeutic techniques, including chiropractic, aim to restructure their patients' attitudes and behaviors with a new set of socially and culturally consonant meanings and activities.

CRITERIA FOR EVALUATING HEALER'S EFFICACY

Naturally, the goal of any therapy is to relieve symptoms and suffering. Along with a new cognitive orientation, certain criteria are framed for judging the efficacy of the healer. In psychotherapy, criteria for judging a therapist's efficacy are not generally known to the patient (Harwood 1987:140). In spiritism, to show her ability the medium manipulates therapeutic objects, talks to and exorcises spirits, and reveals the identity of persons committing sorcery, among other things (Harwood 1987:100).

The chiropractor, from the initial encounters with a new patient, sets up visible, tangible standards by which to judge the efficacy of treatment and the progress of the patient. A diminishing frequency of treatments is programmed, and changes in status of pain and mobility are carefully monitored, measured, and fed back to the patient as continuous progress reports. Expected results of treatment also provide tangible evaluative criteria.

The D.C. promises the patient that he will do everything in his power to get the patient well as soon as possible. Thus, visits will have to be frequent at first, up to six times a week for initial care of acute episodes (e.g., patient cannot stand or walk from a fall) and will gradually decrease—depending on the rate of improvement—to three times a week, then two times, then once, then once every ten days, etc., dropping to once a month for maintenance until the problem is completely healed. Treatment frequency changes with patient improvement, (e.g., "OK, we're going to stretch it out to ten days this next time").

The D.C. initially tests, then periodically retests a patient with a battery of pain tolerance and range of motion exams. He states the new degree of pain and range of motion and compares them to the previous degrees. If there has been improvement, he reminds the patient how bad it had been before. This quantitative assessment, he states explicitly, is better than using perceived reduction of pain intensity as a measure. This is because one quickly blocks out memories of previous pain and may not realize the actual pain reduction unless it is compared against a tangible standard, such as how far one could bend over, rotate the neck, whether lower back pain had been mild, moderate, or severe, etc. Also, the D.C. asks the percentage of improvement at the beginning of each session: "You were 60 percent better. What are you at today?" ("60 percent" meaning one had regained 60 percent of pre-illness functioning).

The "hoped-for" as compared to the "expected" results add to the perceived efficacy of a therapeutic technique, as Young (1976) has pointed out. If certain routine, or expected, results of medical treatment are fulfilled apart from the hoped-for results, patient commitment to a form of therapy might be increased. In chiropractic, while the veritable relief from pain is hoped for, the clicking noises bones make during an adjustment is an anticipated event of the treatment procedure. This sought after result ("did I get it?," "there it went," "did you feel that?" "I heard it pop") gives cognitive satisfaction to both healer and patient that the treatment is working (effective).

Such nonfalsifiable hypotheses tend to reinforce beliefs and practices in a particular method, regardless of whether the successful completion of one procedure actually leads to pain reduction or not (Young 1976). Thus, chiropractic appeals to the mechanistic aspect of our culture (Coulehan 1985). Direct mechanical manipulation of the bone and muscle structure tends to create certain highly predictable results. The D.C. visibly works on the problem in a way tangible to patients of all classes. He does "something...which gives the patient a prolonged experience of something happening to the body" (Coulehan 1985:388).

REVIEW OF PAST HISTORY

An extensive review of a patient's past history is another technique common to all three therapists. Formally during intake and informally during treatment sessions, a chiropractor acquires a detailed account of a patient's personal as well as medical history. This includes information on personal habits, accidents, a psychological inventory, interpersonal problems, and more. This archeology of a person's past allows anxiety-provoking feelings and emotional conflicts to surface, as Harwood has also recognized in spiritism (1987:195).

D. Physical Contact

One additional technique for which certain therapies have an advantage over all other forms of care is their utilization of the power of touch with the patient. The laying on of hands helps to build trust in the practitioner, release tension, and frequently, unleash a stream of communication or emotion from the patient (see Pratt and Mason 1984). That healing energy is actually transmitted from healer to patient is often claimed (Fishman 1979:14; Jackson 1980) but difficult to verify.

Psychotherapists are enjoined on ethical grounds from physical contact with patients. In spiritism, individual attention is called for in the most serious cases. In these cases, massage, or the laying on of hands, is utilized. (Magnetic healing is used for the same purposed in Christian prayer healing [Fishman 1979:1214]).

During treatment the chiropractor is manually involved in treating the patient almost constantly. Approximately 90 percent of the session time is spent with the D.C. palpating, positioning, massaging, and manipulating the patient's body. The therapy calms and relaxes the patients, at times putting them into a trance-like state. Working in physical contact with the patient presents an ideal opportunity to connect affectively as well. The prone position of the patient has the same function of having a client recline on a couch in classical psychoanalysis. Thoughts flow freely without the eye contact and nonverbal cues of the therapist interfering. Even before and after actual treatment, the D.C. usually touches the patient several times, either for therapeutic purposes or simply as a friendly gesture. Thus, the chiropractor's practice of physically working on the patient is especially suited for a patient who needs to talk.

TRANCE INDUCTION

Spiritists clearly do, and psychotherapists usually do not, induce trance states in their patients. In the case of chiropractic, the situation is not as clear-cut. Although a full trance is not achieved, patients many times experience a trance-like, hypnagogic state from the pre- and post-treatment physical therapy, such as diathermy and ultrasound, as well as from the actual laying on of hands and deep muscle massage and manipulation.

In an effort to keep patients from waiting long in the outer waiting room, a chiropractic assistant ushers each into one of the seven treatment rooms, gives them a fresh gown, has them lie down and begins physical therapy until the doctor is available. This flexible waiting period is then used to "work" on the patient instead of having them unproductively, anxiously waiting and watching the clock in the reception area. It has the net result of calming the patient tremendously. So-called alpha states are most likely reached, much like in meditation. Often times the patient has dozed off or is very "spacey" by the time the D.C. arrives.

E. Practitioner-Patient Relationship

A healthy, communicative relationship with a patient is actively sought by psychotherapists as well as spiritists and chiropractors. They recognize the vital importance of a good relationship as a basis upon which rests trust, and subsequently, effective treatment. A patient's self-esteem is boosted by a doctor's concern for and empathy with the sufferer, as it communicates to the patient that he or she is worthy of the doctor's efforts.

Certain positive personal characteristics of the therapist and culturally accepted symbols of practitioner competence have long been touted as aiding in arousing the patient's hope, self-confidence, and trust in the therapist (see Frank 1961). These therapeutically important attributes of the practitioner-patient relationship are positive transference and countertransference, tolerance, respect, support, guidance, empathy, and warmth (Shapiro 1964; Frank 1974). Certain patients faced with the long-term prospects of chronic disease will need more empathy, reassurance, and supportive care. Also, if a condition is irreversible, the patient will need the therapist's guidance in learning to accept this and still lead the fullest life possible.

The D.C., like the spiritist medium, shows a remarkable degree of warmth, concern, optimism, genuineness, and empathy; and he does not withhold hope. The promise of recovery is always given (Oths 1985; Harwood 1987:140). The tone of his conversations with patients is friendly and informal, often humorous (see Oths 1985). The D.C. makes each patient feel special, with his hearty greetings (e.g., "Heeey Mike! How's it going buddy?") and with attention to details of their personal life.

In fact, the D.C. has a social relationship outside the office with many of his patients. (D: "Where are you working now? I never see you anymore." P: I'm working in the (franchised health club) in Akron now.") If 100 percent recovery is not likely, then the D.C. encourages a patient as much as realistically possible and constantly supports the patient that he is improving. (e.g., "we'll do what we can for you," "you've improved tremendously!" "keep up the good work.")

Often patients expressed their gratitude for having helped them, with a few even dubbing him a "miracle worker." He gains the confidence and trust of his patients through his clinical manner and through the strong personal faith and conviction he has in his own practices. When patients express disbelief, he counters, "you don't have to believe in it. It will help you anyhow." By having the confidence to deny the patient's need to believe, he reveals the depths of his own faith, which in turn helps convince the patient.

LONG-TERM RELATIONSHIP

Certain characteristics of chronic disease, which set it apart from acute disease, give its therapist a unique role. As chronic problems range from longlasting to permanent, this affords a practitioner the opportunity to build a strong, trusting relationship with patients. Psychotherapists, spiritists, and chiropractors alike challenge the "detached concern" of biomedicine by actively fostering a communicative, interpersonal relationship with the client, supplying what is usually absent from overly logical, rational, and clinical care (Frank 1961:115; Harwood 1987:187; Oths 1985).

This type of relationship follows from Frank's minimal definition of a psychotherapeutic relationship as one which necessarily involves systematic contacts between the healer and client (Frank 1961:2). In contrast to the episodic and infrequent visits of regular biomedical care, a relatively durable, long-term—sometimes lifelong—relationship is the usual form with any of the three therapists being discussed here. Lengthy practitioner-patient contacts are essential for psychotherapeutic means to be effective, although relationships for crisis intervention are sometimes short-term, as Garrison found for spiritist clients (1977:88).

Especially at first, the chiropractor encourages his patients' visits to be intense, that is, frequent but short in duration. They can be as often as daily during critical phases, ideally working down gradually to a monthly maintenance visit, which can be continued indefinitely. The average number of visits made by patients in the study sample was forty-nine, ranging from two to 112, and were made over a median time period of 8.5 months.

The keeping of appointments is enhanced by the D.C.'s frequent reminders not to miss, because "if you're not here, I can't help you and it won't be my fault." Office assistants who book the appointments are party to this strategy and pleasantly, yet insistantly, repeat to patients the need to follow their treatment schedules. Assistants regularly call patients who miss appointments, gently reprimanding them in order to get them rescheduled. (Patients are not charged for missed appointments.)

F. Rituals and Symbols

Ritual or ritual object use is evident to some degree in almost all clinical settings (Walker 1964). Ritual, or the observance of an established or patterned practice or procedure, has a powerful effect on a patient. Such activities validate and reinforce the natural or supernatural powers of any healer. Culturally meaningful rituals generate hope and the expectancy of cure, which bring about positive changes in attitude and behavior, according to Frank (1961). The more symbolically relevant to the patient's culture are the therapies, the more powerful they will be (see Comas-Diaz 1981:641).

Symbolic ritual objects identify and reinforce the healer's status and power. They are found in abundance in all three therapists' settings. The spiritist *reuniones* in which they contact the spirits are highly ritualized and they manipulate many symbolic therapeutic objects, such as candles, flowers, *agua florida*, clothing, and statues of saints (Harwood 1987:62). The chiropractor uses medical and mechanistic symbolism to increase the patient's faith and acceptance of chiropractic.

MEDICAL SYMBOLISM

Chiropractors and psychotherapists alike, as doctors, utilize the clinic, couch/adjusting table, white lab coat, framed academic diplomas, scientific terminology, and more. Chiropractors additionally use apparently scientific objects and technology such as scale models, ultrasound machines, diathermy, galvanic currents x-rays, and blood tests. As both psychotherapists and D.C.s to a great extent behave as do biomedical physicians—with all the symbolic power such behavior confers—they can imitate or duplicate modern medical practices in a way spiritists cannot. This appeal to scientific respectability influences members of the dominant United States culture, who are conditioned to respond to and even idolize biomedical symbols, even while at the same time looking for an alternative to biomedicine.

The use of medical symbols adds the legitimacy to chiropractic required to impress the mainstream American. In fact, 10 percent of the patient sample in my study were biomedically trained health care providers (four nurses, one dentist, and one medical lab technician.) The invocation of medical appearance is not simply affected, but rather is due to four rigorous years of chiropractic training emphasizing state boards as physicians in the basic sciences. Training standards have been steadily upgraded over the years to improve their status as professionals as a response to mainstream public demands (Manbar 1978).

MECHANISTIC SYMBOLISM

Chiropractic theory and symbolism is consonant with the mechanistic conceptual system of industrialized societies. Structural misalignment, nerve impingement, muscle tone, and vertebral readjustment through manual manipulation are easily understandable and culturally compatible mechanical explanations for musculoskeletal pain, as Coulehan has also noted (1985:387). Because of the mechanistic nature of chiropractic care, D.C.s have an advantage in that they can more easily demonstrate pathophysiology to a patient than can a physician. They make use of charts, x-rays, and scale models whenever they are explaining the skeletal system, slipped disc, scoliosis, etc. For a physician, it is more difficult to demonstrate microscopic and abstract entities such as germs, heart attacks, effects of tranquilizers, and the like.

A D.C. gives patients one of the things they most need for chronic, sometimes debilitating musculostructural problems: support. This support comes in verbal, physical, and symbolic forms. The D.C. never withholds hope and encouragement from the patient, always predicting one can get better, if only partially, through adherence to the treatment regimen. Physically, the chiropractor manipulates the muscles and vertebrae with his own flesh and bones in order to structurally realign the body so it can better support itself and be mobile.

Most significantly, the chiropractor often sends the patient away from the office with a constant and visible symbolic reminder of his clinically based support—the usual neckbrace, or maybe a knee, leg, or back support. The device, which a patient is instructed to wear even in public for what seem like inordinate lengths of time and for sometimes ostensibly minor problems, is a potent symbol conveying the message that the emotional support and concern of the D.C. and his staff remain with the patient in the outside world. There, understanding and sympathy for one's problems is sometimes lacking, especially given the common attitude that chiropractors are quacks with malingerers for patients. The support, then, legitimizes the patient's sick role.

It can be assumed that the neck support reinforces commitment to the D.C. For example, a patient wearing a neckbrace to work and receiving the standard response, "ah, I see you've been to the chiropractor," will be put in the position of defending chiropractic or else suffering cognitive dissonance. Thus, one's psychological investment in the treatment is probably increased by wearing a neck support in public.

Another therapeutic component of treatment is the enhancement of patients' sense of control over themselves and their environment, brought about by giving patients a participatory role in therapeutic rituals—a primary objective of spiritist, chiropractic, and psychotherapeutic practices. Both spiritism and chiropractic sessions are ritualized, though spiritism unquestionably more so (Harwood 1987:57). But following Harwood's use of Turner's definition, we can see that D.C.s, too, use stereotyped sequences of activity involving gestures, words, and objects designed to influence the therapeutic outcome.

In chiropractic, participatory rituals in the clinic include, for example, eliciting patients' childhood history, feelings, emotions, or problems; giving the patient a role in decision making; and, having the patient self-apply physical therapy. Ritual tasks assigned to be performed at home include reflection, prescribed diet and exercises, and special home treatments (Oths 1985). Such participation serves to divert the sufferer's attention from pain, increase the amount of interaction with the healer, and mobilize the expectation of cure.

The form and content of chiropractic ritual, after first exposure, soon become routinized and predictable, very consistent with the United States' mechanistic, techno-industrial pattern of living and working. People learn their particular treatment routine quickly, and once it becomes established, they begin to run through the paces together with an evident ease and familiarity as soon as the D.C. enters.

For example, the D.C. might interject a directional phrase into the midst of an ongoing conversation and continue to talk and adjust at the same time: (patient) "...and I didn't have anything bothering me"; (doctor) "So it's not really fair to ask you, is it? You didn't have time to get bad again. Let it in...let it out...the big hug...Remember when I first started doing this how tender it used to be?..." "The big hug" is an adjustment maneuver to adjust the upper back. The patient will move into the prone position, arms crossed, inhale and exhale while the D.C. lifts the patient in with few commands or prompting.

As a reflection of dominant cultural beliefs which have little to no tolerance for the supernatural and unexplainable, the demeanor of my D.C. informant is not the least bit mystical, nor are his rituals overdramatic. His rituals are simple, routine, and pragmatic, similar to those experienced, and thus expected by, a participating productive member of a highly motivated and time-conscious work-oriented society.

It is, therefore, no coincidence that the chiropractor places the greatest amount of psychological emphasis on the patient's job and family roles. While working manually on a patient, the D.C. makes an effort to find out about and keep updated on the intricacies of each patient's social, economic, and familial roles, but he does so discreetly through amiable chatting, not intentional psychoanalysis. It was a rare session that the D.C. did not inquire about the patient's job or home responsibilities with leading questions reflecting prior conversations. (e.g., "How's work?" "Did you change shifts yet?" "Did you get your raise?" "Are they cutting your hours back?" "Is your daughter back in school yet?" "How were the holidays?" "Did you talk it over with your wife?") He approaches topics of greatest concern and potential problem and lets the patients talk about what is troubling them (see case study below).

As a cultural norm, one eye is always on the clock; mainstream Americans are preoccupied with time, especially promptness (see Hall [1959] for a full account of North American time concepts). The D.C. respects the popular attitudes towards time. When a patient wanted to discuss insurance paper problems with the chiropractor after his session on a busy day, the D.C. postponed the talk to the next available time slot, insisting that he could not keep patients waiting.

Instead of lengthy séances or couch sessions, the time-conscious D.C. assures his patients that, "usually you'll be in and outta here in forty minutes. You're not going to have to wait around." He attends to appointments promptly and promises to spend as little of one's time per day as necessary, while still insisting that in healing chronic problems is a long-term commitment (e.g., "it's going to take time, be patient. That's why they call me 'doctor' and you 'patient'!").

G. Attitude and Behavior Change

If one's attitude is related to one's physical state, a positive change in attitude can bring about a complementary change in health status. One method of facilitating attitude change, commonly seen in psychotherapy as well as the other two approaches, is to encourage insight into the patient's life:

one tells a psychotherapist one's "whole story," confesses in a spiritist session, and gives a detailed personalized account of one's problem in chiropractic.

All three types of therapist engage in operant behavioral conditioning (see Frank 1961). Wittingly or not, all therapists have a tremendous capacity to influence a patient through verbal as well as nonverbal messages. By reinforcement of desired behavior, a healer can subtly guide a patient away from unacceptable behaviors. The more coercive this influence is, however, the more likely a patient will resent the therapist and resist changing. Chiropractors benefit from their lack of overt manipulation of psychotherapeutic techniques, as patients are not made defensive by having to admit a psychosomatic connection to their ailment, which could be misinterpreted as "delabeling," or, "there's nothing wrong, it's all in your head" (Helman 1985).

LOCUS OF RESPONSIBILITY

All therapists described here expect an attitude and behavioral change on the part of the patient. However, where each places the locus of responsibility for the cause of the condition and for its cure differs from one therapy to the next.

Glick classifies the cause of sickness into instrumental, efficient, and ultimate categories, which respectively answer the questions what, who, and why (1967). Psychotherapy sees past unresolved conflicts as the instrumental factor, individual behavior and attitudes as the efficient cause, and social factors such as society and the family as the ultimate cause. Spiritism holds that the instrumental cause is spirits, which may do harm in the form of *envidia* (envy), *brujeria* (sorcery), etc. The efficient cause are evil-meaning enemies and the ultimate cause is the forces of the supernatural world.

In chiropractic, the instrumental cause for illness is a spinal subluxation, or misalignment, which pinches nerves and restricts blood flow. The efficient cause is some accident or improper movement on the part of the patient. The ultimate cause, as in psychotherapy, is societal. Blame is usually concentrated primarily on work (strenuousness, overwork, stress) and secondarily on M.D.s, who are seen to compound existing problems through inappropriate treatment. Nature can also be implicated in the case of genetic problems such as scoliosis.

Unlike psychotherapy, which places blame in the client's mind and behavior, or spiritists, who don't label the client as sick but rather as a victim of suffering from an attack by a disembodied spirit, the locus of control in chiropractic lies midway between the two extremes of internal and external. The responsibility is not focused on the patient, but is attributed in part to society and nature as well.

As for the responsibility for obtaining a cure or relief of symptoms, psychotherapy expects the patient to achieve results with the guidance of the therapist. Spiritists expect a client to behave correctly and solicit help from and obey the supernatural, but the benevolent protective spirits which the medium contacts are the chief architects of healing. In chiropractic, the D.C. assumes a major role of responsibility for patient recovery, yet insists that the full cooperation of the patient is necessary for success. He says:

> We have a 90 to 95 percent chance of helping you if you follow my instructions and do exactly what I ask you to do. If you don't...I won't have much chance of helping you at all, so don't waste your time and money, OK?...If you miss any treatments, then obviously if you're not here, I can't help you, OK?

Emphasizing his own role in recovery, the D.C. says, "Yeah. Gotta get this under control for you and then we've got to keep it there." But he denies total responsibility: "I'm not God. I'll do what I can for you."

Pointing out the joint responsibility for cure he and the patient have, he states to a young woman with reverse lordosis in the cervical region:

> What I do for you here is helping it. What you do is going to either help it or aggravate it...If you aggravate it more than I'm helping it, you're going to lose.

To a male patient with a herniated disc:

> If you keep this under control with once-a-month adjustments, you'll have a better chance of fighting this thing off. But I will tell you this...you're going to have to learn to work around your back, to lift properly, not to sit too long, to change your lifestyle. Because if you don't, no matter what I do for you, you're going to limit the effect I have on you tremendously.

We see then that the onus of responsibility for cure is squarely on the patient's shoulders in psychotherapy, almost completely removed from the patient in spiritism, and is more equally shared in chiropractic between healer and patient.

Harwood believes that psychotherapy's emphasis on individual responsibility stems from the Protestant ethic, whereas spiritism's metaphysical beliefs are rooted in the folk Catholicism from which it originated (Harwood 1987:190). Chiropractic's locus of responsibility assumes a joint effort between actors. The emphasis on cooperation reflects its Midwest, working class-oriented origins: the ideals of everyone pitching in, and of helping out one's neighbors. Chiropractic was effectively rediscovered for the Western world in Davenport, Iowa, in 1895 when a magnetic healer successfully treated a janitor for hearing loss believed to be caused by nerve impingement from a displaced vertebra (Cowie et al. 1975:27). Today, the Midwest continues to have one of the highest chiropractor-to-population ratios, at 15:100,000 (U.S. Dept. of Health and Human Services 1986).

TRANSFER OF THERAPEUTIC LEARNING TO NEW SOCIAL ROLE
AND USE OF GROUP PSYCHOLOGY

The goal of all three therapies, in which their patients are complicit, is to try to separate the client from maladaptive behaviors in order to restore the patient to the fullest functioning realistically possible. One chiropractic patient sensing a need to reestablish her former role identity remarked, "How do you know when you're ready to go back to being a person again."

In addition to restoring a patient to his or her former role capacity, spiritism often utilizes healing as a transition rite to help the patient attain a new social role within the cult, such as spirit medium, which promotes healing by boosting the personal status and esteem of the client. This new role can be attained while at the same time regaining one's old role status in the family and society. In contrast, given the structure of their practices, it is not the aim of psychotherapy nor chiropractic to incorporate patients into new supporting healer roles in their offices (although I did hear the D.C. suggesting to a patient that he ought to consider chiropractic as a profession).

Chiropractic stops short of providing new roles for patients as a means to overcome their psychological difficulties, in contrast to more overtly cult-like traditional psychotherapies such as spiritism, whose patients can become mediums (Harwood 1987:183). Clients also become *tang-kis* (shamans) in Taiwan (Kleinman 1980), temple healers and assistants in Mexican spiritualism (Finkler 1985), *Morita* therapists and *shinkieshitsu* hospital directors in Japan (Reynolds 1976), and church ministers in Christian faith healing (Fishman 1979). However, the main aim of chiropractic therapy is to restore a person to the adequate performance of former roles. In a manifest way, this is done by curing the body, i.e., eliminating pain and pathology, and in a more implicit way by alleviating the psychological stressors.

The D.C., while not providing a new status role for his patients, was himself a role model of healthy behavior. He is a dynamic, superbly fit man, who does not smoke and drinks little. He works out at a number of gyms regularly and teaches and takes marital arts at another set of studios, all from which he draws several of his patients.

Unlike spiritism, where group membership in a religious-like worship provides a new identity for the participant, chiropractic is neither a subculture nor a cult (Harwood 1987:35, 182), although the chiropractor can deliver his teachings with the fervor of a preacher. Sessions are always individual with one patient and attending family. Chiropractic never makes use of group psychology as a psychotherapeutic technique. Commitment to chiropractic tenets does not construe a distinct identity on anyone with the exception of the practitioner himself. In spiritism, all participants—medium, client, supporting family members—are practitioners in the sense used to denote the followers, or congregation, of religious teaching. In contrast, in chiropractic, to the extent that one's conceptual world is realigned with a new set of beliefs, values, and cause-and-effect relationships, it pertains to the world of sickness only. It realigns one's general worldview indirectly, if at all, and certainly not supernaturally or metaphysically. That is, chiropractic teachings do not provide sociocultural meaning outside of the illness context.

In sum, there are many possible types of therapeutic techniques to use in the treatment of patients. Not all therapists utilize all the possible techniques, yet many of the very aspects of psychotherapy which make it a viable tool for patient self-improvement and alleviation of suffering, are equivalent to those aspects of spiritist and chiropractic therapies which make them effective. Each treatment type contains various psychotherapeutic elements, but as in any cross-culturally applicable taxonomy, some characteristics will have more salience than others depending on which are culturally consonant and effective.

Improvement of emotional distress may be due to: the patient's acceptance of pain, mastery over it, improved understanding of it, and a plan for its management; increased physical activity; withdrawal from prescription drugs; and/or alteration of biochemical states by physical or psychological means, among other things (Kramlinger, Swanson and Maruda 1983). Non biomedical therapists alleviate the suffering of their chronically ill patients by using psychotherapeutic techniques to achieve these goals. Regardless of what circumstances lead an individual to the nonbiomedical options discussed above, one can be certain that when they arrive, psychotherapeutic techniques will be called into play, perhaps in conjunction with physical therapy, to alleviate the stress causing or abetting the somatic disorder.

Resort

We have seen that psychotherapists, spiritists and chiropractors have much in common in their treatment of sick people. What then accounts for the patient's decision to visit one over the other? Why do people choose the therapist they do?

Recourse to all three types of practitioners is similar. Usually they are resorted to after all biomedical options have been exhausted without success. Patients are discouraged and apprehensive about their problem, yet continue to harbor hope for eventual cure or remission of symptoms. They are likely to be either people with chronic complaints, usually with a psychological overlay, or with psychological problems often masked by somatization.

Fit Between Practitioner and Patient

Patients often choose a practitioner because of a link or "fit" between their respective worldviews, that is, they share certain social and cultural

assumptions about sickness that makes them more compatible and accepting of each other in the clinical situation (see Kroeger 1983:152). Both Garrison and Harwood show this very capably in their findings on Puerto
Rican spiritism. In the case of chiropractic, however, there may be a sociocultural match of therapeutic expectations but not of ideological ones. The
latter link usually follows and is secondary to an initial match-up on the
grounds of the D.C.'s therapeutic speciality. After all, it is common knowledge that a chiropractor mechanically treats muscle and skeletal aches and
pains. But beyond this, prior knowledge or experience is usually limited at
best regarding chiropractic ideology, which contains a unique theory of disease etiology and an antimedical perspective. Therefore, the ideological fit
either occurs or fails to occur after one or more visits. The point is that
whereas the two types of fit between therapists and patients may occur
before the first visit when a patient is already acculturated to the therapist's chiropractic worldview, generally, the therapeutic fit occurs before
resort and the ideological fit afterwards. This is why the chiropractor finds
it necessary to go to such great lengths to educate new patients to his subluxation theory (see above).

Psychiatrists are not usually sought by Puerto Ricans for problems of
living but only as a last resort when a person is seriously mentally ill, or
demonstrably "crazy." Harwood (1987:184), Garrison (1977:163), and
Rogler (1961) all find that, in addition to seeking help for interpersonal
problems and short-term crises, people who frequent spiritists are those who
have not been fully satisfied or "cured" by professional biomedical treatment (also see Fishman 1979:4). In Garrison's study, 86 percent of the spiritist clients had seen a physician within the past two years, and 56 percent
had done so within the past month for psychiatric and somatic complaints
(1977:180–1).

Many researchers have made similar claims about chiropractic
patients, stating that people use D.C.s when standard biomedical care for
their sickness yields few successful results (Cobb 1954; Elder and Acheson
1970; Freidson 1961; Koos 1954; Oths 1985; Schmitt 1978; Weil 1983). In a
study by Kelner et al. (1980), 56 percent of D.C. patients had already
sought medical help for their chief complaint, and 85 percent of them had a
family physician. In my chiropractic sample, at least 46 percent of the
study patients were visiting the chiropractor after experiences with a
biomedical doctor for their current complaint; 70 percent of these patients
have a family doctor. Apparently, they were going to the D.C. for something they were not receiving from their regular physicians (Oths 1985).

Coulehan (1985:385) found that there were four categories of chiropractic users. The first and largest group consists of those with acute musculoskeletal symptoms who are there because of past experience or on
referral from acquaintances. The smallest group consisted of those seeking

preventive care. The second and third largest groups, together representing about half of the patient load, consisted respectively of those with unresolved chronic problems, i.e., "difficult cases" who had repeatedly unsuccessfully sought biomedical help for their problems, and those with ill-defined "functional" problems such as headache, dizziness, tension, constipation, etc. The symptoms of both groups two and three, i.e., chronic and functional, are often found to be psychosomatic. It is the type of patients found in these two groups which will most likely find the D.C.'s psychotherapeutic techniques of primary benefit.

Psychotherapy, spiritism and chiropractic alike appear to be helpful for those with problems of living, and minor to moderate psychological and emotional conflicts. I conclude that certain patients with psycho-social-emotional components to their problems may end up on the nonbiomedical alternative end of the medical care system—in a D.C.'s clinic, in a spiritist or other cult-like healing session, or else in the psychotherapist's office—depending on several considerations, some of which I list below.

In general, sociocultural differences between patients shape the illness experience and affect practitioner choice. A therapist who shares a cultural and symbolic system similar to that of the ill person will more likely be the latter's treatment of choice (Harwood 1987; Comas-Diaz 1981:641). Referring back to Table 1, there are some characteristics which hold for all three therapies. These include number 6—meaningful cognitive framework, 9—strong practitioner-patient relationship, 10—long-term relationship, 11—ritual object use, and 12—behavior and attitude change. Though common to all therapies, these characteristics will still influence treatment choice because of the variation in the cultural content of each.

In addition to the general relevance of the cultural form and content of each psychotherapeutically oriented practice, specific sociocultural, economic, and cognitive factors which appear to play a major role in determining a person's choice of therapist deserve to be highlighted. These include degree of somatization, stigma (associated with going to a particular therapist), cost of treatment, and individual personality.

Somatization

The degree to which a patient somatizes emotional problems helps predict whether a patient chooses a psychologizing, spiritual, or a mechanistic-type therapy. Psychiatric and physical symptoms may be alternative responses to similar stressors, and the degree to which one expresses his or her disvalued state in somatic or psychic terms depends on the cultural, psychological, and social factors which shape a person's illness experience (Katon and Kleinman 1982).

"Somatization" can been defined simply as a process in which individuals express psychological complaints in an idiom of physical symptoms. It is by now commonly recognized that physical complaints can be, either wholly or in part, the result, or a secondary consequence of, psychological stressors (see Cassel 1976). As an examples of this, several authors have each cogently shown how depressive affect is articulated and expressed in physical terms (Gaines and Farmer 1986; Kleinman and Good 1985; Good 1977).

Social Stigma

Social stigma or the fear of being labeled "crazy" may keep some from seeking psychotherapeutic care (Rogler et al. 1961:17; Harwood 1987:200), while others equally stigmatize alternatives as "quacks" and see psychotherapy as sophisticated. Also, to some, psychotherapy is associated with the conventional medicine that they have become disenchanted with and, therefore, is not regarded as worth pursuing.

Cost

Especially for a patient without insurance, the prospects of paying $50–100/hour for a visit to an analyst makes the $20–40 fee for a chiropractic session much more attractive. For this reason, chiropractic has sometimes been referred to as "poor man's therapy" (Cowie et al. 1975). However, for a truly low-income person, chiropractic is not affordable without public or private insurance. Spiritists rarely charge more than $10 per session, and usually much less (Harwood 1987:95). Culture and society can be held accountable, in general, for the distribution of occupation, resources, jobs, etc. which create costs.

Personality

Personality types may also help predict choice of a compatible therapist. The personality of a patient attracted to a particular practice may be one on whom placebos work best, or it may be one with weaker integration of the self, and thus greater susceptibility to a new belief system (see Frank 1961). Persons seeking psychotherapy may tend to see their problems as a result of personal inadequacy. Spiritists and chiropractic users may be prone to blame external sources (Kadushin 1969). As with cost, personality is in part due to one's sociocultural heritage.

In sum, a particular resort occurs when there is a fit between person and therapy, that is, a match-up of expectations, thought, and behavior along sociocultural, economic, cognitive, and personality dimensions. (See Figure 2).

Chiropractic will be chosen by many patients with unresolved chronic physical and physiomorphized complaints because it answers certain sociocultural imperatives, i.e., it provides a tangible, work-oriented explanation

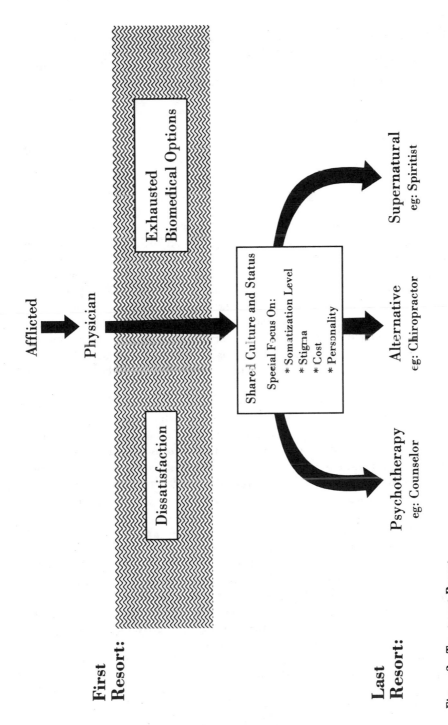

Figure 2. Treatment Resort

of problems. The psychotherapeutic aspects of treatment do not stigmatize, as its use does not directly admit that problems are compounded by emotional-psychological factors. Problems are dealt with indirectly, in conjunction with physical treatment, through chatting and physical contact, rather than making them the object of concern through direct counseling, as do psychotherapy and spiritism. In essence, each therapist deals with a unique configuration of physical and psychological problems in a unique manner, but all to some degree or another use some combination of the commonly identified techniques of psychotherapy to do the job.

Conclusions

My interest here has been in exploring the psychotherapeutic aspects of chiropractic and identifying the factors which draw people to use this particular healing modality. This model of treatment resort is presented as a framework for investigating the treatment choice of those disenchanted with biomedicine. The foregoing is not meant to imply that all patients of chiropractic have problems that psychotherapy would benefit, but simply that, beyond what is presently assumed, people with certain ailments, after exhausting biomedical options, end up at the other end of the system and are well treated by nonmedical therapies such as spiritism and chiropractic, for problems similar to those which psychotherapists are known for, and capable of, treating.

Chiropractors appeal to the productive, if oppressed and exploited, middle to upper socioeconomic level of people who value their work and mobility and can afford to pay moderately well for appropriate treatment. It is left for us to wonder what happens to the socioculturally mainstream low-income individuals when they have emotional-psychological problems. To whom do the unemployed and disenfranchised turn in times of crisis when family members are not enough? Are there other providers of implicit psychotherapeutic care who have not been identified, professional or otherwise? Clergy and bartenders might be of assistance, but trained therapists likely are not available. This issue requires further study, to be sure.

The observations made herein have substantial implications for understanding medical service utilization and patterns of resort in this society. An estimated five million people a year receive chiropractic treatment (Consumer Reports 1980:180). Not coincidentally, the rise in chronic disease has paralleled the rise in utilization of alternative medical therapies. Given the projected increase in the elderly population—those most plagued with chronic disease—the resort to alternative therapies will undoubtedly continue to escalate. Why these unorthodox practices are so attractive is a question we must reckon with if a comprehensive understanding of our medical care system is to be gained.

Notes

1. There has been much debate recently about the proper terminology to use when discussing the occurrence of a differential locus of disvalued states in particular social and culture groups (see Kleinman and Good 1985; Katon and Kleinman 1982; Ohnuki-Tierney 1984; Scheper-Hughes and Lock 1987). That some people tend to experience symptoms as originating alternatively in the psyche or the soma is indisputable and well-documented. Whether one uses the term "physiomorphize" or "somatize," I do not see a problem. Using "somatize" does not indicate a hidden bias suggesting where the symptoms ought to be located any more so than does "psychologize" imply that that locus is faulty or ill-perceived. Nor does "physiologize" correct the problem, if there really is one.

References

Ackerknecht, E. H.
1946 Natural Diseases and Rational Treatment in Primitive Medicine. Bulletin of the History of Medicine 19:467–497 .

Adler, H. M. and V. B. O Hammett
1973 The Doctor-Patient Relationship Revisited: An Analysis of the Placebo Effect. Annals of Internal Medicine 78:595-598 .

American Chiropractic Association
1978 Doctor of Chiropractic: Occupational Description. Department of Public Affairs (pamphlet), July.

Anderson, R. T.
1980 Chiropractic: Recognized But Unproved. New England Journal of Medicine 302:353–4.
1984 An Orthopedic Ethnography in Rural Nepal. Medical Anthropology 8(1):46-59.

Barsky, A. J.
1981 Hidden Reasons Some Patients Visit Doctors. Annals of Internal Medicine 94:492.

Ben-Sira, Z.
1976 The Function of the Professionals Affective Behavior in Client Satisfaction. Journal of Health and Social Behavior 17:3–11.

Bernstein, B.
1964 Social Class, Speech Systems and Psychotherapy. In Mental Health of the Poor. F. Riessman (ed.). New York: Free Press.

Blumer, D. and U. Heilbronn
1981 The Pain Prone Disorder: A Clinical and Psychological Profile. Psychosomatics 22:395–402.

Brill, N. and H. Storrow
1960 Social Class and Psychiatric Treatment. Archives of General Psychiatry 3:340–344.

Cassel, J. C.
1976 Contributions of the Social Environment to Host Resistance. American Journal of Epidemiology 104:107–123.

Cmich, D. E.
1984 Theoretical Perspectives of Holistic Health. Journal of School Health
      54(1):30–32.

Cobb, B .
1954 Why do People Detour to Quacks? The Psychiatric Bulletin 3:66–69.

Comas-Diaz, L.
1981 Puerto Rican *Espiritismo* and Psychotherapy. American Journal of
      Orthopsychiatry 51:636–645.

Consumer Reports Books, eds.,
1980 Health Quackery. Mt. Vernon, New York: Consumers Union.

Cornacchia, H. J. and S. Barrett
1982 Shopping for Health Care: The Essential Guide to Products and Services. St.
      Louis: C.V. Mosby Co.

Coulehan, John L.
1985 Chiropractic and the Clinical Art. Social Science and Medicine 21:383–390.

Cowie, J. B. and J. B. Roebuck
1975 An Ethnography of a Chiropractic Clinic. New York: Free Press.

Duffy, D. L., D. Hamerman and M. A. Cohen
1980 Communication Skills of House Officers: A Study in a Medical Clinic. Annals
      of Internal Medicine 93:354–357.

Elder, R. and R. M. Acheson
1970 Social Class and Behavior in Response to Symptoms of Osteoarthritis. Mil-
      bank Memorial Fund Quarterly 48:449–502.

Engel, G. L.
1961 "Psychogenic" Pain. Journal of Occupational Medicine 3:249–257.
1977 The Need for a New Medical Model: A Challenge for Biomedicine. Science
      196:129–135.

Fábrega, Horacio
1990 personal communication.

Finkler, K.
1985 Spiritualist Healers in Mexico. South Hadley, Massachusetts: Bergin and Gar-
      vey.

Fishman, R. G.
1979 Spiritualism in Western New York: A Study in Ritual Healing. Medical
      Anthropology 3(1):1–22.

Frank, J. D.
1961 Persuasion and Healing: A Comparative Study of Psychotherapy. Baltimore:
      Johns Hopkins Press.
1974 Therapeutic Components of Psychotherapy. Journal of Nervous and Mental
      Disease 159:325-342.

Freidson, E.
1961 Patient Views of Medical Practice. New York: Russell Sage.

Gaines, Atwood D. and Paul E. Farmer
1986 Visible Saints: Social Cynosures and Dysphoria in the Mediterranean Tradi-
      tion. Culture, Medicine and Psychiatry 10:295–330.

Garrison, Vivian
1977 Doctor, *Espiritista* or Psychiatrist?: Health-Seeking Behavior in a Puerto Rican Neighborhood of New York City. Medical Anthropology 1(2):65–191.

Glick, L. B.
1967 Medicine as an Ethnographic Category: The Gimi of the New Guinea Highlands. Ethnology 6(1):31–56.

Good, Byron J.
1977 The Heart of What's the Matter: The Semantics of Illness in Iran. Culture, Medicine and Psychiatry 1(1):25–58.

Gursslin, D., R. Hunt and S. Rosch
1964 Social Class and the Mental Health Movement. In: Mental Health of the Poor. F. Riessman, J. Cohen and A. Pearl (eds.). New York: Free Press.

Hahn, Robert A. and Arthur Kleinman.
1981 Belief as Pathogen, Belief as Medicine: "Voodoo Death" and the "Placebo Phenomenon" in Anthropological Perspective. Paper presented at Society for Applied Anthropology meetings, April. Edinburgh, Scotland.

Hall, Edward T.
1959 The Silent Language. Greenwich, Connecticut: Fawcett.

Harwood, Alan
1987 Rx: Spiritist as Needed: A Study of a Puerto Rican Community Mental Health Resource. Ithaca, New York: Cornell University Press (orig. 1977).

Helman, Cecil
1985 Disease and Pseudo-Disease: A Case History of Pseudo-Angina. In: Physicians of Western Medicine. Robert A. Hahn and Atwood D. Gaines (eds.). Dordrecht, Holland: D. Reidel Publishers.

Houpt, J. L., C. S. Orleans, Linda K. George and H. Keith H. Brodie
1980 The Role of Psychiatric and Behavioral Factors in the Practice of Medicine. American Journal of Psychiatry 137(1):37–47.

Jackson, R.
1980 Holistic Massage. New York: Sterling.

James, R., M. Fox and T. Guity
1983 Who Goes to a Natural Therapist? Why? Australian Family Physician 12(5):383–384.

Kadushin, C.
1969 Why People Go to Psychiatrists? New York: Atherton Press.

Kaplan, S. R. and M. Roman
1973 The Organization and Delivery of Mental Health Services in the Ghetto. New York: Praeger.

Katon, Wayne and Arthur Kleinman
1982 Depression and Somatization. American Journal of Medicine 72(1):127–135.

Kelner, M., O. Hall and I. Coulter
1980 Chiropractors. Do They Help? Toronto: Fitzhenry and Whiteside.

Kiernau, T.
1974 Shrinks, Etc: A Consumer's Guide to Psychotherapies. New York: Dial Press.

Kiev, Ari
1964 Magic, Faith and Healing. New York: Free Press.

Kleinman, Arthur
1980 Patients and Healers in the Context of Culture. Berkeley: University of California Press.

Kleinman, Arthur, Leon Eisenberg and Byron Good
1978 Culture, Illness and Care. Annals of Internal Medicine 88(2):251–258.

Kleinman, Arthur and Byron Good, eds.
1985 Culture and Depression: Studies in the Anthropology and Cross-Cultural Psychology of Affect and Disorder. Berkeley: University of California Press.

Kleinman, Arthur and L.H. Sung
1979 Why do Indigenous Practitioners Successfully Heal? Social Science and Medicine 13B:7-15.

Koos, E. L.
1954 The Health of Regionville. New York: Columbia University Press.

Koss, J.
1975 Therapeutic Aspects of Puerto Rican Cult Practices. Psychiatry 38(2):160–171.

Kotarba, J. A.
1983 Social Control Function of Holistic Health Care in Bureaucratic Settings. Journal of Health and Social Behavior 24:275–288.

Kramlinger, K. G., D. W. Swanson and T. Maruta
1983 Are Patients With Chronic Pain Depressed? American Journal Psychiatry 140(6):747–749.

Kroeger, A.
1983 Anthropological and Socio-Medical Health Care Research in Developing Countries. Social Science and Medicine 17:147–161.

Landy, David
1983 Medical Anthropology: A Critical Appraisal. In: Advances in Medical Social Science, Vol. 1. Julio Ruffini (ed.). New York: Gordon and Breach Science Publishers, Inc.

Leonard, G.
1976 The Holistic Health Revolution. New West 1(10):40–49.

Lévi-Strauss, Claude
1963 Structural Anthropology. Garden City, New York: Doubleday.

Luborsky, L., B. Singer and L. Luborsky
1975 Comparative Studies of Psychotherapies. Archives of General Psychiatry 32:995–1008.

Manbar, M. M.
1978 Chiropractors: Pushing for a Place on the Health Care Team. Medical World News 19(25):57.

Marquis, M. S., A. R. Davies and J. E. Ware
1983 Patient Satisfaction and Change in Medical Care Providers. Medical Care 21(8):821–829.

Maslow, A. H.
1963 The Need to Know and the Fear of Knowing. Journal of General Psychology 68:111–125.

McCorkle, T.
1961 Chiropractic: A Deviant Theory of Disease and Treatment in Contemporary Western Culture. Human Organization 20(1):20–22.

McLemore, T.
1981 1979 Summary: National Ambulatory Medical Care Survey. Advance Data 66:5.

Moerman, D. E.
1983 Physiology and Symbols: The Anthropological Implications of the Placebo Effect. In The Anthropology of Medicine. Lola Romanucci-Ross, D. E. Moerman and L. R. Tancredi (eds.). New York: Praeger.

Murphy, Jane M.
1964 Psychotherapeutic Aspects of Shamanism on St. Lawrence Island, Alaska. In Magic, Faith, and Healing. A. Kiev (ed.). New York: Free Press.

National Analysts, Inc.
1972 A Study of Health Practices and Opinions, #PB210978. Philadelphia, PA: NAI. June.

Ohnuki-Tierney, Emiko
1984 Illness and Culture in Contemporary Japan. Cambridge: Cambridge University Press.

Oths, Kathryn
1985 Practitioner-Patient Interaction in a Chiropractic Clinic. Paper presented at the American Anthropological Association meetings, Washington, D.C.
1991 Treatment Choice and Health Outcome in a Peruvian Village. Unpublished Ph.D. dissertation in Anthropology. Case Western Reserve University. Cleveland, Ohio.

Palmer College of Chiropractic
1983 Palmer College of Chiropractic Bulletin 1983–84. Davenport, Iowa: Palmer College of Chiropractic.

Pratt, J. W. and A. Mason
1984 The Meaning of Touch in Care Practice. Social Science and Medicine 18(12):1081–1088.

Pratt, L., A. Seligman and G. Reader
1957 Physicians' Views on the Level of Medical Information Among Patients. American Journal of Public Health 47:1277–1283.

Prince, Raymond
1969 Psychotherapy and the Chronically Poor. In Culture Change, Poverty, and Mental Health. Joseph Finney (ed.). Lexington: University of Kentucky Press.
1980 Variations in Psychotherapeutic Procedures. In Handbook of Cross-Cultural Psychiatry; Volume VI: Psychopathology. Harry Triandis and Juris Draguns (eds.). Boston: Allyn and Bacon.

Reich, J., J. P. Tupin and S. I. Abramowitz
1983 Psychiatric Diagnosis of Chronic Pain Patients. American Journal of Psychiatry 140(11):1495–1498.

Reynolds, David K.
1976 Morita Psychotherapy. Berkeley: University of California Press.

Rogler, L. H. and A. B. Hollingshead
1961 The Puerto Rican Spiritualist as a Psychiatrist. American Journal of Sociology 67:17–21.

Scheper-Hughes, Nancy and Margaret Lock
1987 The Mindful Body: A Prolegomenon to Future Work in Medical Anthropology. Medical Anthropology Quarterly (n.s.) 1(1):6–41.

Schmitt, M.
1978 The Utilization of Chiropractors. Sociological Symposium 22:55–74.

Shapiro, A. K.
1964 Factors Contributing to the Placebo Effect: Their Implications for Psychotherapy. American Journal of Psychotherapy 18(Supp 1):73–85.

Sirott, L. and H. Waitzkin
1984 Holism and Self-Care. In Reforming Medicine. V. and R. Sidell (eds.). New York: Pantheon Books.

Stoeckle, J., I. K. Zola and G. Davidson
1964 The Quantity and Significance of Psychological Distress in Medical Patients. Journal of Chronic Diseases 17:959–970.

Swanson, D. W.
1984 Chronic Pain as a Third Pathological Emotion. American Journal of Psychiatry 141(2):210–214.

Szasz Thomas
1957 Pain and Pleasure: A Study of Bodily Feelings. New York: Basic Books.

Thompson, T. L., A. Stoudmore, W. D. Mitchell and R. L. Grant
1983 Underrecognition of Patients' Psychosocial Distress in a University Hospital Medical Clinic. American Journal Psychiatry 140(2):158–161.

Torrey, E. Fuller
1972 The Mind Game: Witchdoctors and Psychiatrists. New York: Emerson Hall.

U.S. Department of Health and Human Services
1986 Supply and Characteristics of Chiropractors. PHS, HRSA, Bureau of Health Professions Bulletin. August.

Waitzkin, H. and J. D. Stoeckle
1972 The Communication of Information About Illness. Advances in Psychosomatic Medicine 8:180–215.

Walker, V. H.
1964 Ritualism and Its Effects on Patient Care. USPHS Grant No. GM08544. Indianapolis U. Medical Center.

Wardwell, W.
1972 Limited, Marginal, and Quasi-Practitioners. In Handbook of Human Sociology. H. Freeman, S. Levine and L. Reeder (eds.). New Jersey: Prentice Hall.

Weil, A.

1983 Health and Healing: Understanding Conventional and Alternative Medicine. Boston: Houghton Mifflin.

White, M. and J. K. Skipper

1971 The Chiropractic Physician: A Study of Career Contingencies. Journal of Health and Social Behavior 12:300–306.

Young, Allan

1976 Some Implications of Medical Beliefs and Practices for Social Anthropology. American Anthropologist 78:5–24.

Zborowski, Mark

1952 Cultural Components in Response to Pain. Journal of Social Issues 8(1):16–30.

Zola, I. K.

1966 Culture and Symptoms: An Analysis of Patients' Presenting Complaints. American Sociological Review 3:615–630.

5

The Affliction of Martin: Religious, Clinical, and Phenomenological Meaning in a Case of Demonic Oppression

Thomas J. Csordas

Introduction

To say that "the glass is half empty" or "half full" is to give an existential account of an objective circumstance: the level of fluid is at the midpoint in the glass. To say that an individual is afflicted by "demonic oppression" or "psychopathology" is to give a cultural account of an existential circumstance: a person is suffering. The methodological gulf between the two kinds of accounts is vast. One can appeal to the objective circumstance of fluid in the glass to understand the derivation of optimistic and pessimistic accounts, but how can one define an existential circumstance prior to the elaboration of a cultural account? Equally as important, if one were to develop such an existential language, would it be of value in understanding the cultural logic that distinguishes divergent cultural accounts?

This chapter examines the cultural and existential relation between religious and clinical understandings of human suffering. It is popular to note that what in previous centuries was understood as demonic possession is in the present era understood as psychopathology. Recent work, such as Kenny's (1986) study of multiple personality, suggests that as now, in the nineteenth century the discovery—or perhaps creation—of psychiatric disorders was deeply imbued with cultural meaning (see Gaines, Nuckolls and Swartz, this volume). Kenny shows that the experience of individuals who were the prototypical cases of multiple personality in the United States embodied cultural conflicts associated with the nature of personhood, and that their experience was framed alternately as religious and medical. Even more striking is the tragic case documented by Goodman (1981) of the young German woman who died in 1975 after a conflict-laden interaction between religious exorcism from demonic possession and psychiatric medication with anticonvulsant drugs. The fact that the case ended in the court system indicates not only the currency of religious paradigms for understanding distress, but the continued social inability to translate between sacred and psychological interpretations of human reality.

The ethnographic backdrop for our approach to the problem is Roman Catholicism in the contemporary United States. Three active traditions of healing exist within Catholicism: healing through prayer to saints, who themselves must be credited with posthumous miracles in order to achieve that status; healing by the Virgin Mary, typically at shrines such as that at Lourdes in France; and healing of one believer by another, typically accompanied by the laying on of hands, as popularized in the Charismatic Renewal movement. The latter originated within the wave of spiritual interest of the 1960s that included the "new religions," the "new age," and "neo-Pentecostalism" (McGuire 1982; Csordas 1983, 1988). Catholics influenced by this movement participate in the late twentieth-century shift among Christians from emphases on suffering and self-mortification as an imitation of Christ, to emphases on the possibility and benefit of divine healing practiced by Jesus in the gospels (Favazza 1982).

We begin with a phenomenological narrative of intense spiritual, physical, and emotional suffering of a young man and the attempt by a Catholic religious healer to "deliver" him from the influence of an evil spirit. The narrative is based on conversations with the protagonists over the course of two and one half years. The story and subsequent analysis is one of winks upon winks (Geertz 1984) and of multiple perspectives within divergent cultural accounts. The key informant is the healer, whom we shall call Peggy. As often happens in families of the severely mentally disturbed, she became the one to adopt the role of spokesperson for the afflicted young man, whom we shall call Martin. This situation, combined with the facts of their parallel forms of suffering, and that Martin could not bear to be interviewed himself (was present only at the first interview), made analytic separation of their experiences a near impossible task. Therefore, the narrative must be understood as a text produced in the interviews with Peggy, rather than as a case study of Martin's experience.[1] What follows is a discussion of the cultural logic in two accounts of the case based on commentaries by mental health professionals and charismatic healing ministers. Finally, a phenomenological analysis of bodily experience provides the grounds for showing how both accounts are cultural objectifications of meaning that is already inherent in basic sensory experience.

The Affliction of Martin

At the time of our first meeting, Peggy was forty-two years old, a mother of three (another child died at birth). She had been married to a successful professional for twenty years. She had long been interested in things spiritual, having practiced yoga since age fourteen, and having out-of-body experiences and visions of figures of Catholic devotion such as Thérèsa of Lisieux. She completed two years of college in math and chemistry, and early in her marriage worked as a laboratory technician, but had been a housewife for the past seventeen years. She and her family are practicing Catholics; her husband is an active layman and plays a role in adult religious training (catechesis) in their parish. He is aware and somewhat supportive of her activities as a healer, but in practice remains aloof; he never participated in our interview sessions, which Peggy intentionally scheduled for times when he was away from the house, and he never participates in her healing sessions.

Although it is not strictly required among Catholic charismatics that a healer experience his or her own healing in order to pray for others, Peggy made a surprisingly strong claim of never having felt a need for any healing because her past had been without trauma (this is in spite of the loss of a child at birth) and because her relations with her parents had always been smooth. Nonetheless, she claimed specific experiences to validate her self-definition as a healer, including having heard a voice that said, "You will heal for me."

Peggy already had experienced this ability to heal when, at age thirty five, she encountered the Catholic Charismatic Renewal. Her husband had heard about a local prayer group and suggested that she might be interested. She attended the movement's standard initiatory program (Life in the Spirit Seminar) during which she heard God say, "Come follow me," and received the gift of tongues (glossolalia). Following this experience she attended both the Catholic prayer group and a nondenominational Pentecostal group, and reports becoming recognized as a healer in both. In the Catholic group, healing was always prayed for in a collective prayer, and conflict arose when one woman asked Peggy for a private, one-on-one healing session. The group regarded this as potentially dangerous, and as a result Peggy left. She continued her individual healing prayers, but at the time of our first meeting had not been involved in a group for four years.

Peggy's methods of healing are somewhat unorthodox vis-à-vis the mainstream of Catholic Pentecostal healing. Although her principal methods (Healing of Memories and Deliverance) are those recognized by charismatics (Csordas 1983, 1988), she began healing independently of, and prior to, her involvement with the movement. She has not had any guidance from other healers or read any of the movement's substantial literature on healing, but states that her training comes directly from God. She always prays about whether to accept someone as a supplicant in healing, but does not always work through prayer; if the person is not particularly religious, she may not even speak about God in healing.

Her diagnosis of a person's problem is based on her "psychic" gifts:

she "becomes" the other person in the sense that she knows their subconscious mind and their past, and she conducts a "mini-scan" of the supplicant by means of visionary "seeing," although she always respects the person's privacy by never probing deeper than she can feel the person wants her to. She also reads a person's "aura," and interprets the meaning of light glowing around each of a person's *cakras* (i.e., *shakras*) (Peggy's version of a Hindu concept of energy centers within the body). She makes astrological determinations when she deems them appropriate, experiences precognitive dreams, interacts with good and evil spirits, utters words of prophecy, and also gives nutritional counseling. She occasionally consults with non-Christian psychics to assist or confirm some course of action in her own work.

Peggy has a close friend in Randy, a man of about thirty years of age. They share the same spiritual orientation and interests, and often attend visiting evangelists and healers. Randy often spends the evening with Peggy and her family, visiting or watching television. Three years before our interviews, Randy convinced his housemate to see Peggy for spiritual healing. This young man, Martin, was twenty-two at the time, but his story, by his own and Peggy's account, begins much earlier, when he was nine.

During his childhood, the relation between Martin's parents had not been smooth. He remembers his father as rather cruel, fighting with his mother and being physically and verbally abusive to him. He believes his parents had virtually no sexual relationship. His mother suspected that something was wrong with her husband, but the family doctor did not think it too serious. Then, when Martin was nine, his father committed suicide by shooting himself in the head. Martin heard the shot and found the body. Soon after this event, his mother had a "nervous breakdown" and was committed to a mental hospital; she has been hospitalized several times since.

Martin and his brother (five years his junior) were committed to an orphanage. Later they were assigned to the care of foster parents, adherents of a strict form of evangelical Christianity. Martin's brother eventually rebelled against this environment and moved abroad, severing contact with his mother and Martin as well as with his foster parents. Martin did not rebel overtly, and remembers always being eager to please his foster parents. Peggy believes that the fear of God inspired by their upbringing prevented him from committing suicide during his darkest moment of suffering.

Martin began having sexual fantasies at age thirteen, but these were apparently not of an obsessive nature. He also reports "seeing colors" at that time. At age fifteen, he had an experience that he described as feeling like a net descending over his head and enclosing it; at that time he developed a chronic headache that has been with him constantly for the past ten years. Also at that time, he began experiencing vivid erotic images that were so pervasive and uncontrollable that (in retrospect) he perceived "pornography as a state of being within me." He also began to hear a voice that offered him friendship and companionship, at the same manipulating him and "making deals" with him.

As a freshman in college, Martin developed a terrible guilt about his sexual obsessions, knowing that they were in conflict with the upbringing given by his fundamentalist foster parents. Despite increasing discomfort, he successfully graduated from the nearby state university Phi Beta Kappa in chemistry and mathematics (Peggy made a point of reporting that he has an IQ [intelligence quotient] of 140). Following graduation, he experienced uncontrollable convulsions, but was able to take a laboratory job in biochemistry, and he worked successfully for a year. He experienced increasing difficulty in learning things for his job, with chronic headache and stomach pain accompanying his "fuzzy thinking." A neurologist found no sign of a tumor and recommended biofeedback for his headache, indicating that it was a physical handicap that he must learn to live with. Aspirin and prescription drugs provided no relief. Martin became almost completely disabled and had to leave his job. In the sixty days before he met Peggy, he apparently had almost reached the point of convulsions again. Peggy reports that he "had not slept" during this two-month period and his housemate, Randy, observed that he was "wandering around the house like a zombie."

When Peggy first met Martin, his condition had deteriorated to such an extent that she had him move into a spare room in her house until he could get past the crisis. At this point he had lost considerable weight and was very "dense" in conversation. As he regained some of his physical strength, Peggy began the process of Healing of Memories, retracing the events of Martin's life and praying for the healing of resultant emotional scars or "brokenness."

In the course of Healing of Memories, Peggy felt that Martin successfully overcame a great deal of anger toward his suicidal father, and that his attitude toward his natural mother was also substantially ameliorated (she resides in federally subsidized housing in a neighboring city, living on income from social security and stock investments). Whereas previously he could hardly treat her with civility, he became able to talk to her, tell her he loved her, and to treat her with compassion. Martin grew stronger physically and emotionally, and regained lost weight. He moved back to his own house, although he still could not work, and spent many of his days at Peggy's house. Given his state at their first encounter, Peggy, Martin, and Randy all agreed that the healing experience literally saved his life. But Martin was not yet healed.

Although he "worked through" a lot of anger toward his father, Martin still felt "more anger than he would like to." (In Healing of Memories, sincere forgiveness of past wrongs is a major component of successful healing). In addition, he still experienced the full complement of chronic, intractable problems to be described below. Although Peggy at first thought that Healing of Memories, by resolving Martin's "brokenness," would eliminate these problems, she became convinced that they were due to the influence of an evil spirit. In effect, Martin had reached a plateau. Peggy saw him as emotionally "back together" in the sense that, intellectually, he knew what he *wanted* to feel, but was blocked from experiencing it by the evil spirit.

It was God, states Peggy, who told her that she was dealing with an evil spirit or demon. She had thought that she was telepathically "picking up" some of Martin's thoughts, but now realized that it was the spirit speaking. God told her (through inspiration) to "confront" the spirit to determine its identity. When she discovered its presence, it reacted violently with the telepathic message that it was going to "knock Martin out." Peggy tried to get him to sit down, but suddenly he fainted.

The exchange between Peggy and the demon had been silent, and Martin had not anticipated passing out or known anything was "going on." This occurrence was one confirmation of the spirit's presence. Peggy then demanded its identity, and discovered it was a Spirit of Pornography, or alternatively a Spirit of Abnormal Sexuality.[2] This name was "confirmed" in a phone conversation with a local psychic of Peggy's acquaintance, and through several incidents involving Randy and an out-of-town house guest.

Although Peggy thought at first that the spirit was external to Martin, oppressing and harassing him from "outside," she became convinced through its intransigence and degree of influence that it had taken up residence "inside" him, while still not achieving absolute "possession" of his personality. Yet this Spirit of Pornography is itself vassal to a more ominous spirit outside of Martin, but lurking silently nearby. Peggy and Randy succeeded in catching visionary glimpses of this spirit. It appeared as a silent male; tall with dark hair, cloaked, dignified, and exuding a cool power. They discovered its name to be Andronius, but reported no special significance to that name other than that it indicates a high rank in the demonic hierarchy. The role of this spirit was ambiguous, but its presence made Peggy's task as a healer more formidable, and increased the drama of the situation.[3]

Critical to the understanding of therapeutic process in many forms of religious healing is the manner in which life events and symptoms are reinterpreted and made consistent in terms of religious themes (Bourguignon 1976; Monfouga-Nicolas 1972). In the present instance, a double reinterpretation occurred. The first was intrinsic to the Healing of Memories, where Martin was reconciled to the overwhelmingly traumatic events of his early childhood. Themes of brokenness, forgiveness, and the invocation of the healing presence of Jesus within the memory of traumatic events are essential to this reinterpretation. With the lack of success in this healing, the discovery of a demon's presence motivated a second reinterpretation. The evil spirit became a link between the traumatic life events and the genesis of Martin's symptoms.

Specifically, in the Catholic Pentecostal healing system evil spirits are thought to prey upon the vulnerability created by such events. Thus the spirit began hovering around Martin at age nine, after his father's suicide. While in the orphanage, Martin had participated in a séance with some other children, during which he "saw things moving around in the room." While this event had had little relevance to him, it was now recalled and attributed significance as an incident of involvement with the "occult" that allowed the demon to increase its purchase on Martin's "personality." His recollection of "seeing colors" was interpreted by Peggy in terms of the emission of light from the *cakras* (this is Peggy's idiosyncratic borrowing from Hinduism and is not typical of Catholic charismatic thinking) as the spirit took over different parts of his body.

Thus, the ostensibly normal sexual fantasies that began at age thirteen became obsessive by age fifteen as the spirit, which had now entered Martin in earnest, took advantage of the natural erotic drives of an adolescent. Peggy was able to see a "gray mass" engulfing Martin's head, apparently a visionary analogue of the "net" he had felt descending over him at age fifteen. The voice Martin hears sometimes represented itself as three separate voices, although Martin was convinced that it was really only one spirit. Peggy explained this trickery as an example of typical demonic "deception" (Satan is the Father of Lies), and the three-in-one motif as a "blasphemy" on the part of the spirit in diabolical mockery of the Holy Trinity. The difficulty in separating one's own thoughts from those of the spirit demonstrates how the spirit gradually "inches you away," taking over one's personality in incremental stages.

The Sensory Organization of Suffering

Given this narrative account of Martin's early life, his crisis, and Peggy's initial attempt to heal him, let us turn to a more detailed description of the nature of his suffering. We shall not frame the description either in terms of pathological symptoms or of demonic manifestations, but instead organize it based on the observation that all of Martin's sensory and cognitive modalities are engaged and enveloped in suffering.

The auditory modality is dominated by a voice experienced as audible; however, Martin does not exactly claim to "hear a voice," instead, he "hears thoughts." He described the way the voice would manipulate him in earlier years. He believed it "knew everything about me." It would make deals with him, such as agreeing not to talk about his father if he did certain things it wanted. It would discuss religion with him; on one occasion, by "outwitting" him in such a discussion, it was able to "get deeper into his gut." It would also make jokes about Martin's foster mother. About his natural mother it would say, "My mother left me" instead of "Your mother left you," in such a way that he tended to lose consciousness of the voice's separateness from himself. The change of grammatical person, "makes you think it's your own thought." In a separate auditory experience not involving the voice, a loud crackling sound occurs when the voice temporarily "releases" its hold.

The pornographic obsession engages Martin's visual modality with compelling eidetic imagery. This imagery can arise spontaneously at any time, even awakening him from sleep. Martin is typically "bombarded" with sexual pictures. The images move rapidly from one scene to another. They often begin with heterosexual pictures but progress to homosexuality, bestiality, sex with children, and sex that includes pain and violence. The pictures are accompanied by almost overwhelming sexual feelings, making resistance (to masturbation) very difficult. These feelings are, in turn, accompanied by equally powerful feelings of acceptance and desire to yield to the influence of the images. It feels "good" and "right" to give in and, at such moments, the voice's presence feels like a kind of friendship and companionship that it is difficult to forego. If there is some weakening of his will in response to the onslaught of pictures, his omnipresent head pain is somewhat diminished. If he begins again to resist, the pain reintensifies. Martin is not always successful in his resistance, and sometimes succumbs to the desire to masturbate. He is concerned that the trajectory of his experience is in the direction of seeing his world exclusively in sexual terms, but continues to struggle against this.

The tactile modality of Martin's experience is dominated by his intractable headache, the pain of which diminishes somewhat if he slackens his resistance to the images. The feeling of a knot in his head accompanies the episode of imagery. This knot remains even when the pain moderates. He often feels a "yanking" and "pulling" in his head, often in response to situations with spiritual content or import, but this experience is only infrequently visible to others in the form of a tic. Periods of maximum affliction are evident by glazing over of Martin's eyes and a thickening or swelling of his eyelids. He also experiences periodic pain in his joints, and varying degrees of pain in his stomach and groin areas. The sensations in his stomach and groin also include yanking or pulling, e.g., his testicles are sometimes yanked. These sensations occur at unexpected times, and he often experiences them as sexually stimulating. Martin also feels a yank in his gut any time his father is mentioned. He periodically feels great heat in his body, and his body temperature fluctuates. Sometimes his body feels "like jelly"; there is a "fluid movement" within him, "as if another person were trying to embed its personality" in his body. This configuration of physical sensations is capped by a generalized heavy feeling, as if he was weighted down, and a constant drain of energy. Finally, in one instance during his association with Peggy, he suddenly fell as if violently thrown to the ground.

The gustatory modality is engaged as a terrible taste in Martin's mouth, and at times his food tastes bad. His saliva sometimes thickens, particularly when he first wakes in the morning. Martin's sense of olfaction is not directly affected, but instead he exudes odors that repel others, including extreme halitosis and body odor. These are so strong that, hours after Martin had left after spending a night in a spare room at Peggy's house, her young daughter observed that the room "smelled just like Martin's mouth."

Specific distortions of thought and emotion are also woven into this configuration of affliction. Martin has extreme difficulty maintaining concentration, especially on religious topics. When he accompanies Peggy and her family to church on Sundays, he finds it difficult to pray. His regular religious reading "blurs out" in front of him. From our own analytical viewpoint, his experience appears to conflate concentration and attention with intensity of feeling and religious faith, for along with these examples Martin included the observation that while he was reading through the Catholic exorcism rite, "I was not sure I was believing it while I was doing it." In addition, only with great force of will can he carry on normal activities such as conversation or computer work. As with his attempts at religious reading, if conversation turns to theological matters his concentration will slip, his eyes glaze over, and his eyelids will visibly thicken.

Among emotional distortions he reports experiences of anger in situations where it is, in retrospect, either inappropriate or a clear overreaction to a minor irritation. He also experiences powerful feelings of anxiety and fear. Martin summarized the overall effect of his tribulation as creating "panic in his body," and the feeling that he was "running from himself."

Martin's sleep patterns are also disrupted. It will be recalled that he had severe insomnia for two months before entering his healing relationship with Peggy. At the time of our interviews, he was still subject to periodic insomnia and was sometimes awakened in the night by a stream of pornographic thoughts and images.

In a phenomenon she described as "psychic mirroring," Peggy began to experience many of the same forms of suffering as did Martin. In general, she feels that through experiencing the pain of others, she can absorb and neutralize that pain. With Martin, however, she acknowledged that the situation "got out of hand," and the demon began to attack Peggy herself at her own "weak points." She reported all the same symptoms as did Martin, with the exception of pain in the joints, and halitosis and body odor. Often their bouts with the evil spirit were simultaneous, though their content was not necessarily the same.

Peggy reported beginning to feel some degree of head pain as soon as she heard of Martin, three years before our interviews. The spirit began "jerking her head around" and attacking her in other ways as soon as God told her its identity and she "confronted" it. Later the pain became constant for her and at such an intensity that she had difficulty meditating, and her capacity to remember things was compromised.

The evil spirit also attacked her verbally, screaming, cursing, and calling her "every name in the book," for example screaming "You bitch!" as if from very far away.[4] She stated that this visionary tongue lashing meant that the spirit felt threatened by her because she was the one who uncovered its presence. The demon also tried to deceive and threaten her, saying, for example, "God has abandoned you, you love *me* instead," or "Give me to someone else and I will leave" (demons must be "sent" to Jesus or to hell, never to afflict another person). It may threaten her family with something of a sexual nature or saying it will throw them into the fire. Another rhetorical trick (regarded as typical of demons) is condemnation. If she feels tired in the morning, the spirit might say, "Go have a cup of coffee." If she had one, the spirit would deride her, saying "You know more about nutrition [than to use such an unhealthy substance]."

The evil spirit's sexual assault on Peggy included both visualization and physical sensation such as tugging at her ovaries and sexual probing of her vagina and breasts during the night. Her visualizations were "like a TV show," with a story of sexual episodes accompanying the images. At first these visualizations were somewhat abstract, but they began to include real acquaintances. The visualizations sometimes flowed in a constant stream, coming on almost like a hypnotic state, a state of preoccupation in which thinking clearly was extremely difficult. There was a kind of "pressure" on her eyes that induced her to look at people only sexually. She says, "You feel like you *are* pornography." The visualizations occur with no warning, day or night, sometimes awakening her from sleep. In the midst of one of our interviews, for example, Peggy reported that the vivid image of a woman's vagina had appeared across her field of vision, although she could at the same time still see us.[5]

Peggy reported being especially susceptible to the pornographic imagery when she lost her temper and when she was tired. The spirit also directly caused anger and the urge to utter vulgarities (coprolalia). Although she felt that she "has a temper" from her ethnic background, the spirit intensifies it. The spirit also controlled her facial muscles, drawing them into an expression of anger, and thereby trying to deceive her into feeling angry even when she knew subjectively that she was not.[6] Still, Peggy felt she had more control over her experiences than did Martin, in that she could still find some relief and mystical connection to God through prayer in spite of the intractable pain. She also felt better able to distinguish a thought or emotion of her own from one provoked by the spirit. For example, several times she said she felt anger at my presence, but realized it was the spirit's anger.

That is, the spirit perceived a threat, and its anger therefore indicated that we should continue the interviews. On the other hand, Martin was only able to attend the first of our three interviews; the demon had persuaded him that his participation would literally be too painful.

Peggy interpreted her own suffering as essential to Martin's deliverance from the evil spirit. God "told her" that her pain would remain till it departed from Martin; that would be her sign that he was free. She felt that she was only an indirect target for the evil spirit, and that God wanted her to serve in this way as a "barometer" of Martin's suffering so she could understand its dynamic and so speak for Martin. She would not need a deliverance herself, she felt, but would automatically be freed when he was freed. God also indicated that psychiatrists would be of no help in this process.

Randy also felt that he had a role to play. He only peripherally felt the presence of the evil spirit, sometimes having insomnia when Peggy and Martin had it, sometimes feeling unusual sensations of heat and cold (head hot while feet are cold). Sometimes during a sexual scene in a film he felt an external heat around his head, though this was "not explicitly sexual heat." Aside from these minor experiences, Randy felt that his situation paralleled Martin's in that his own career plans were adrift and at a standstill. He came to regard this apparent stagnation as part of God's plan in the situation so that he could, in a sense, keep Martin company insofar as the latter feels anguish about a life that has for several years been mired in disability. Randy felt that God would allow his own life plans to mature once Martin was healed.

The Struggle for Integration

Peggy made several tentative attempts to obtain outside help, but felt that a general reluctance on the part of others to deal with problems of demonic origin, as well as the recalcitrance of the spirit itself militated against success. Three times Martin was in the presence of a highly reputed Catholic healer who conceivably could have helped. The first instance was when Peggy and Randy took him to a public healing service in a nearby city, conducted by a nationally known healing priest from New England. Martin became upset and angry; he left without receiving an anointing (with blessed oil) and was vocally angry at Peggy on the drive home. They regarded this as behavior entirely controlled by the evil spirit, whose interests were at great risk in the healing session.

Formal channels within the Church were not effective in obtaining help either. Peggy's parish priests claimed unfamiliarity with demonic phenomena and declined to become engaged in the situation. The local bishop responded that he did not understand such things, and referred them to a Jesuit priest who was respected as a counselor in the diocese. According to

Peggy, this priest acknowledged the reality of her healing gifts but was not convinced of the need for deliverance or exorcism in Martin's case.[7]

Peggy took only one step in the preliminaries to formal exorcism, a mandatory interview with a psychiatrist. It is noteworthy that she and not Martin made this interview. Peggy reports that after listening to her account of the prayer for Healing of Memories applied to the emotional scars of Martin's past, the psychiatrist concluded that Peggy had already done what she herself would do in therapy, and that it would only be a matter of time before Martin improved. Peggy's detailed presentation of symptoms caused by the spirit apparently made little impression on the mental health professional, either with respect to convincing her of the demonic attribution or in suggesting the need for further therapeutic intervention. However, the psychiatrist reportedly did note that after three years of becoming almost a part of Peggy's family, the difficulty of separation might be creating an obstacle to Martin's improvement. Peggy acknowledged this possibility but also expressed confidence in her ability and motivation (cessation of her own pain) to see the situation to a conclusion. Thus, in isolation and in a painful stalemate with the devil, Peggy, Randy, and Martin faithfully continued to wait for God to determine the moment of deliverance.

Peggy believed that Martin had great internal strength, and that it was increasing. She believed that, "he will do God's work powerfully at some point in the future." Indeed, this strength made him an important target for Satan. During the second year in which I followed his case, Martin decided to enter training as a Catholic catechist and was baptized a Catholic at Easter of the next year.[8] Peggy reported that after his baptism, Martin began to find temporary relief in the sacraments of the Catholic Church in the sense that the demonic oppression "lightened" from its usual "heaviness." Nevertheless, going to church was difficult because of the spirit's resistance, and Martin's mind typically became "foggy" just before approaching the altar to receive the Eucharist. However, Martin made a choice to go ahead with his life. He said, "I can remain immobilized or go forward," and he chose to go forward. He enrolled in courses in automotive repairs and computers at the local technical college and soon began to repair cars for Peggy, her husband, and one of his housemates. He also took a course in theology from a priest at the local university, in spite of persistent mental "fogginess" that required him to read and reread his textbooks, and in spite of his persistent pain and uncontrollable sexual imagery. However, according to Peggy, Martin's small successes bolstered his will and strengthened his ego.

In the face of continued tribulation, Peggy claimed to achieve a deeper level of meditation than ever before, in which she found at least temporary refuge. People still came to her for healing, although at one point she had felt so exhausted from her struggle with the evil spirit that she had expressed the intention of retiring. After more than four years of struggle, the encounter with an evil spirit appeared to have settled into a way of life without further dramatic incident. Unable finally to free themselves from the spirit's influence, they concluded that they must, in Peggy's words, "learn to live with the appearance of absolute normality."

Just before Christmas in the year following Martin's baptism, Peggy described the changes that had occurred and the improvements over his previous state as being "on the miracle side." He had completed technical school training in automotive mechanics and continued his computer training. However, most of the basic problems persisted, including slowness, heaviness, dullness, and a weight on his entire body, especially his head, pain in other parts of his body, and spontaneous imagery. He no longer experienced fluidity and dissolution of his body because, said Peggy, he now "knows the truth" about his problem. Nevertheless, his problems created difficulty in the school environment.

Particularly bothersome were uncontrollable sexual fantasies about classmates, apparently both male and female. The individuals who attracted his attention were not necessarily ones who "would normally appeal" to him, and he found it "annoying to look at some three-hundred-pounder and want to go to town." Peggy explained that the spirit "sees through his eyes," so that although he does not see anyone who on the "real" level appeals to him, on the "other" level, he wanted to "jump everything that moves." Peggy confirmed that Martin had in college stayed away from girls because of his problem, suggesting that he did not date because of difficulty "controlling his feelings." He currently had no female friends, and Peggy felt that this would not be advisable unless it was someone of the same spiritual orientation with whom he could be open about his thoughts.

Martin was also afraid that others would be able to perceive the demonic activity through his behavior. In particular, there was a "motion in his eyes" that Peggy could perceive because she is psychic. She said it looked, "almost like another eye behind his eye," but could elaborate no further: she did not know whether the spirit really has eyes of its own or not, but her perception of the hidden eye conforms to her interpretation that the spirit saw through Martin's eyes. She observed, however, that this manifestation occurred only when he was "weak," and often when they were out in public. She qualified this as no more than an exacerbation of a "natural nervousness" associated with going out and felt that other people perceive the demonic manifestations in Martin only as "a little nervousness." He was nevertheless concerned, and she found it necessary to "help keep him focused on the fact that no one can tell."

Peggy herself continued to be afflicted and was concerned about her own anger, worrying particularly that a situation might arise where she would "lose control." Her experience remained linked to Martin's in that whenever he lost a degree of personal control, she was affected. For example, while he was elsewhere working on someone's car, she suddenly felt a tightening in her head, her mind switched to sexual thoughts, and images began to flood in. At the same time, Martin had become frustrated in tightening a bolt and, when he "loses his balance," the evil spirit "releases its personality, which is pornographic." A second example was an instance in which Martin was at school while Peggy had the puppy out in the yard. She suddenly felt a "drop in a sexual place as if my stomach dropped down, *whump*." She learned later that the same thing had been happening to Martin in his class, a sexual reaction to being surrounded by men and women.

By late summer, despite a continuing "block on his head" and mental "haze," Martin continued to increase his level of social functioning. Peggy's husband assisted with a reference in helping Martin obtain a half-time job working with computer applications of statistics in a division of the local university. In preparation for this, Peggy had spent all of May in "heavy prayer," reciting three rosaries per day, and was "told" by the Virgin Mary that the power of prayer would move the demon. Still it "applied pressure" to prevent Martin from beginning work, causing pain, fear, a turmoil of low self-esteem as it attempted to weaken him in its "emotional grip." Martin and Randy stayed awake praying the entire night before his first day of work. Peggy thought the whole effort would be unsuccessful because the spirit "does have a definite degree of control over him," but she was impressed at Martin's ability to maintain himself with little sleep.

One morning during his first days at work she once again commanded the spirit to depart, and Martin's chest "went *whump*" while she saw it pushed outward from the inside as if there were a "fist from inside, punching." In spite of this demonic harassment, Martin had settled into his work for the two months prior to my final interview with Peggy. His weekly routine included school every morning and work every afternoon. Following work he frequently swam in the faculty pool, which Peggy reported as having a beneficial "cooling" effect given the continued intensity of his suffering. Every night he ate dinner with Peggy and her family, and given that his computer was set up at their house, spent a good deal of his free time there. He had been visiting his mother every Friday for a year until she "slipped" and went off her medication for bipolar depressive disorder. On Sundays he regularly attended mass and communion. Randy, who had formulated a plan to live as a writer and support himself with a low-stress civil service job, typically joined the family for Sunday dinner.

The principal difference Peggy saw in Martin is an increased ability to "discern" his own thoughts and reactions from those of the demon. She elaborated by saying that he at one time had lost sight of his own pain, distancing himself from it and therefore having less sensitivity and feeling in his body. Martin reportedly stated that when the affliction first began he could distinguish between his own self and the alien presence, but that he had lost this ability as the demon progressively merged with his self. He now appeared to be regaining that ability, and could at times say "that is not my thought." He still sensed the pornographic images clearly, but also regarded them as alien. He expressed, according to Peggy, a desire for "freedom" and had become able to utter the prayer of "command" that the spirit depart from him. A principal difficulty that remained is that he had little or no contact with his emotions—no "heart feeling," according to Peggy—for example being unable to distinguish between "love" and "sex." In spite of this isolation from his emotions, he had been learning to conduct his life through an "intellectual" understanding of what is "good or right."

Peggy's interpretation of the situation at this time was that though the evil spirit was rather high-ranking in the demonic hierarchy (as indicated by its mysterious name), the persistence of their prayers had succeeded in denying it access to help from other higher spirits such that it was isolated and (presumably) on the defensive. Martin still at times exuded the "odor of a sickroom," either in his breath or as a body odor, and Peggy could still psychically perceive a gray aura around him indicating "unhealthiness"; she could see as well the spirit "moving behind his eyes." Thus, the problem was still there, but Martin was "moving on despite enormous odds" because "you go on with life."

Religious and Psychiatric Meanings

In order to generate culturally competent accounts of Martin's affliction from within two distinct healing systems, a detailed case description was prepared based on fieldnotes that covered the period up to Martin's baptism as a Catholic. The case description was given to five charismatic healing ministers with whom I had worked in a study of therapeutic process in religious healing. All five were recognized as legitimate healers in the local charismatic movement. The description was also given to five mental health professionals, all of whom have substantial experience in both research and clinical practice. The text examined by these ten individuals was essentially similar to that presented above, such that the reader may formulate his or her own reading of the data in relation to the charismatic and clinical accounts.

The Charismatic Account

The five Catholic Pentecostal healing ministers included two nuns, a priest, another priest who works as a team with a lay woman, and a lay woman assisted by a team of five other women. Each (referred to hereafter as numbers 1 to 5) is recognized within the movement, though their reputations range from local to regional to national. One priest has professional training in counseling and psychotherapy; aside from the background in pastoral counseling acquired by priests and nuns as part of their religious training, the knowledge of the others stems solely from their practice of charismatic healing. Like the mental health professionals, they were told that the purpose of their comments was to "help separate religious and psychiatric meanings" of the case. In accordance with the principles of their healing system, they were asked not for their "diagnostic and dynamic impressions" but for their religious "discernment" of whether or not an evil spirit was present in the case, for an interpretation of what was wrong, and of why the healing seemed not to be effective.

The most striking result of this exercise is the uniform agreement that the healer is a source of the problem, while the issue of presence of an evil spirit appears secondary and is, in fact, the subject of some disagreement among the consultants. These two observations are linked by an important characteristic of the healing system. That is, the knowledge brought to bear on this case by the participating healers is *empirical* knowledge, based on concrete experience in healing encounters and systematized through sharing *via* media such as conferences and publications.

In evaluating the case description, there was less ambiguity in the healers' application of their empirical knowledge to the practices and experiences of their fellow healer than in their determination of the presence of an evil spirit which, ideally, requires face-to-face interaction with the afflicted person. More than this, however, the healers implicitly assume that if one is gifted and competent to identify evil spirits and to know how to deal with them, then one can use the more or less routine spiritual technique of commanding the demon's departure through invocation of a divine power that is, by definition, greater than that of the demonic. Hence, before elaborating the healing ministers' comments on the issue of demonic presence *per se*, we must elaborate on their critique of Peggy as a healer.

None of the commentators questions Peggy's motivation to help people as a healer, but the validity of her "calling" to act in that role is explicitly questioned by healers 1–4 and implicitly by 5. They attend closely to the details of the story of her beginning to heal. What appears as an archetypal motif of the prophet's or healer's call, "I heard the voice of God and tried not to pay attention, but the call was insistent and I had to obey," is challenged not on grounds that such calls never occur, but on grounds that it may not be valid in her case. One commentator wants to know *why* she resisted and, it is pointed out, the voice she heard might not have been the voice of God.

Likewise, it is not denied that the "prophecy" she heard at a prayer meeting in confirmation of her healing gift could have occurred; the challenge is that God never "makes" anyone attend an event against their will and that the prophecy she heard at that prayer meeting could have been a message intended for someone else. Even more suspect to the commentators is her statement that she never felt a need for healing in her own life; in the logic of the healing system, not only do healers often experience their own healing in the process of becoming channels of divine power, but the person in general who needs no healing "does not exist."

Peggy's healing practice is also suspect because of her isolation, both in terms of learning and of ongoing support for her work. The healing system is a social system embedded in the Catholic Charismatic movement, which is itself a "movement" of the Holy Spirit; that is, it is understood to be instigated by God. For a healer to say that all her knowledge comes directly from God is then, questionable, not because this is impossible and not because it has never happened, but because the resources for learning through books, tapes, conferences, and the experience(s) of others has been made available by God, and is, therefore, meant to be used.

Again, "gifts" of healing are granted for the sake of "ministering" to and building Christian communities, and are used appropriately only in such contexts. At the same time healing requires guidance, support, and prayer from members of such a community both for success and for the protection of the healing minister who in the nature of the enterprise is exposed to harmful influences. Thus, Peggy's alienation from both charismatic groups with which she was involved casts further doubt on her validity, and bodes ill for the success of her work in the view of the five healers.

Largely as a result of this isolation, healing ministers 1 and 3 explicitly judge Peggy to be "incompetent" as a healer. That is, her marginality does not place her outside the healing system: her practices are in general recognized by the commentators, and even at some points affirmed, but she is regarded as beyond her abilities, unable to handle the situation because she is ignorant of how things really work. Thus, both healing ministers 1 and 4 draw attention to the "empirical fact" that God never requires a healer to *confront* a demon to demand its identity. God knows its identity and may reveal it, or one may command in the name of God that the spirit state its name (through the voice of the afflicted person), but one is never left to face a demon on one's own. Without her isolation she would have known that God does not work like that and would not have committed an error of technique. Likewise, although the healer may at times feel another's pain, it simply "does not happen" that such suffering is necessary for a healing to occur or that the healer's release is contingent on the deliverance of the afflicted. Were she not so isolated, she would have known that this is not acceptable; it would have been prevented or she could have obtained help and been saved the consequences of an error of interpretation.

The final criticism of Peggy's healing practice from within the logic of the charismatic healing system is her use of "occult" practices in combination with, or in place of, healing prayer (healing ministers 1, 4, and 5).

Peggy herself explicitly equated her psychic abilities with "what the charismatics would call discernment." In the perception of charismatic healing ministers, however, a distinction is drawn between the divine gift of "discernment" and "psychic powers," the former is a gift from God, the latter is inspired by Satan. In at least one instance, the commentaries were not in complete agreement about all of Peggy's practices in this respect. Minister 1 grants plausibility to Peggy's feeling that a higher spirit may lurk behind that of Pornography, and that the healer could gee it, but suggests that Peggy may be allowing herself to be carried away and should "keep both feet on the ground." Healing minister 4 questions whether Peggy has the spiritual gift of discernment that would allow her to have a visionary glimpse of the spirit, and, more forcefully, argues that unless such knowledge has some clear purpose in the healing, it is a psychic knowledge, the work of the devil.

However, other of Peggy's practices such as astrology, reading of auras, and examining the "*cakras*" are invariably proscribed and seen as occult, or Satanic, in origin and purpose. Healing minister 4 specified that although some of the *techniques* of the Eastern religions could be used in abstraction from their philosophical underpinnings, acceptance of their basic principles, regarded as contradicting those of Christianity, constitutes involvement in the occult and cannot be tolerated. Therefore Peggy, whether or not she knew it, was inviting demonic influence by the very nature of the practices in which she was engaged.

Given the above critique of Peggy as a healing minister from within the logic of charismatic healing, one could readily conclude, "No wonder she was unsuccessful in her attempts to heal Martin, and no wonder she was herself susceptible to demonic attack." Yet within the commentaries, the presence of an evil spirit is by no means a yes or no issue, and we must now sort out the healing ministers' own ethnopsychology of the interaction between demonic and psychological forces. Given that most of the healing ministers hesitated to make a definitive judgment about demonic action, their commentaries reveal three areas of divergent interpretation: relation between demonic action and mental disorder, relation between evil spirits and emotions, and suggestions for therapeutic intervention.

The first area is most clearly exemplified in contrasting healing ministers 1 and 4. The former is a nun with no professional mental health training but extensive experience in Deliverance, and the latter a priest with a doctorate in psychology, but who also has extensive experience in Deliverance. Healing minister 1 concludes that Martin's problem is primarily religious and spiritual and requires Deliverance, though psychiatric follow-up could be necessary or beneficial. She suggests that Martin is "obsessed" by the spirit, which means that it has taken up residence within him while not yet fully "possessing" his personality. Healing minister 4 explicitly labels

Martin's symptoms psychotic, specifically schizophrenic and obsessive, using the latter term in its clinical, as opposed to religious, sense. Insofar as demonic symptoms can be identical with those of psychosis, however, and insofar as evil spirits are inherently deceitful and will hence attempt to disguise their identity, their presence is not ruled out. Yet the very fact that the powerful prayer of Deliverance—a divine command that evil spirits must obey—has not been successful is taken as evidence that a psychological problem exists. This problem is labeled *folie à deux*, referring to the enmeshed relationship among the protagonists. Healing minister 4 concludes that *if* there is an evil spirit, Martin and Peggy are both in a position to be manipulated by it, but that the foremost need is for psychiatric evaluation of both Martin and Peggy.

The contrast between the spiritualizing and psychologizing religious perspectives, as we may call them, is best illustrated by comparing the evidence marshaled in these two commentaries. Healing minister 1 cites early involvement in the occult, i.e., participation in a childhood séance, difficulty praying, loss of concentration in theological conversations, insomnia, being wakened by pornographic images, inability to tolerate presence of a tested religious healing minister, a voice screaming and cursing which is yet unable to utter the name of Jesus, anger, anxiety, and fear. When entertaining the semidynamic hypothesis that the latter three emotions could be linked to developmental issues from Martin's childhood, she again spiritualizes: the problem may not be with a demonic spirit, but with the restless spirit of Martin's father. Healing minister 4's enumeration of psychotic symptoms includes visualization, the disembodied voice, auditory hallucinations, intractable headache, disabling anxiety, sleep disturbance, yanking and pulling sensation (visceral sensations indicating rage at his father), undifferentiated sexuality, bad taste of food, body odor, twinges of pain indicating autosuggestion and autohypnosis.

While these two sets of evidence are not in themselves sufficient to contrast two logical styles, several provocative points can be made. First, a great deal of overlap exists between evidence for evil spirits and psychopathology: visual and auditory phenomena, insomnia, anger, anxiety. However, the more spiritualized account pays much greater attention to content than to form of symptoms. Thus, it is important not only that there are visual phenomena, but that these are pornographic, and not only that there are auditory phenomena, but that the voice screams and curses. This emphasis on content may be related to the apparent emphasis on action over somatic sensation; thus healing minster 1 emphasizes attending a seance, prayer, conversation, reaction to the presence of another person while healing minister 4 mentions pain, bad taste, body odor, yanking and pulling sensations.

Further research may succeed in specifying the different styles of spiritualized and psychologized religious approaches within this healing system, but for the present it will suffice to stress that demonic influence and psychopathology are not mutually exclusive. Thus, between the more clear-cut examples of 1 and 4, healing minster 3 specifically acknowledged a high degree of "spirit activity," while simultaneously suggesting that Martin suffers from schizophrenia. Healing minister 5 summarized the problem as one of imbalance between the demonic/spiritual and psychological/emotional aspects of the case.

More light is shed on the logic of the healing system by consideration of the relation between evil spirit and emotion. In Catholic Pentecostalism it is rare, though not unheard of, for demons to bear names such as Andronius in the present case. Typically, they bear the name of sins (Lust, Gluttony), negative behaviors (Self-Destruction, Rebellion), or negative emotions (Anger, Fear). This leads to a systematic ambiguity in distinguishing where human emotion and behavior leave off and the influence of evil spirits begins. Healing minister 1 does not explicitly label Martin's anger, anxiety, and fear as demons, but does call them "hallmarks of Satan." At the same time she links anger to chronic problems rooted in Martin's childhood. Healing minister 2 indicates that Martin is oppressed by disobedience, rebellion, and rejection. This term is used technically to designate a specific level of demonic influence; recall that healing minister 1 felt Martin was obsessed, indicating a higher degree of influence. However, she says, without an actual healing encounter, it cannot be discerned whether these are demons "in the strict sense" of intelligent but evil spiritual entities.

Healing minister 3 identifies homosexuality, guilt, self-hatred, and poor self-image as specifically psychiatric, rather than demonic, problems, but acknowledges that there is some spirit activity that must be dispelled. Healing minister 4, whom we have already identified as the most psychologically oriented, mentions rage, anxiety, and undifferentiated sexuality, but only insofar as they appear as symptoms of psychopathology. Healing minister 4 never rules out the possibility of demonic activity. Healing minister 5 does not name specific emotions or behaviors, but distinguishes demonic/spiritual from psychological/emotional aspects of the case.

Whether or not the emotions and behaviors identified by healing ministers are granted the ontological status of evil spirits or human attributes, they indicate a shared therapeutic style of identifying pragmatic issues dealt with in the healing process: anger, rage, anxiety, fear, disobedience, rebellion, rejection, homosexuality, guilt, self-hatred, poor self-image. These are issues whose concrete content can be explored in the life of the afflicted person, and stand at an intermediate level between Peggy's abstract Andronius and symptomatically superficial Pornography. In the logic of the healing system, when one cannot resolve anger through Healing of Memories or Inner Healing, one may conclude that a spirit of Anger or another spirit is present. When Peggy reached this impasse in her attempt at healing Martin, anger became not symbolically concrete Anger, but a mystically abstract Andronius.

The issue of human versus demonic in attribution of emotion is important for the more orthodox healing ministers in that it determines the preference for further treatment. Healing minister 1 recommends charismatic Deliverance from evil spirits as the treatment of choice. Healing minister 3 recommends a combination of psychiatric care and charismatic healing. Healing minister 5 recommends psychotherapy completely removed from a spiritual emphasis, feeling that the situation is already overspiritualized. At the same time, both 3 and 5 suggest that the exorcism prayer within the Catholic sacrament of Baptism should have the effect of releasing Martin from evil spirits if he is properly disposed and has a spiritual relationship with God. Thus the relation between discernment and diagnosis, demon and disease, deliverance and psychotherapy, remains inherently ambiguous. The healing system allows for interpretation of a situation as demonic influence *instead of* psychopathology, but also allows demonic influence as a *qualification* of psychopathology.

The Clinical Account

Five mental health professionals were presented with the case materials. These included three psychiatrists and two psychologists; one of the psychologists is female, the others are male. All are university-based and have both clinical and research experience. The initial assumption of this exercise was that the clinical interpretation of Martin's difficulties would be in terms of diagnosable psychopathology. Methodological difficulties exist in that the ethnographic description does not fulfill all the requirements of a definitive diagnostic interview, which can only be conducted in a face-to-face encounter between clinician and patient. Thus, what follows are not true differential diagnoses but diagnostic and dynamic impressions offered by clinical consultants. In this light, it must be stressed that the purpose of the exercise was neither to make a definitive diagnosis of Martin and/or Peggy, nor to compare the different schools of psychotherapy represented. It was instead to elaborate a composite clinical interpretation of an atypical case that could stand in contrast to a composite religious interpretation by the clinicians' counterparts in the charismatic healing ministry.

In creating a composite clinical understanding from these commentaries, caution must be exercised with respect to disagreements that might occur due to (a) the limitations of the data, and (b) clinicians' adherence to different psychotherapeutic schools. The principal example of the former is the possible diagnosis of schizophrenia. The data allow this diagnosis to be entertained by consultants 1, 2, and 5, and rejected by consultant 4, with consultant 3 refusing any label more specific than psychotic. Based on the written description, both consultants 1 and 5 felt that a diagnostic criterion of schizophrenia, "deterioration in functioning" was present, while consultant 2 saw insufficient deterioration to warrant the diagnosis. Likewise, there was disagreement as to whether Martin's visualizations were true hallucinations, pseudohallucinations, or "possible" hallucinations.

An example of the second consideration is the tendency of the psychiatric consultants to comment on disease concepts, while the two psychological consultants emphasized personality disorder or personality structure. This represents neither an inadequacy in the data nor an issue that can be synthesized into a composite interpretation, but a difference in disciplinary emphasis between clinical psychology and psychiatry. Differences among therapeutic schools are reflected in the consultants' various recommendations for family as opposed to individual therapy for the principal actors in the situation.

Given these limitations, the validity of the exercise based on clinical commentaries depends on not overstepping the bounds of the task. Only with such caution can certain differences among consultants be shown to be grounded in commonalities of clinical thought rather than inadequacies in the data. Likewise, even though consultants explicitly stated that the case was unusual, only with the necessary caution can interpretive ambiguities be shown to stem from the atypicality of the case rather than from different approaches of clinical disciplines or schools.

This situation is further complicated by the fact that differential diagnosis is a complex process of discrimination among disorders that may have certain symptoms in common, or may differ only in time of onset or duration relative to other symptoms. Yet while differential diagnosis in medicine operates primarily by excluding possible in favor of more likely diagnoses, it also allows for the simultaneous and overlapping application of more than one category in the final analysis. This is particularly likely in the case of a person as severely disturbed as Martin. In addition to limitations in the data and atypicality of the situation, diagnosis is complicated by the presence of multiple disorders. Nevertheless, it is possible to examine the clinical logic of the consultants' suggestions based on the American Psychiatric Association's *Diagnostic and Statistical Manual* (DSM-III) (1980).

As discussed above, it appears that "schizophrenic disorder" is a likely candidate as a label for Martin's condition. The commentaries of the mental health professionals also frequently mention depression or severe affective disorder, but the problem here is that major depressive disorder and schizophrenia are mutually exclusive. In addition, the long-term treatment outcome of depression is typically considered better than that of schizophrenia. The DSM-III system, however, includes ways to hedge between these mutually exclusive diagnoses. For example, "depression with mood-congruent psychotic features" would include "delusions or hallucina-

tions whose content is consistent with the themes of either personal inadequacy, guilt, disease, death, nihilism or deserved punishment" (DSM-
III:215), a description consistent with Martin's sexual preoccupations and
early experience of family trauma. Again, the DSM-III system allows for the
possible diagnosis of an admittedly ill-defined schizoaffective disorder if the
clinician cannot distinguish between schizophrenia and affective disorder.

In this case the chief concern of differential diagnosis would be to
determine whether the affective symptoms preceded the psychotic symptoms; if so one would tend toward depression, if not one would tend toward
schizophrenia. The early history of Martin's life is not clear enough to determine this. We know that Martin's father committed suicide, often associated
with depression, and that Martin's mother has been diagnosed with bipolar
affective disorder (also called manic-depression). The latter fact may suggest
a genetic factor predisposing Martin to depression and, at the same time, the
double loss of parents is precisely the kind of bereavement that has also been
associated with depression (Brown and Harris 1978). On the other hand, the
abusive family environment which Martin must have endured in his childhood often suggested to be typical for those who develop schizophrenia at
about the same age as the onset of Martin's troubles.

To further complicate the diagnostic picture, some physicians have
argued for the existence of a disorder which they call "chronic pain syndrome" (Black 1975) or "learned pain syndrome" (Brena and Chapman
1985). In the sense that Martin's pain has no objectively determined source
and that he has learned to associate it with certain situations and thought
patterns, this category might appear relevant. This is in accordance with
our consultants' mention of somatization (consultant 1) or displacement
(consultant 2) of traumatic experience into pain. The neurologist, who originally told Martin that his pain was something he must learn to live with,
apparently had something like this in mind. It can be assumed, however,
that in the clinical encounter no mention was made of voices or spontaneous
visualizations, for it is possible that at that time Martin regarded them as
side-effects of the head pain itself. On the other hand, it must be noted at
least in passing that the chronic headache with blurring of consciousness
and strange visual manifestations could also suggest migraine (Sacks 1985).

Whether such a thing as chronic pain syndrome exists as a clinical
entity is currently a topic of debate among physicians. A subtopic of this
debate is the relation between chronic pain and depression (Turner and
Romano 1984; Bouckoms et al. 1985; Gupta 1986). Depression here is associated both with losses suffered by Martin in his childhood (cf. Brown and
Harris 1978) and with chronic entrenched feelings of guilt and anger that
are not uncommon among patients with chronic pain. Depression is commonly associated with anxiety, a feature mentioned explicitly by only one
consultant, but the evidence for anxiety and panic is complicated by cur-

rent research suggesting that obsessive-compulsive disorder be included among anxiety disorders (Insel et al. 1985).

In line with the above considerations, the DSM-III also requires obsessive-compulsive disorder to be ruled out in making the differential diagnosis of schizophrenia. The distinction here is that in obsessive-compulsive disorder what appear to be delusions are frequently recognized in a conscious way as irrational and quite unpleasant. It indeed appears that Martin's bizarre and intrusive thoughts are of an obsessive nature and are in addition associated with rigid moral compunctions of a religious nature. Here it is relevant to recall the commentaries' mention of dissociative disorders, and especially the epidemiological observation by consultant 2 that obsessive and dissociative features may co-occur more frequently than previously thought. Following this line, diagnostic logic could lead to a conclusion independent of either depression or schizophrenia as principle diagnoses.

The question of possible personality disorder raised by two of the consultants requires two observations. First, DSM-III requires a diagnostic distinction be made between these disorders and schizophrenia, because they can sometimes include transient psychotic symptoms. In severe paranoid personality disorder, the distinction is based on intensity and severity of paranoid ideation and distortions in communication and perception. The issue of paranoia leads directly to the second observation, in which consultant 5's suggestion of dependent personality structure can be related to the reference by consultant 2 and 3 to *folie à trois*, which is technically defined as a "shared paranoid disorder." This raises a variety of issues simultaneously, all having to do with shared aspects of the situation.

Perhaps Martin is afflicted with a major form of psychopathology, or perhaps the maladaptive characteristics of his personality are exacerbated by the relationships in which he finds himself. In either case, consider the comment by consultant 3 that an apparent predisposition to florid symptoms is exacerbated by the expectations of the system. The question here is whether the beliefs and experiences of the afflicted persons are delusional. In this case, it is critical to distinguish the two. Between consultants 1 and 2, on the one hand, and 3 and 5, on the other, there is some disagreement about whether the religious beliefs themselves are delusional. Consultant 2 points out that beliefs are not delusional if they are shared by a cultural group, but still uses the term *folie à trois*. This is not an inconsistency, but rather an implicit recognition that particular experiences may be delusional even though religious or cultural beliefs used to make sense of them are not.

This is an important consideration when we raise the question of whether Peggy herself has a diagnosable psychopathology. Consultants 1 and 2 appear to think not, while 3, 4, and 5 recommend therapy for Peggy as well as Martin, with 3 suggesting the entire healing career may be a "depressive system" and 4 suggesting histrionic personality. Beyond the issues of a shared delusional system and a possible individual diagnosis for Peggy, the consultants seem to share a consensus that Peggy is overly dominant and controlling, and that Martin would benefit by independence from her. The consultants describe this critical aspect of the situation with terms such as "family pathology," "enmeshment," "mutual dependency," "undifferentiated family ego mass," and "interpenetration."

Indeed, Martin's definition of the situation is singularly dependent on Peggy and Randy. They both suggested that because the evil spirit has been harassing Martin since the time of his father's death at age nine, he has nothing with which to compare his present state; that is, he remembers no state of consciousness that was not influenced by the demon, and cannot always distinguish his own thoughts from those of the demon. Martin acknowledges that "all he knows" is what Peggy has taught him, thus giving Peggy a powerful role as arbiter and interpreter of his experience. In one instance, for example, when Martin recalled that at an early period in life he felt a psychic connection with his mother, Peggy was quick to add that Martin by himself has no "real psychic power." In addition, and as something of a contradiction, while Peggy claims that Martin has "worked through" a lot of anger and other emotion, she reports that he cannot experience his emotions. This report could be interpreted as indicating either a symptom of schizophrenia, i.e., blunted or flat affect, or the emotional dullness of depression. In the present context, however, the fact that he only knows intellectually what he wants to feel but cannot have any emotional experience must be related to the degree of Peggy's control in teaching him what he should be feeling. Both consultants 1 and 3 comment that in effect Randy and Peggy have symbolically agreed to become Martin's parents themselves. Experience of the spirit's "resistance" to outsiders' offers of healing could then be understood as resistance by Martin in order to remain in the dependent relationship.

Interestingly, in the only formal contact with a mental health professional reported in this episode (see above), the psychiatrist suggested to Peggy that the "difficulty of separation might be creating an obstacle to Martin's improvement." Peggy's confidence in her motivation (cessation of her own pain) to see the situation to a conclusion was not shared by the consultants, who noted that Peggy's own emotional needs were apparently being satisfied by the tight bonds among Martin, Randy, and herself. Consultants 1, 2 and 4 explicitly define these bonds as sexual as well as emotional.

Characterization of the trio's bonds as sexual and emotional raises the issue of Peggy's rather aloof husband and the nature of their relationship. The consultants appeared to be in consensus on this issue; and consultant 3 was especially emphatic. He suggested that the entire healing enterprise represented a depressive reaction to the frustrations of the marital relationship, and he perceived a weakness in her example of "intimacy" between husband and wife (e.g., weekly two-hour car rides during which they never faced each other but talked while looking ahead out the window).

Peggy admitted that her uncontrollable pornographic fantasies affected her sexual relationship with her husband in the sense that she sometimes became distracted from lovemaking. He was not fully aware of this, however, and they do not talk on a daily basis about her experiences. Peggy herself acknowledged no long-term problem in the relationship, but admitted that early in the three-year trial of Martin's affliction, their relationship was strained by the demands of the situation. She claimed that since then her husband had "grown," accepting the reality of the situation, and waiting and hoping for a resolution. Yet Peggy's approach is never to complain to her husband about her own suffering but to try instead to "be smiling" in his presence.

Meanwhile her husband leads a busy professional life about which she knows little. A newspaper write-up listing his awards and achievements left her surprised that he is so renowned; she never accompanies him on his many travels because she, "doesn't want to leave the kids when the youngest is still ten." In light of data on this topic, the situation suggests not so much an estranged husband, but one who sacrifices intimacy to the demands of professional life and is also somewhat leery of probing too deeply into his wife's spiritual affairs.

What can be concluded from this brief diagnostic exercise is not primarily that the data are inadequate for diagnostic purposes, nor that Martin's situation is too complex to be easily diagnosable. Instead, the exercise suggests that the very diagnostic categories available are fluid, overlapping, and more or less vaguely defined. Martin may have one or a number of serious forms of psychopathology; what appears clear in the diagnostic logic is that the situation is serious, involves psychopathology, and requires psychiatric intervention. Whether Peggy is herself diagnosable hinges in part on whether her religious beliefs and symptoms are related as part of a delusional system, whether her symptoms are a logical consequence of religious beliefs admitted as culturally acceptable, or whether she has made a pathological adaptation to culturally normal religious beliefs. Beyond the attribution of individual psychopathology, the diagnostic logic extends to issues of sexual and emotional relationships characterized by dominance, dependency, lack of fulfillment and frustration, possible shared delusion, spirituality, and isolation. Isolation, along with the persistence and severity of the situation, led consultants 1 and 2 to suggest that as a healer, Peggy may be deviant even in terms of the religious system; consultant 3 observed that Peggy appeared to combine elements of Charismatic Christianity and New Age spirituality. These culturally perceptive comments, in fact, conform to some of the responses of the religious healers noted above.

Convergence and Divergence

The most striking contrast between commentaries of mental health professionals and charismatic healing ministers is perhaps not that the latter include the influence of evil spirits, but that they focus on Peggy and technical flaws in the therapeutic process rather then on Martin and his symptoms and pathology. For the healing ministers, Peggy is a "fringe" practitioner of a kind warned against in Catholic Pentecostal teaching and literature on healing: poorly informed, of questionable competence and legitimacy, lacking the support of a community, and hence "in over her head" in trouble. Partly for this reason, but partly because of the nature of her relationship with Martin, Randy, and her husband, Peggy, too, is afflicted and needs healing, or even psychotherapy, herself.

While the mental health professionals point to the same dynamic and interpersonal issues, they tend to reserve judgment about Peggy out of a desire to respect her religious beliefs. Culturally shared beliefs are not delusional, and Peggy's bizarre experiences are based on these beliefs; therefore Peggy is probably not diagnosable. Lacking the cultural information about the low degree to which Peggy's beliefs and practices are in fact shared by the most logical reference group, they tend to emphasize Martin's symptoms and pathology. This tendency is, of course, only a relative one, for the mental health professionals certainly identify patterns of enmeshment, *folie à deux*, family pathology, and dependency.

The point is not that the two groups of commentaries reach different conclusions. The point is that different sets of cultural knowledge brought to bear on the problem lead to different emphases and explanations within analyses that are pragmatically similar. Several of the mental health professionals suspected Peggy's lack of orthodoxy. On the other hand, the healers' critique of Peggy's practice as isolated anticipate a clinical judgment of enmeshment among the protagonists. For the therapists, the kind of person who becomes enmeshed may be the kind of person perceived as marginal by her cultural reference group; for the healers, the kind of person who is marginal may be the kind who may become enmeshed.

In order to appreciate fully the interaction of worldviews in this case we must insert Peggy's religious interpretation between that of the clinicians and the healers. The religious critique of Peggy can be summarized as follows: if there is an evil spirit, she is not handling it properly and, if not, she should acknowledge the need for psychiatric care. There is a chance that both therapy and Deliverance are needed, and she is incompetent in both areas. The fact that the healing ministers pay surprisingly little attention to Martin's own problem is probably because, initially, Peggy's approach and interpretation were not incompatible with theirs and neither was it incompatible with psychotherapeutic interpretations. When at the outset Peggy refers to Martin's "brokenness," she has in mind the traumatic early events leading to his father's suicide, Martin's discovery of the body, loss of his mother, and subsequent assignments to an orphanage and foster parents. For Peggy and other charismatic healers these early experiences create a vulnerability to demonic influence, while for the clinicians they create a vulnerability to psychiatric disorder. Her focus on resolution of anger and guilt, which includes encouraging concrete steps toward reconciliation between Martin and his mother, is so unobjectionable as to remain unmentioned by both clinicians and healing ministers.

Peggy's subsequent "discovery" of demonic presence was closely associated with recognition that Martin still felt "more anger than he wanted to" toward his father. Indeed, discovery of a spirit is an acknowledgment that a deeper level of unresolved problems exists. Conversely, reaching a therapeutic impasse can be construed as evidence for the presence of an evil spirit—but these are by no means necessarily the same thing. The healing system assumes that a block to change exists within the afflicted person and infers that this block is caused by an evil spirit. Clinical consultant 3 suggested that, at least in this case, the block was the limit of effectiveness for a "transference cure," which could be achieved by a clinically untrained religious healer but which left unresolved deeper conflicts accessible only to a highly skilled psychotherapist.

Whether or not the block is "within" the afflicted person or "between" the person and the healing minister, discovery of a spirit is a rhetorical strategy for transcending the block and bringing the problem out in the open in such a way that it can be challenged with the support of divine power: the lonely and isolated individual is no longer alone because his struggle is now part of a cosmological struggle of universal scope, the spiritual warfare between God and Satan (Csordas 1983; also see Dow 1986, Tambiah 1977). But transcending and bringing out in the open appear to go necessarily hand in hand; transcending alone can be dangerous. For, as noted above, according to some healing ministers Deliverance is easy, because a prayer commanding it to depart, or the exorcism contained within the rite of Baptism, *must* work due to God's inherent power over Satan. It is perhaps important that this is not the only approach to Deliverance, but emerged within the movement as an antidote to practices emphasizing struggle against evil spirits that could last for agonizing hours and include shrieks, vomiting, and writhing on the floor; Peggy may have expected and needed this kind of approach to be convinced of divine empowerment.

Thus, the conventional rhetorical strategy backfired. By positing a source of affliction external to Martin, Peggy made herself vulnerable as well; instead of psychic mirroring of Martin's symptoms, a situation was created in which the evil spirit could attack her directly "at her own weak points." In psychiatric terms, the cool, dignified figure of Andronius became an opaque metaphor of Peggy's uncontrolled countertransference, the impenetrable "humanity" in which the protagonists were enmeshed, and the universal pitfall shared by psychotherapists and exorcists of whatever tradition (Henderson 1982; Good et al. 1982). Thus, the sexual fantasies that began at Martin's puberty, and were exacerbated when the evil spirit took advantage of his unresolved developmental crisis of intimacy, find their parallel in sexual fantasies that reflect Peggy's ambiguous relationship with her husband and her role as housewife/mother, her close spiritual relationship with Randy, and her dominant/dependent relationship with Martin.

The Existential Ground of Demon and Disease

Comparing medical and sacred realities in this way throws some light on their different properties as systems for organizing experience and some light on the nature of suffering and healing. However, it leaves an essential problem untouched. That is, how is it possible in the first place for such accounts to have so much in common yet be so different; what in fact is the nature of the experience for which they account? We must now turn to this question.

The comparative study of plural healing systems coexisting within an overarching cultural tradition suggests that underlying continuities of process and structure can be found among such systems (Rhodes 1980). In our comparison of North American Catholic charismatic and psychiatric systems, the principal continuity is the mutual emphasis on residual effects of events in the afflicted person's past, and the principal divergence is the role of spiritual practices and demonic entities. The different ways in which these systems elaborate the implications of these issues may paradoxically contribute to the possibility of their coexistence. That is, insofar as they represent, as it were, intersecting planes in the field of experience, they can be complementary rather than contradictory; an afflicted person is much more likely simultaneously to seek help from a religious healer and a psychotherapist than simultaneously to seek help from a psychoanalyst and a cognitive therapist. Although practitioners in either system may reject the validity of the other (as the healer in the case discussed here rejected any psychiatric interpretation), in principal they are often regarded as complementary and in practice sometimes even actively integrated. At the same time, Christian psychotherapists may reject certain competing forms of therapeutic practice as incompatible not only with each other but with principles of religious healing (Csordas 1990a).[9]

We have just now introduced the metaphor of intersecting planes to describe the relation between two readings of Martin's experience. This intersection can be understood in two senses, the cultural and the existential. In the first instance, both readings share a North American cultural proclivity for formulations in strongly *psychological* terms. That is, the interpretations of Martin's experience in both healing systems are predicated on cultural assumptions about emotion, self, and person that begin and end in predominantly psychological understandings. In the second instance, it remains the case that despite our ability to formulate distinct accounts of his experience, there is ultimately only one Martin, in a unique existential situation. I will argue that the common existential ground from which the two accounts are abstracted is his suffering as an *embodied* human being, for whom any distinction among somatic, cognitive, or affective pain is experientially irrelevant.[10]

Specifically, I would argue in favor of bodily experience as the starting point for cultural analysis, the existential ground for divergent cultural elaborations of illness experience and therapeutic intervention (Csordas 1990b). Borrowing our terminology from the existential phenomenology of Merleau-Ponty (1962), we must try to describe Martin's preobjective world of distress and the thematization that creates the possibility for objective entities such as demon or disease to be posited as accounts of that distress. By "preobjective" we refer not in a temporal sense to Martin's experience before he came under the influence of a religious healer but to the manner in which he spontaneously engages the cultural world of everyday life, or on the other hand the degree to which he has lost his hold on that world. Merleau-Ponty would argue that cultural objects such as demons or diseases, no less than natural objects such as rocks or trees, are the end products of a process of abstraction from a perceptual consciousness wherein the sentient human body is an opening on an indeterminate, open-ended, and inexhaustible field: the world.

Critical to our purpose is the understanding that in normal perception one's body is in no sense an object, but always the subject of perception. One does not perceive one's body; one is one's body and perceives *with* it both in the sense that it is a perfectly familiar tool (Mauss 1950) and in the sense that self and body are perfectly coexistent. To perceive a body as an object is thus to have performed a process of abstraction from perceptual experience. When we turn to Martin's situation we are struck first of all with the manner in which all sensory modalities are in crisis. Martin's senses do not give him an immediate grip on the world. In a way he must go through his senses to the world rather than perceiving with them; they are in the way, standing between him and the world such that his perception is not faced with an open horizon but with a wall. This inability to engage the world is thematized in the language of each of the senses, and we must now take a closer look at that language.

The voice Martin hears knew everything about him, would make deals with him, discuss religion, make jokes about his foster mother, cast aspersions on his natural mother, offer friendship and companionship. In short, the voice was thematized as a rather cruel friend, a source of both intimacy and irritation. It is unclear whether, prior to Peggy's identification of the voice with a demonic entity, he perceived the voice as evil, and whether it is legitimate to suggest that Martin was already denying unpleasant thoughts by projecting them onto an alien being. Peggy's reinterpretation of this theme of the cruel friend was that the demon was of the type of the "familiar spirit" (in the sense of the "witch's familiar" and not that of a "family spirit"). Only after the voice was objectified as an evil spirit did it make sense in cultural terms for Martin to say that "it" was able to get deeper into his gut, that it was imitating being three instead of one, or that it "inches you away by merging with your own consciousness." One can only wonder what the consequences might have been if Martin had truly let the utterance, "Your mother left you" become, "My mother left me" in such a way that he was forced to live through his anger and rage about his feelings of abandonment.

In the visual domain the language used to describe the sexual imagery appears curiously contradictory. Martin is "bombarded" with images in rapid succession, with content of increasing perversion and violence, and the sexual impulse is "almost overpowering." Yet it feels good and right to give in, and giving in is accompanied by feelings of friendship and companionship. Is Martin giving in to purely sexual impulses, or to the anger and rage mentioned above and sexually thematized as bombardment with violent content? Relevant here is Merleau-Ponty's (1962) argument that just as sexuality is an atmosphere permeating our lives as human beings, sexual perception itself is modulated by and fully integrated with the other perceptual functions of our bodies. In the present case, there appears to be a phenomenal interrelation between vision and hearing in Martin's experience of imagery and voice as cruel friendship.

This line of thinking is strengthened by considering the language of touch or bodily sensation in Martin's affliction. Pain occurs primarily in his head, but also in his joints, stomach, and groin. It is described as yanking and pulling, with a knot in the head and an occasional release accompanied by a crackling sound; the yanking and pulling can be sexually stimulating if in the genital area. Any mention of his father will also be answered by a pain in his "gut"; this word also appeared in the interviews in the context of the spirit "getting deeper into his gut." If we bracket the idea that these sensations describe the intentional gripping action of a demon, we can see that they in fact isolate body parts in a way phenomenologically parallel to the experience of religious healers who can sense when one of their followers is healed of a heart problem by a spontaneous painful sensation in the chest (Csordas n.d.). Whereas for the healer each pain is thematized as an index of the outside world to be read in her body, Martin's pains alienate him from the parts of his body in a way more akin to dismemberment. The inner integrity and unity of his body is compromised. In addition, however, the pain is thoroughly integrated with visual and auditory phenomena. Unlike chronic pain patients whose pain is thought to modulate almost mechanically with varying levels of stress or relaxation, there is a distinct conative dimension to Martin's pain. It modulates directly in relation to his response to the voice and to sexual imagery. If he bears down in resistance he can be assured the pain will increase, and if he gives in it invariably eases.

Description of Martin's bodily sensation includes feelings of heat coursing through his body, his body becoming like jelly, and the sense of a fluid movement through his body. Here is a sense not so much of dismemberment but of *dissolution* of body boundaries. The overall effect is described as creating panic in his body, and the feeling of running from himself. When these sensations are objectified in terms of demonology, the experience is one of feeling an attempt to embed another personality in his body. This must be compared to the image of getting deeper into his gut and the image of being inched away in his interactions with the voice. Each image corresponds to a particular mode of sensory experience, but note especially that the image of being inched away prompted by the more cognitive interaction with the voice is equally as physical as those associated with pain and corporal dissolution.

In addition to the sensations that isolate parts of his body in pain and those that indicate a dissolution of his body as an integrated being in the world, the interviews include a constellation of descriptions including a net descending over Martin's head, visualization of a gray mass around his head, thickening of the saliva, thickening of his eyelids and glazing over of his eyes when his thinking blurs out, a thickness in conversation, feeling heavy, weighted down, or drained of energy. It can be argued that the bad taste in Martin's mouth, along with his halitosis and body odor, be included in this constellation of meanings revolving around heaviness and thickness. The overall theme of these "heaviness" words appears to be that of *immobility*. Note that this immobility can be objectified as the kind of slowness symptomatic of clinical depression, or as a literal manifestation of oppression by an evil spirit. For Martin it was thematized in the recognition that he could "remain immobilized or go forward."

A cultural phenomenology (Csordas 1990b) of the existential situation exhibited in this language of the senses can be summarized as a radical narrowing of the horizon of perception and experience. Whereas the unafflicted person in everyday life can ceaselessly continue to explore the world, for Martin the world's horizons have become opaque and impenetrable. The image of dismemberment refers to the inner horizon in which the parts of one's body mutually imply one another or communicate with one another in an experientially undifferentiated and taken-for-granted way, here closed

off by the thematization of individual body parts in pain. The image of dissolution refers to the horizon that is the boundary of one's body with the
world. In this case, it cannot be said that the horizon is sealed off, but that
there is no horizon, no foreground or background of personal reality, neither a direction to explore nor any discrete self to do the exploring. The
image of immobility refers to the horizon of action in the world, where one
can formulate an unlimited number of open-ended life projects, but which
for Martin is sealed off by the total preoccupation with affliction. The voice
experienced in the auditory modality participates in all three insofar as
what it says is directly connected with pain, makes it difficult for Martin to
distinguish his own thoughts from alien ones, and prevents him from engaging in his preferred activities.

The constant barrage of sexual imagery, on the other hand, has its
existential significance in opening up an *artificial horizon* of an inex-
haustibly sexual world. In this respect the key phrases are that Martin is
impelled to see the world exclusively in sexual terms and that he feels
"pornography as a state of being" within him. These are not to be distinguished as respectively cognitive and physiological but as alternate phras-
ings of the same underlying stance toward the world. To recall Merleau-
Ponty's (1962) notion of the radical contingency of sexuality as a
component of all human experience, it can be said that Martin's coming
face to face with this reality is coterminous with the closing of other horizons, such that the truth of sexuality as a state of being within everyone was
distorted by appearing as the only transcendent or open-ended modality of
experience. Martin's moment of crisis came in the episode of anorexia and
insomnia immediately prior to his initial encounter with Peggy. The near
absolute collapse of the world and its horizons around him was graphic in
his inability to eat, understandable as the inability to allow the world inside
himself, and his inability to sleep, understandable as the inability to allow
himself an exit from the frozen immediacy of affliction.

Critical to my argument is the recognition that what might appear as
distinctly cognitive or affective distortions of Martin's experience are at one
with the language of bodily experience. The blurring of Martin's consciousness and his inability to concentrate are closely bound up with other
aspects of heaviness and thickness. The special association of these effects
with religious content is tied not only to the preoccupation with an evil spirit but to religiously motivated sexual guilt that preceded this preoccupation.
Feelings of friendship, companionship, goodness, and rightness are also
associated with yielding to sexual temptation and modulation of pain. Panic
and fear are inseparable from feelings of bodily dissolution. Inappropriate
and exaggerated anger, including anger toward his parents, are associated
with promptings of the alien voice, but if we are allowed to apply Peggy's
personal report to Martin's parallel experience they are also associated

with feelings of one's body being manipulated into the expression and posture of anger. Thus, cognition and affect are not to be understood in
abstraction from bodily experience. They are equally components of what
Schilder (1950) called the "postural model" that is subject to transmutation
in a variety of situations, most notably those of affliction.

A parallel description could be made of Peggy's experience with reference to her own acknowledgment that the evil spirit attacks her at her own
weak points. In brief, there are three key differences in her experiences: l)
she hears the voice primarily as screaming, cursing, condemning her and
threatening her family, and concurrently provoking coprolalia in her; 2)
sexual images appear in episodes like a television show and have developed
from anonymity to inclusion of real people (Martin persisted for some time
in the mode of anonymous sexual violence); 3) absence of halitosis or body
odor. The first two features can be understood as concrete representations
of conflicts between her role as Martin's healer and her role within her family, and conflicts over sexual intimacy. The third represents the absence of
at least one dimension of the heaviness (the olfactory) which for Martin
constitutes an obstructed experiential horizon.

This, then, is our approximate reconstruction of Martin's preobjective experience of distress and his initial thematization of that distress,
prior to objectification of his experience in the accounts of religious healing
or psychiatry. My argument is that each system presupposes this experience, and that its account is in that precise sense an abstraction (see Fig. 1).
Each account thematizes preobjective experience according to its own principles. In the religious system, the relevant principle is *moral*, and can be
stated as the contradiction between good and evil. In the psychiatric system, the relevant principle is empirical, and can be stated as the dichotomy
between body and mind. Based on these principles, the systems posit either
a demon or a disease as an objective entity.

The nature of these cultural objects is directly related to variations in
the definition of the person in the two systems. The Catholic Pentecostal
person is a tripartite composite of body-mind-spirit, in contrast to the conventional contemporary Western mind-body. The domain of spirit is equally as empirical as mind and body, and equally susceptible to both positive
and negative influences. Evil is ontologically real and is embodied in active,
intentional beings, i.e., the evil spirits. Thus, the term "entity" directs analytic attention to the ontological claim by healers and clinicians that demons
and diseases are empirically real things in the world. In their respective
systems, the demon is a spiritual substrate of distress, and the disease is a
biological substrate of distress.

In recent years, scholars have questioned the status of disease as an
empirical entity (Campbell 1976: 50–51) and reinterpreted it as a symbolic
or conceptual form in terms of which clinicians organizes their interpreta-

Religious Account	Psychiatric Account
Moral principle: Good/Evil	Empirical principle: Body/Mind
Origin: Occasion	Origin: Cause
Entity: Demon	Entity: Disease
Evidence: Manifestation	Evidence: Symptom? Syndrome

First-person Process:
    Oppression/Struggle
	Third-person Process:
	    Disorder/Somatization

Figure 1. Cultural Accounts as Objectifications of Experience

tion and their patients' experience of affliction and distress (Kleinman 1980, 1983). In this view, the substrate is the phenomenology of affliction, or the experience of illness, and the status of the disease as an entity is made problematic. It is in this sense, and on this level, that the diagnostic logic of disorders and the logic of discernment in the religious healing system are generated in the two sets of commentaries presented above.

The categories of disease and demon organize the understanding of how the distressful condition comes about quite differently. A disease has an underlying *cause* in the strict sense, understood as some kind of infection, degeneration, trauma, genetic abnormality, biochemical imbalance, etc. A demon, by contrast, has an underlying *occasion* or circumstance by means of which it can gain a purchase on a person through certain vulnerabilities. The occasion can be a traumatic event or the existence of sin. Sin in turn can be the personal sin of the afflicted person, a sinful environment to which the person was exposed, or the general cosmological condition of original sin that permeates the world. This is specifically an occasion and not a cause, for the evil spirit that is thus "allowed in" is, properly speaking, itself the cause of the problem. The evil spirit then accounts for a variety of manifestations that constitute the person's affliction.

This disjunction accounts for the different way the two categories name the problem and the way they are posited as entities. A disease is more than a summary label for a constellation of symptoms, as a demon is more than a summary label for a constellation of manifestations. A disease names a third-person process that has a specifiable course, natural history, or range of predictable outcomes. A demon typically names a behavioral trait or affective state and posits it as a first-person process, endowing it with intentionality and, hence, precluding the possibility of either a completely circumscribed set of symptoms or a completely specifiable natural history. It is precisely by endowing the behavioral trait or affective state with intentionality that the religious system establishes the demonic entity as a cause rather than as something that is caused. In the psychiatric system the equivalent traits and states are objectified not as ontologically real entities but at the more specific descriptive or attribute level of symptoms.

Thus, although the phenomena of preobjective experience are treated or thematized by both systems as a kind of evidence for the posited objective entity, the epistemological status of this evidence is different in each instance. On the religious side a vision of light is a *manifestation* of a demon possessing one's *cakras*; pain is the manifestation of a being who will punish one for resistance to its will; dull-mindedness is a manifestation of a being intent on interfering with one's performance of the work of God. On the psychiatric side peculiar gustatory sensations are *symptoms* of temporal lobe epilepsy; insomnia, weight loss, and poor concentration are symptoms of depression; hearing thoughts and experiencing visual imagery are symptoms of atypical psychosis. Given this formulation it can be suggested that one of the difficulties in Peggy's attempts at healing was precisely a preoccupation with phenomena as evidence, and a consequent inability to deal adequately with the task of healing. In her isolation from like-minded individuals she became so intent on proving her diagnosis that she cultivated the very phenomena she hoped to eliminate.

However, the relation among manifestations of a demon need not be as systematic as those among symptoms of a disorder. It is true that specific spirits are sometimes identified by specific manifestations (Csordas 1990b), but my point is somewhat different. In a psychosomatic model, emotions can be understood as causing physical distress. Thus, in Martin's case, clinical consultant 1 suggests that "chronic entrenched feelings of guilt and anger" are directly associated with experience of chronic pain. Charismatic healing ministers' familiarity with popular psychology includes the concept of psychosomatic distress, and in practice they tend to integrate it into their work. However, positing an evil spirit preempts the direct connection between pain and affect: the spirit causes them both, or different spirits cause them. I suggest that Peggy's strict adherence to the logic of demonic causality prevented her from seeing the interrelation of features of Martin's distress in any other way. The manifestations have no inherent relation among themselves as do symptoms; they are related only as items in a list of problems caused by the demon.

Once the entity of demon or disease is objectified, it in turn becomes the trope by means of which experience is organized, interpreted, and thematized. This leads to rather different consequences in the two accounts. A demon is posited as an *oppression* of the afflicted with the intent to achieve control of a person's soul, initiating a powerful existential *struggle*. Negative experiences are thematized as forms of oppression. In the strongest formulation of this logic, there would appear to be no compelling reason to look for a relationship of causation or influence between thought and emotion on the one hand and sensory disturbance on the other. Suffering is cumulative, each form being just one more way that the person is hurt, one more channel of demonic harm, one more area of life under siege.

The process of psychiatric disease, however, is posited not as oppression but as disorder. Experiences thematized under the trope of disorder are those which can influence one another, rebound upon one another, and especially mask one another *via* mechanisms such as dissociation, obsession, and somatization. Of particular interest with respect to lived body experience is the concept of somatization, which in psychiatry and anthropology is variously defined as presentation of physical symptoms in the absence of organic pathology, amplification of organic physical symptoms beyond physiological expectations, presentation of somatic symptoms as an alternate expression of personal or social problems, and a mechanism by which emotions give rise to somatic signs and symptoms (Kirmayer 1984). In the present case, although organic pathology in the form of temporal lobe epilepsy or biological (hereditary) depression are not ruled out, somatization can be understood as a transmutation of cognition and affect.

The relationships among evil spirits are markedly different than the relationships among illnesses. Differential diagnosis is precisely a process of differentiation, whereas the discernment of evil spirits is additive. Temporal lobe epilepsy may be ruled out in favor of schizophrenia in Martin's case, meaning that symptoms originally suggesting epilepsy will appear in a different configuration and carry different connotations with regard to the expected course of the illness. The healer does not rule out the presence of particular evil spirits, for discernment of a spirit's presence carries with it an apodictic certainty. It is almost never a question of reorganizing the manifestations in a more satisfactory way under the name of a different demon, although the presence of additional spirits may be discovered.

It is, however, common for evil spirits to gather in clusters and "work together" and, in addition, to be under the hierarchical coordination of a single "master" or "manager" spirit. By itself, this clustering might seem analogous to the patterning of symptoms into a syndrome, but to make this analogy would be to err from the analysis that demon is to manifestation as disease is to symptom. A more accurate parallel is as follows. Insofar as the differential diagnostician is left with more than one apparently confirmed diagnosis, the diseases are superimposed and understood as complicating one another, but very likely they will be analyzed into primary and secondary diagnoses, such as schizophrenia with secondary anxiety and somatization. Similarly, the Catholic charismatic healer might discern a principal spirit of Self-Destruction, with attendant spirits of Rebellion, Hatred, and Anger.

We have already suggested that positing a demon is in one sense a rhetorical strategy, and there are indeed a variety of intriguing analyses of sickness as rhetorical process (Frankenberg 1986; Chesebro 1982). Can it be said that making a diagnosis is a rhetorical strategy in the same sense or on the same level of analysis as discovering a demon? Superficially they

have in common that they name the problem, and we can concur with arguments that naming may both offer a sense of control and the reassurance of
knowing what is wrong, and may limit the choices for treatment and shape
the course of an illness. From the perspective of labeling theory, it can also
be argued that demon and disease both insinuate themselves into the very
being of a person, not only accounting for symptoms but transforming a
person's identity and experience of self. What makes these parallels superficial is that the way demon and disease name a problem and the way they
exist as entities bespeak two different culturally constituted ways of organizing experience in a therapeutic process.

A more significant sense of the parallelism between demon and disease
as rhetorical strategies can be made clear by being specific about what the
charismatic discernment of evil spirits is *not*: itself a symptom of psychopathology. Henderson (1982) discusses "demonological neuroses" as
they appear for psychiatry, giving a case of Freud's along with one of his
own. He argues that the phenomenon can be understood in terms of internal object relations theory and as an indication of psychodynamic processes
of introjection and incorporation. However, the cases he discusses are ones
in which the presence of a demon is the patient's presenting complaint, and
hence part of the patient's pathology. In the case of Martin, and in most situations of Deliverance among Catholic charismatics, the presence of an evil
spirit is not given but discovered or discerned by the healer. Even when the
evil spirit names itself through the voice of the afflicted person, it usually
does so only on direct questioning by the healer.

Catholic healers themselves have encountered cases like those discussed by Henderson. One healer told of a man who had contacted several
priests in vain in the belief that he was being tortured by evil spirits. After
spending several sessions with this man himself, the healer concluded that
he could be of no help. He indicated that the man probably had serious
emotional problems rather than demonic oppression, and suggested to him
that the reason he had gone from priest to priest was that none would validate his self-attribution of demonization. We see here that care must be
taken to distinguish between evil spirits as a symptom of psychopathology
and as the religious equivalent of a diagnostic category. Whereas in Martin's case it may be legitimate to describe the voices he hears in terms of ego
introjection, the evil spirit must itself be described in terms of externaliza-
tion in roughly the same sense as is a disease.

Yet where these two entities diverge the most is precisely in their
rhetorical properties or possibilities. The fact that an evil spirit is a first-
person process with an intentional history rather than a third-person process with a natural history means that it can be questioned and commanded. Hence, it can be manipulated in its intimate relations with the afflicted
person. Moreover, the form of this intervention is the same whatever spirits

might be discerned to be present, and the healing is culminated when the evil spirit is ritually commanded to depart. The psychiatrist does not command schizophrenia or depression in the same way as the healer commands an evil spirit, but intervenes in it as in an event or against a thing. If the psychiatric patient acknowledges the presence of a disease it is something he "has" rather than something vicious that is attacking him, or something he already "is" ("I guess I'm crazy") rather than something that is not him but wants to possess him.[11] Moreover, because each disease implies a different natural history, it also implies a different treatment; the psychiatrist is much less comfortable in saying that psychotherapy is appropriate for all psychiatric disease than the healer is in saying that Deliverance prayer is appropriate for all instances of demonic oppression.

Again, because a demon is a first-person entity, it can play an immediate rhetorical role as an actor in the healing process, although some charismatic healing ministers refrain from informing supplicants that they have discerned a demonic presence, preferring to cast it out silently and thus avoid disruption and histrionic display. On the other hand, because a disease is essentially a third-person entity it can still more easily be thought of as treatable without, for example, the psychiatric patient ever knowing that it is called schizophrenia. Yet even here, some advocates of "psychoeducational" programs regard naming and understanding the illness as essential to its treatment. Moreover, in a rhetorical sense, diseases can sometimes be granted at least a metaphorical intentionality, as when cancer is described as a "vicious killer" or an "invader." There is a profound qualitative gap, however, between understanding the hearing of voices as a symptom and as an intentional verbalization. Martin sometimes experienced what seemed to be three different voices. However, he believed that in fact a single spirit was "mimicking" being three. Peggy's religious interpretation was that first of all this was exactly the kind of deception that is typical of spirit behavior, and second that the three-in-one illusion was an intentional blasphemy on the part of the spirit, in diabolical imitation of the godhead of trinitarian Christianity.

If the potential multiplication of Martin's voices can be understood as the potential for dissociation and fragmentation of self, then Peggy's rationale for keeping them unified appears as a kind of spiritual damage control. This is especially the case given the ominous presence of Andronius, the master spirit. Already beyond control, to grant a multiplicity of voices and identities to the spirit would surely have added to the sense of danger in the situation. On the other hand, in more typical cases there may be a rhetorical advantage to having clusters of spirits present, both in that it allows a more complex interpretation of what may be a very complex personal situation, and in that it allows a feeling of incremental progress if demons can be expelled one by one over the course of several healing ses-

sions (cf. Csordas 1983, 1988). There appears to be nothing directly parallel to this in psychiatric treatment, which is not to say that psychiatric diseases do not have rhetorical properties of their own. Certainly doctors and
patients both can construct elaborate discourses ("let me tell you about my
schizophrenia...") about a disease in such a way as to influence the course
of an illness.

The fact that demon and disease are constituted differently and hence
have different properties does not in itself determine their relation should
they both be applied in a particular case. Demon and disease can be completely redundant, accounting for exactly the same constellation of symptoms but applying at different ontological levels: healing minister 4 asserted
that schizophrenia and the effects of demons can be identical, and only with
the spiritual gift of discernment can they be distinguished. They can overlap, including either variations in features or variant interpretations of the
same features, as was evident in the comparison between healing ministers 1
and 4, and in the reference by 5 to spiritual and psychological aspects of
the case. Demon and disease could be judged to coexist as mutually complicating conditions, or be mutually exclusive as strict alternatives. In the
commentaries of the charismatic healing ministers, the principal trope can
be either oppression or disorder, either evil spirit or psychiatric diagnosis.

Conclusion

The cultural comparison I have elaborated highlights the pragmatic
merit of conceiving not only demons, but also diagnostic categories or diseases as interpretive forms rather than as ontological entities. To see psychiatric diagnosis as an interpretive or hermeneutic process (Good and Good
1980) is essential to the development of methods for parallel analyses of religious and medical accounts of distress, wherein convergences and diver-
gences of presupposition and interpretation can be detailed systematically.

The phenomenological description of Martin's affliction as an embodied totality provides the basis for a critique of both these accounts. Disorder and oppression are each processes of an objective entity, either disease
or demon. In proposing that affect and cognition cause bodily sensations
through somatization, or that an internal mechanism transmutes them into
bodily signs, the clinical view misses the unity of somatic and psychic experience that we have demonstrated in the case study. In this way it is subject
to the same criticisms that can be made of any type of mechanistic empiricism (Merleau-Ponty 1962). On the other hand, in proposing that all sensory, somatic, cognitive, and affective manifestation are caused by a demon,
the notion of oppression admits that somatic and psychic experience are all
of a piece by placing them on a par. This notion, however, makes the error
of attributing the unity to an abstract constituting consciousness, namely

the evil spirit, instead of to the essential unity of the human being in which every modality of perception is conditioned by every other. In this way it is subject to the same criticisms that can be made of any type of rationalist intellectualism (Merleau-Ponty 1962).

I have argued that the paradigm of embodiment is useful in comparing different cultural accounts of experience by providing a description of the existential common ground from which those accounts are abstracted. In spite of this advantage, does phenomenological description of embodied experience offer merely another objectification of the same order as demon, disease, or emotion? My necessarily brief answer will be to show how the paradigm of embodiment helps to reveal the embedded themes that are elaborated as cultural objects by following Martin's experience through his eventual return to a moderate level of social functioning.

Let us return to the images of dissolution, dismemberment, and immobility that we found to be themes of Martin's lived body experience. During the final period in which I followed this case, Peggy reported that feelings of fluidity and dissolving no longer characterized Martin's experience, while most other problems remained. It would appear that the reintegration of body image was his critical achievement. Judging by the language of panic and self-alienation in which he described it, this had been the most distressing dimension of Martin's affliction.

Certainly, in a society where the ethnopsychology of the ego ideal is radically individualistic, an integrated body image could be expected to be critical to acceptable daily functioning. From the perspective of embodiment, a bit of data that may otherwise appear as minor emerges as prominent in Martin's move toward engagement in the world of daily life: he had begun swimming almost every day. In her idiom, Peggy interpreted this as beneficial primarily in terms of "cooling" him from the heat of his oppression. In the phenomenological idiom we can suggest that the flow of water over his skin helped redefine body boundaries against dissolution, that the coordinated muscular action helped redefine bodily integrity against dismemberment, and that continuous motion helped redefine the ability to act against immobility. Yet, Martin had no more than reached another plateau, and insofar as he continued to suffer with only the outward appearance of normality, the evil spirit appears as a condensed symbol of his affliction. From a perspective outside the religious definition of reality, a demon from which one can be delivered may be a metaphor of disease; a demon from which one cannot be delivered is a metaphor of chronicity.

Beyond the questions of metaphor, translation, or equivalence of meaning, analysis of religious and psychiatric meanings in this case suggests the fruitfulness of a cultural phenomenology in comparing radically different accounts of experience. A return to the phenomena of preobjective experience reveals the common ground from which such accounts are built, through alternative thematizations that lead to the positing of cultural objects such as demons and diseases. I have attempted to describe the existential ground presupposed by religious and clinical reflection, and in so doing argued that to explain religious phenomena of affliction solely in medical terms is to merely put one view of the world in place of another.

Acknowledgments

Earlier versions of this paper were presented to the Seminar in Clinically Relevant Medical Anthropology at Harvard University, where valuable comments were offered especially by Arthur Kleinman, Byron Good, and Janis Jenkins. A version was presented to the invited symposium on The Dialectic of Medical and Sacred Realities at the 1986 annual meetings of the American Anthropological Association, where valuable comments were added by Jean Comaroff, Stanley Tambiah and Atwood Gaines. The paper was completed under support from NIMH grant 2ROl-MH40473-04.

Notes

1. In all, I conducted three interviews with Peggy during the spring and summer of 1986. These were followed up with periodic phone conversations that continued for two and one half years. Although it was clear that I offered no therapeutic help or direct contribution to the religious resolution of the problem, Peggy remained open to my questions on the grounds that, at the least, the account of Martin's trials could help other similarly afflicted people in the future. On these grounds she also (unsuccessfully) encouraged Martin to complete a standard psychiatric symptom checklist (SCL-90). Although she understood that it was designed to assess symptoms of psychopathology, she was firmly convinced that his was a religious, instead of a psychiatric, problem.

2. In the charismatic religious tradition demons typically have names drawn from the cultural repertoire of negative affects, personality traits, and behaviors (Csordas 1983).

3. Peggy rejected the notion that the spirit could be negotiated with or "converted" on the grounds that it is one of Satan's minions and as such is irredeemably diabolical. She also rejected the notion that the spirit was Martin's deceased father, although such an identification would be acceptable to some Catholic charismatic healers who practice "generational" or "ancestral" healing (Csordas 1988).

4. Nevertheless, in these curses it never directly utters the name "Jesus." This is a notable element of cultural and religious shaping or modeling of the spontaneous audition and can be interpreted according to the belief that Jesus is so powerful that a demon fears to use his name even in a curse.

5. Compare the discussion of superimposition of images in hallucination by Merleau-Ponty (1962:334–45).

6. Compare the theory of emotions proposed by William James (ca. 1890) (James 1967) in which emotional experience is a response to prior biological and physical changes.

7. The formal Church rite of exorcism differs from Deliverance prayer in two important respects. First, it implies a full-blown possession in which the demon is understood to be inside a person and in control of all that person's faculties. In a situation requiring Deliverance, the demon is typically outside the person, "harassing" and "oppressing" rather than possessing him. This distinction in degree of severity is crucial to the claim of legitimacy for Deliverance prayer, which is borrowed from the protestant Pentecostal tradition, within the Catholic setting. It thus bears directly on the second difference between the two ritual forms. That is, exorcism must be performed by a priest with the formal consent of the local bishop, and requires an eligibility procedure in which all other causes, including psychopathology, must be systematically excluded before causality is attributed to an evil spirit. Deliverance prayer, in theory because it is assumed to be less serious, is often performed by lay people. The format of the prayer is much more flexible than that of exorcism, and the presence of an evil spirit is established not through a formal procedure but through the discernment of the healer or healers. (Deliverance prayer is often performed in teams of several healers whose "spiritual gifts" are complementary.)

8. There was no noticeable manifestation of the evil spirit during that portion of the baptismal rite that includes a prayer for exorcism; neither was there any evidence that the spirit's hold was weakened by the rite. Although I questioned Peggy specifically about this, she appeared not to have regarded it as a significant moment. With regard to overt behavioral "manifestations," however, it is noteworthy that the evil spirit made its presence felt in any situation that might have resulted in public embarrassment for those involved.

9. The situation is more complex than is evident from the cases that typically achieve notoriety in which medical treatment is objected to on religious grounds by the parents of a minor afflicted with life-threatening illness (see, for example, Redliner and Scott 1979) .Within any healthcare system, the relation between any two forms of healing may be characterized as compatible alternatives, conflicting or contradictory alternatives, complementary forms addressing different aspects of a problem, or coexistent and noninteracting forms.

10. This integrated approach to pain in American culture is taken up in the recent work of Good et al. (in press).

11. The distinction between "I have" and "I am" in an illness has recently been discussed specifically with respect to schizophrenia by Estroff (1989).

References

American Psychiatric Association (APA)
1987 Diagnostic and Statistical Manual, 3rd Edition (DSM-III). Washington, D.C.: A.P.A.

Black, Richard G.
1975 The Chronic Pain Syndrome. Surgical Clinics of North America 55(4): 999–1011.

Bouckoms, Anthony, R.E. Litman and L. Baer
1985 Denial in the Depressive and Pain-Prone Disorders of Chronic Pain. Advances in Pain Research and Therapy 9:879–87.

Bourguignon, Erika
1976   The Effectiveness of Religious Healing Movements: A Review of Recent Literature. Transcultural Psychiatric Research Review 13(1):5–21.

Brena, Steven and Stanley Chapman
1985   Acute vs. Chronic Pain States: The Learned Pain Syndrome. Clinics in Anesthesiology 3(1):41–55.

Brown, George and T. Harris
1978   The Social Origins of Depression. New York: Free Press.

Campbell, E. J. M.
1976   Clinical Science. In Research and Medical Practice: Their Interaction. Ciba Foundation Symposium 44. Amsterdam: Elsevier.

Chesebro, James
1982   Illness as a Rhetorical Act: A Cross-Cultural Perspective. Communication Quarterly (Fall) 30:321–331.

Csordas, Thomas
1983   The Rhetoric of Transformation in Ritual Healing. Culture, Medicine, and Psychiatry 7(4):333–375.
1985   Medical and Sacred Realities: Between Comparative Religion and Transcultural Psychiatry (Review). Culture, Medicine, and Psychiatry 9(1):103–111.
1987   Health and the Holy in African and Afro-American Spirit Possession. Social Science and Medicine 24(1):1–11.
1988   Elements of Charismatic Persuasion and Healing. Medical Anthropology Quarterly 2(2):121–142.
1990a The Psychotherapy Analogy and Charismatic Healing. Psychotherapy 27(1):79–80.
1990b Embodiment as a Paradigm for Anthropology. Ethos 18(1):5–47.
n.d.   Somatic Modes of Attention. In Meaning, Context, and Experience: Interpretive Violence and the Living Body in a World of Contradictions. Gilles Bibeau and Ellen Corin (eds.). Paris: Mouton de Gruyter. In Press.

Dow, James
1986   Universal Aspects of Symbolic Healing: A Theoretical Synthesis. American Anthropologist 88(1):56–69.

Estroff, Sue E.
1989   Self, Identity, and Subjective Experiences of Schizophrenia: In Search of the Subject. Schizophrenia Bulletin 15:189–196.

Favazza, Armando
1982   Modern Christian Healing of Mental Illness. American Journal of Psychiatry 139(6):728–735.

Frankenberg, Ronald
1986   Sickness as Cultural Performance: Drama, Trajectory, and Pilgrimage: Root Metaphors and the Making Social of Disease. International Journal of Health Services 16(4):603–626.

Gaines, Atwood
1982   The Twice-Born: 'Christian Psychiatry' and Christian Psychiatrists. Culture, Medicine and Psychiatry 6:305–324.

Geertz, Clifford
1984 "From the Native's Point of View." In Culture Theory. R. Shweder and R. LeVine (eds.). Cambridge: Cambridge University Press.

Good, Byron and Mary-Jo DelVecchio Good
1980 The Meaning of Symptoms: A Cultural Hermeneutical Model for Clinical Practice. In The Relevance of Social Science for Medicine. Leon Eisenberg and Arthur Kleinman (eds.). Dordrecht: D. Reidel.

Good, Byron, Henry Herrera, Mary-Jo DelVecchio Good and James Cooper
1982 Reflexivity and Countertransference in a Psychiatric Cultural Consultation Clinic. Culture, Medicine, and Psychiatry 6(3):281–303.

Good, Mary-Jo DelVecchio, Paul E. Brodwn, Byron J. Good
and Arthur Kleinman, eds.
In press Pain as Human Experience: Anthropological Studies in American Culture. Berkeley: University of California Press.

Goodman, Felicitas
1981 The Exorcism of Anneliese Michel. New York: Doubleday.

Gupta, Madhulika A.
1986 Is Chronic Pain a Variant of Depressive Illness? A Critical Review. Canadian Journal of Psychiatry 31:241–248.

Henderson, W.
1982 Healing and Affliction. Boston: Beacon Press.

Insel, Thomas, et al.
1985 Obsessive-Compulsive Disorder: An Anxiety Disorder? In Anxiety and the Anxiety Disorders. A. H. Tuma and J. O. Maser (eds.). Hillsdale, NJ: Erlbaum Publishers.
1982 Exorcism and Possession in Psychotherapy Practice. Canadian Journal of Psychiatry 27(2):129–134.

James, William
1967 The Emotions. In The Emotions. C. Lange and W. James (eds.). New York: Hafner.

Kenny, Michael
1986 The Passion of Ansel Bourne: Multiple Personality in American Culture. Washington, D.C.: Smithsonian Institution.

Kirmayer, Laurence
1984 Culture, Affect, and Somatization. Transcultural Psychiatric Research Review 21(4):160–187, 237–261.

Kleinman, Arthur
1980 Patients and Healers in the Context of Culture.Berkeley: University of California Press.
1983 Editor's Note. Culture, Medicine, and Psychiatry 7(1):97–99.

Mauss, Marcel
1950 Les Techniques du Corps. In Sociologie et Anthropoplogie. Paris: Presses Universitaires.

McGuire, Meredith
1982 Pentecostal Catholics: Power, Charisma, and Order in a Religious Movement. Philadelphia: Temple University.

Merleau-Ponty, Maurice
1962 Phenomenology of Perception. New Jersey: Humanities Press.

Monfouga-Nicolas, Jacqueline
1972 Ambivalence et Culte de Possession. Paris: Éditions Anthropos.

Redliner, Irwin and Clarissa Scott
1979 Incompatibilities of Professional and Religious Ideology: Problems of Medical Management and Outcome in a Case of Pediatric Meningitis. Social Science and Medicine 13(2B):89–93.

Rhodes, Lorna Amarasingham
1980 Movement among Healers in Sri Lanka: A Case Study of a Sinhalese Patient. Culture, Medicine, and Psychiatry 4(1):71–92.

Sacks, Oliver
1985 Migraine (3rd ed.). New York: Simon and Schuster.

Schilder, Paul
1950 The Image and Appearance of the Human Body. New York: International Universities Press.

Tambiah, Stanley
1977 The Cosmological and Performative Significance of a Thai Cult of Healing through Meditation. Culture, Medicine and Psychiatry 1(1):97–132.

Turner, Bryan
1984 The Body and Religion. In The Body and Society. Bryan Turner. Oxford: Basil Blackwell.

Turner, Judith and Joan Romano
1984 Review of Prevalence of Coexisting Chronic Pain and Depression. Advances in Pain Research and Therapy 7:123–130.

6

Medical/Psychiatric Knowledge in France and the United States: Culture and Sickness in History and Biology*

Atwood D. Gaines

Introduction

This chapter initiates an examination of the ontological status of "biology" in French and American biomedicine in the context of an ethnological study. The study considers two aspects of these Western biomedical systems. French somatic disturbances are discussed and their classification within U.S. medicine is considered. These disorders would appear as psychiatric problems in the U.S. The Sickness History of these forms of dysphoric affect then is presented, drawn largely from theology and the history of Latin religion. Then, reversing things, I examine U.S. social classification and patienthood and show the absence in France of the U.S.'s peculiar social classificatory system. Identical research (e.g., epidemiological) and clinical practices are shown to be impossible in the two traditions because of divergent sickness histories and conceptions of biology. Biology here is construed as a key symbol uniting disparate meanings and embodying cultural ideals of science and progress in U.S. medicine. Overall, the paper analyzes two areas of U.S. and French medicine in a way which allows each to serve as a standard of evaluation for the other. The paper represents the beginnings of an ethnology of biomedicines as cultural systems and is intended as a contribution to the anthropologies of biomedicine and of science.

Sickness History

The analysis demonstrates that certain central conceptions are not shared between the two biomedicines. The distinctiveness of the systems, it

---

*The short original version of the present paper, then titled, "Culture and Medical Knowledge in France and America," was read at the American Anthropological Association Meeting in Washington, D.C., December 1985.

is argued, derives from their unique "Sickness Histories," sedimented historical experiences from which have been created conceptions of particular sickness entities and their culturally constructed social contexts (e.g., "races," "classes," genders, age groups, regional or religious groups). Culture histories may be seen as containing, among other things, sickness histories. These are seen here as serving as culturally particular models of and charters for past and present responses (individual and group) to culturally defined sickness events.

Sickness histories, I shall argue, constitute the *conceptual categories* within and through which "local knowledge" (Geertz 1983) is expressed. The expression of this aspect of local cultural knowledge is the stuff from which professional and popular medical knowledge, practice, and organization are constructed. Those elements of medical knowledge and medical systems constructed on sickness histories include personal/cultural cognitive understandings of sickness such as Semantic Illness Networks (Good 1977), Explanatory Models (Kleinman 1980), and "prototypes and chain complexes" (Young 1982). However, sickness histories are categories of cultural thought and hence may be said to structure and to provide the content of medical discourse (Good and Good 1982), to determine a culturally (including scientifically) appropriate array of "core clinical functions" of a local healthcare system (see Kleinman 1980), and to promote the development of local, including biomedical, systems' medical specialties and their sickness categories (i.e., nosologies). Sickness histories are those historical experiences out of which a culture's folk and professional ethnomedicines fashion their understandings of sickness and ascribe meaning to them such that people organize themselves in a culturally sensible way to address their experiences. The notion of sickness history allows us to understand why cultures have distinctive and particular etiological theories, medical organizations, sickness realities, and specific means for diagnosing and treating them.

Perspectives on Medicine

This paper represents a shift in interest from early social scientific interests in health and illness in modern society. That work included the sociological concern for the patient and the physician, primarily in terms of their social roles (e.g., Apple 1960; Koos 1954; Freidson 1961; Parsons 1951). Subsequently, medical training and socialization became foci of research interest (e.g., Becker et al. 1961; Merton, Reader and Kendall 1957). An interest in medicine as a profession developed still later (e.g., Freidson 1975). An anthropological path, first opened by Caudill, Devereux, and Henry (see Gaines and Hahn 1985) and sociologist Renée Fox (see Maretzki 1985), has been retaken with new emphases, perspectives, and tools.

Modern medical anthropological interest has focused on the actual knowledge and practice of biomedicine, rather than employing idealized images, whether positive (e.g., Foster and Anderson 1978; Hughes 1968) or negative (e.g., Baer, Singer and Johnson 1986; Frankenberg 1980; Navarro 1976). Some research endeavors were undertaken as theoretical enterprises while others were directed toward both understanding and improving medical and psychiatric care (e.g., Bosk 1979; Engel 1977; Hahn and Gaines 1985; Kleinman, Eisenberg and Good 1978; Mishler et al. 1981; Young 1980, 1981, 1982).

The key characteristic of most such studies is that they have developed and employed perspectives from modern interpretive social science, itself derived from the work of such scholars as Weber, Schutz, Mead, Dilthey, Husserl, Turner, and Geertz (Rabinow and Sullivan 1979, 1987). Interpretive studies sought to demarcate and focus on biomedical knowledge and practice as culturally constructed and as problematic. That is, medical knowledge was not seen as given in or reflecting an autonomous, independent "nature" (e.g., Gaines 1979, 1982a,b; Gaines and Hahn 1982; Gordon 1988; Kleinman, Eisenberg and Good 1978).

In the late 1970s an aspect of Western medicine, psychiatry, was first defined as a "cultural system" (Gaines 1979, after Geertz 1971, 1973) with the other specialties of medicine becoming so viewed shortly thereafter (Gaines and Hahn 1982; Hahn and Gaines 1985; Hahn and Kleinman 1983). This formulation has been recently restated (Rhodes 1990). A similar approach, derived from the sociology of knowledge and termed *social constructionism*, developed in British sociology (Wright and Treacher 1982a). The term *cultural constructivism* has been proposed more recently to distinguish the anthropological from the sociological enterprise and to label, develop, and distinguish interpretive social science in medicine from empiricist, functionalist critical medical anthropologies (Gaines 1991, chapter 1, this volume).

Especially important has been the demonstration that medicine is both a part and an expression of a particular culture and society. This contrasts with the critical medical anthropological view wherein medicine is seen as constituting a distinct social stratum. This stratum is said to be ideologically distinct and autonomous from the wider society and is set apart and opposed to it. Medicine is said to function as a system of social control (Navarro 1976; Waitzkin 1979) and as establishing hegemony over one society or another (e.g., Frankenberg 1980, 1988). Medicine's function and its being are seen as a "reflection" or "product" of one or another asserted material entity, e.g., a capitalist world system, means, modes, and/or relations of production (Baer, Singer and Johnson 1986; Frankenberg 1988; Waitzkin 1979; also see Rabinow and Sullivan 1987). Such functionalist arguments typically are made by self-labeled "critical theorists" about medicine and other professions.

However, Marxist and critical analyses actually, "hide precisely the quality that endows medicine with such great potential ideological and cultural power. (They) hide its apparent distance and distinctiveness from other social practices" (Wright and Treacher 1982b:11). Critical approaches' use of notions of class and ideology make it quite impossible for us to differentiate medical from any other professional knowledge and any other professional practice such as law or politics. They also assume a homogeneity and universality that cannot be demonstrated ethnographically. These and other functionalist sociological approaches do not make central use of the key tool of modern social science and of the modern anthropological understanding of human events and experience: the concept of culture (Douglas 1979).

The central element in the new research perspective on modern medicine is that it is a cultural medicine, an "ethnomedicine," albeit a professional one. Further, biomedicine is a domain comprised of a system of sociocultural knowledge and practice focally concerned with cultural definitions and notions of self, existence, morality, mortality and morbidity, and of nature (Gaines 1982b, 1992; Hahn 1985; Gordon 1988; Young 1990).

In medicine we find the contrasting "medical model" of sickness. In this model, disorders are constructed in purely biological terms (Engel 1977; Mishler et al. 1981). Those disorders that do not currently fit into this model are assumed to be explicable in biological terms at some future time when biological knowledge, it is assumed, will have increased such that the pathological processes will have yielded to, and/or arisen into, the gaze of medicine and psychiatry (Foucault 1963).

In biomedicine, universal sickness entities are seen as expressed in acultural, empirical, pathophysiological processes and histopathological structures. The model, "assumes disease to be fully accounted for by deviations from the norm of measurable biological (somatic) variables. It leaves no room within its framework for the social, psychological and behavioral dimensions of illness" (Engel 1977:130); nor does it allow for cultural dimensions (Kleinman 1986, 1988) including the sociocultural meaning of "norms" which, for this writer, encompasses the others. The professional ethnomedicine of Western culture may be properly characterized as 'a preeminently, even exclusively, biological medicine' (Gaines and Hahn 1985). Hence, an appropriate designation for this domain of Western cultures is biomedicine.[1]

Analysis suggests that some rather central conceptions are not shared between French and United States biomedicines. The two biomedicines appear not to be simply units or divisions of a universal medical system focused on a universal natural biology and pathology. Distinct medical systems question the notion that one biomedicine is exercising hegemony over all other medical systems of the world(e.g., Singer 1986; Frankenberg

1988). Rather, these professional ethnomedicines appear as distinct symbolic systems which, like world religions, are locally received and constructed and, through local history, create and (re)interpret central symbols (e.g., biology). The distinctiveness of biomedical systems derives from their unique sickness histories which incorporate theological and social historical elements and from their particular medical/social histories (e.g., see Lesch on the emergence of experimental physiology and its method in France in the last century [1984]).

Culture history provides the semantic richness, the polysemous character of sickness experiences. Culture history contains sickness histories which serve as charters for subsequent personal and group responses to contemporary illness experiences. Below, I present data on sickness entities in France that are considered somatic disturbances. These would be classified, if they existed, as psychiatric problems in the United States. The sickness history of these forms of dysphoric affect is presented. It largely derives from theology and the history of Latin religion (see also Gaines [1991] from which this is drawn). The unique sickness history explains why these diseases/illnesses are not found in United States biomedicine or dominant popular culture. Such conditions are, however, widely found in industrial and nonindustrial Mediterranean traditions and their daughter Latin traditions in the New World.

Then, reversing things, I examine "racial" classification and patienthood in United States psychiatry and there indicate the absence in France of that peculiar system of social classification. It is shown how identical research (e.g., epidemiological) and clinical practices are, therefore, impossible in the two traditions. Overall, the paper analyzes two areas of U.S. and French medicine in a way which allows each to serve as a standard of evaluation for the other in one domain. This arrangement allows us to view two areas of each medicine in a brief report and prevents the use of one form of biomedicine as an implicit, unexamined and idealized, standard of comparison as has been the case in much of medical anthropological writings (Gaines and Hahn 1985), e.g., Foster and Anderson (1978) and Hughes (1968; 1990). The paper concludes with some explanations for the maintenance of the cultural ideal of a purely scientific, biologically-based biomedicine in the face of much contrary evidence. Biology is there construed as a *key symbol* uniting disparate meanings and embodying cultural ideals of science and progress (Ortner 1974).

Sickness in France

Spasmophilie

The last twenty years or so have seen a growing popular cognizance in France of a disease entity called *spasmophilie*. Spasmophilie, first noted in the French medical literature in the late 1950s, represents a new professional ethnomedical diagnostic entity. In the last decade or so, it has increased dramatically as a diagnosis, increasing some sevenfold in the decade between 1970 and 1980 (Payer 1990:38). Because both professional and lay persons recognize spasmophilie as a form of affliction, it is both an illness and a disease (Eisenberg 1977; Kleinman, Eisenberg and Good 1978). It is constructed as a medically and socially significant disorder; therefore, it is also a sickness in Young's (1982) sense. As we show that professional medicine's diseases are cultural constructs, the once useful distinction between disease and illness dissolves.

In the public media (in 1980 and 1983 in the author's experience) physicians and contemporary news reports suggested that as much as 35 percent of the adult French population may be affected annually. It is one of a number of diagnoses in France that are unknown in other Western countries (Gaines 1986a, b; Gaines and Farmer 1986; Helman 1990; Payer 1988). And we note that there are a number of diseases found in other Western countries that are unknown in France.

The condition of spasmophilie appears to be related to several other sickness entities found in France. These include *fatigué*, "tired, fatigued" (Dodier 1985) and *triste (or fatigué) tout le temps* ("sad [or tired/weary] all the time"), both discussed below. Spasmophilie has been accepted by the general population as a valid and recognizable illness. Informants stated that one could easily recognize the condition, making self-diagnosis possible. The public use of the label indicates the cultural sense which the condition makes, though its prevalence and incidence are as yet poorly understood.

The disorder is marked by a number of nondiagnostic symptoms such as mild fatigue, bodily aches, mild nausea, listlessness, loss of appetite, sleep disturbances, and distractibility. No particular symptomatic picture is asserted to be common to all cases; no identifiable, stable syndrome is asserted to exist. Symptoms vary from case to case as does their severity. Although U.S. physician informants can translate the term and even locate it in medical dictionaries, the term here refers to various forms of hypersensitivity, they have no knowledge of or reference for the term as a specific disease with a known etiology.

The diagnosis of the disorder, seen as a physical, medical problem and not a psychiatric one, actually depends upon the social state of the person. The disorder appears to the U.S. psychiatric observer as an expression of dysphoric affect expressive of an existential problem, not a syndrome of bodily aches and pains. In fact, it is common for one to be labeled as having a susceptibility to the disorder (one then is a *spasmophile*) in the *absence* of any symptoms at all. *Stress*, an idiomatic term recently applied to an historically ubiquitous French experience of life as wearing, difficult, and burdensome, and "mineral deficiencies" appear to be the most common etiological hypotheses (lay and professional) for the rather ill-defined malaise of spas-mophilie. A physician may prescribe magnesium, acupuncture but also rest and the seeking of care, specifically and especially in a secure surrounding, i.e., at one's family home, even if at far remove (see Payer 1990). The latter suggestion derives from a culturally constituted notion of vulnerability seen as characteristic of those away from home. In another Mediterranean cul-ture, a similar vulnerability of travelers or migrants is expressed as the sus-ceptibility to the affliction of "fright illness" among Iranians (Good and Good 1982). The contrasting but overlapping etiological hypotheses and treatment regimens suggest that social information and demeanor, rather than specific, pathognomonic physical symptoms, are central to diagnosis.

In this regard it is perhaps noteworthy to point out the typical promi-nence of social features in the diagnoses of disorders in the Mediterranean culture area and its Latin New World daughter cultures. These conditions are exampled by fright illness and "heart distress" among Iranians (see Good and Good 1982), the Italian evil eye (Foulks et al. 1977), Moroccan she-demon possession (Crapanzano 1973) and, in Latin America, *susto* (Rubel 1977), *tristitia* and *pena* (Tousignant 1984). (Scheper-Hughes [1988] incorrectly describes these latter forms as "wasting diseases" in her effort to categorize them as related to problems of hunger in Brazil.) (For a delin-eation of the Mediterranean culture area, see Davis 1977; Gaines 1978, 1982a; Gaines and Farmer 1986, Gilmore 1982; Peristiany 1966; Pitt-Rivers 1963, among others.) It is possible that the disorder is a new, modern label for an old idiom of distress, that of being *fatigué*, a condition described below.

Fatigué

Another disorder, labeled simply *fatigué*, used as an adjective and expressed as, *"je suis fatigué"* (I am tired (or fatigued)) or *"je me sens fatigué"* (I feel tired) is quite widespread in France. The expression refers to a state of being, an illness state, and may be contrasted with another experience of *la fatigue*, which expresses a sense of lassitude caused by work that is too difficult or too long (e.g., *Malgré la fatigue, j'écrit*— Despite fatigue, I (continue to) write).

In an article on sickness and its moral justification in the French workplace (Dodier 1985), "being tired" was shown to be a common sick-ness, in fact, one of the most common experienced by both blue- and white-collar workers. Diagnosis, treatment and management of this condition by physicians in France is usual, expected, and appropriate. Leaves of absence for "rest" ranging from a matter of days to a month or more are regularly prescribed by physicians and are deemed appropriate (morally justified) by both employers and co-workers.

The condition is not a symptom of another or other disorders. Rather, in this context, it refers to a specific disorder. One notes, though, that it is also the means by which the French express all manner of other illness states in terms of degree, ranging from "*un peu fatigué*" to "*bien fatigué*" to "*fatigué tout le temps*" ("a little tired," "very tired," "tired all the time") (for example, see Wylie 1957). Colloquially, the terms mean "mildly ill," "very ill," and "seriously ill." Only the first two terms may or may not also refer to other diseases recognized by biomedicine. The etiology of fatigué as a disorder is not overwork or lack of a few nights' sleep, both causes of *la fatigue*. Rather, the etiology of being *fatigué* is a perceived burdensome life situation. This condition may appear at any time and does not necessarily derive from a specific, unusually stressful period or noxious event in one's life. All aspects or phases of life are seen in France as difficult, burdensome, and taxing. One's day-to-day life is seen as a constant "struggle," which periodically simply weighs one down. In France, it is deemed appropriate to have a view of life as tragic or sad. To view life otherwise is an indication of immaturity and of a shallow personality (Gaines 1982a, b; Wylie 1957). This connection, of maturity and personal validity with the understanding of and appreciation for sadness and the tragic, is also integral to the cultural psychology of other areas of the Mediterranean including Iran (see Good 1977; Good, Good and Moradi 1985), Italy (Cornelisen 1971), Greece (Blue 1991; Campbell 1964; Lee 1959), and North Africa (Abu-Lughod 1986).

In France, medical leaves for fatigué are viewed routinely by employers, colleagues, and physicians as appropriate when other signs are present (drawn appearance, irritability). The disorder is widely recognized and morally sanctioned in popular and professional circles. We note also that the notion of tiredness as a common, morally justified, medically recognized and treated disease was entirely unproblematic to the French author Dodier (1985). However, such would clearly be problematic to U.S. clinicians, researchers, and lay readers. In U.S. folk and professional ethnomedicine, tiredness is a *symptom* of a number of disorders; it does not constitute a disorder in and of itself. In Dodier's work, he sought not to find a disease behind being tired, because being tired is the disease.

Triste/Fatigué Tout le Temps

A third disorder is known both in French professional and folk ethnomedicine; it is therefore both a disease and an illness as are spasmophilie and fatigué. This disorder is *triste (or fatigué) tout le temps* ("sad (or tired) all the time"). This disorder is a chronic version of fatigué with similar complaints and behavioral manifestations, but, it differs in two very important ways. It has a specific precipitating event, generally a personal loss or great disappointment, and it is chronic, which is to say of very long duration, ranging from years to a lifetime (Gaines and Farmer 1986; Gaines 1986a).

Informants queried in Paris and Strasbourg all knew of the disorder, could describe it and its various possible symptoms.[2] Each could relate a tale of one or more people personally known to them who had the disorder, many of whom had seen physicians. This and other research indicates that individuals will seek medical help for the disorder's symptoms and/or for exacerbations of the condition if not specifically for the disorder.

The symptoms of this French disorder are many and various and include chronic disturbances of vegetative signs, such as sleep and appetite, as well as problems of concentration and memory, sad affect, sometimes psychomotor retardation, chronic tiredness and weakness, distractibility, and other, but again nonspecific, multiple symptoms. "Sad (or tired) all the time" is a syndrome with a widely varying symptom picture. Its origins appear to lie in reactions to some form of perceived traumatic event, such as a miscarriage, the death of a child, spouse, or close friend, or the termination of an important relationship. *Parisien* and *Strasbourgeois* informants (in 1982 and 1983) also suggested that the precipitating event may not be a loss but a failure to achieve some important personal goal such as entrance to a favored school or winning an important sporting contest. Examples of both can be found in the literature and films of France (e.g., the film, *La Femme à Côté*, and the 1980s novels *Élise ou la Vrai Vie* and *Les Enfants du Siècle*).

An attempt to apply U.S. psychiatric nomenclature to the condition, sad/tired all of the time, would meet with failure, though it is in this domain of medicine that U.S. diagnosticians would turn immediately with the presentation of the variety of symptoms associated with this disorder. Taking the descriptive approach championed by the third *Diagnostic and Statistical Manual* of the American Psychiatric Association (1980), or its revision (DSM III-R, 1987), one could construct a label for the disorder, e.g., "chronic, reactive depression." In U.S. psychiatric theory and practice, however, such an entity is not only unknown; it is also impossible. A person with a normal premorbid personality, psychiatric colleagues assure me, could not develop a chronic reactive depression.[3] In Latin American and Mediterranean countries *nervios* appears in chronic reactive form as well, and the term is employed for what U.S. psychiatrist would label schizophrenia (Jenkins, this volume) or depression (e.g., Dugan 1988). (Although Dugan, we note, does not recognize the incompatibility of clinical depression with a chronic reactive syndrome labeled *nervios*.) The same folk and professional disorder is found in Greece as *Nevra* (Blue 1991).

Individuals afflicted by the illness are not in the least unable to care for self and others. The use of psychodiagnostic instruments employed do indicate the presence of clinical depression among these exemplary people, these dramatic embodiments of the conception of life as difficult and tragic. Because of their presence in the community of the living, rather than the past of the martyred saints, I have called these people "visible saints." They are referred to by friends and neighbors (but less often by their families) simply as "saints."

Ethnographic research, including the noting of the saint's social functioning and activity levels, easily disconfirmed the diagnosis of clinical depression, despite the subjects being easily moved to tears, exhibiting slight psychomotor retardation from time to time, frequent sad affect and the self-reporting of depressive symptoms ("symptoms" in terms of U.S. psychiatry). (See Gaines and Farmer [1986] for a detailed case history, cultural and historical background and context for visible sainthood, and psychodiagnostic test results.)

Though this problem is recognized widely, active interventions to alleviate the condition appear to informants as inappropriate. Informants see the condition as a reasonable response to misfortune. Significant others do not regard the condition as requiring immediate remedial medical action though it can and does have mild to profound effects on behavior and activity. In this the French show the cultural basis and "logic" of the idea that sickness conditions *necessitate* action to eliminate them (Parsons 1951). This sociological (and Northern European) perspective misses the cultural validity and value of illness in some cultures, such as the Mediterranean area, and suggests a cultural voice of social theory.

The primary response to the condition is to allow more-than-usual rest for periods that may extend for months or years. An attitudinal response of commiseration from significant others is appropriate. No cure is expected, just a modicum of relief from episodic exacerbations of the basic chronic picture. A reaction to single trauma, a loss or frustration, thus, can produce a chronic, even lifelong, sickness that alters mood, affect, and cognition as well as behavior. The response becomes a whole style of self-presentation and being in the world, i.e., the elements (cognitive, somatic, affective) are not distinct.

While manifested in the soma, these three disorders have neither a somatic seat nor etiology. Each sickness in its own way reflects culturally specific French views of the self (Gaines 1982a) and the nature and positive meaning of suffering in life. The latter is commonly manifested as a culturally expected "rhetoric of complaint," an aspect of local discourse which communicates the suffering and misfortune and, therefore, the worthiness of the speaker (Gaines 1982a). The illnesses also demonstrate the patterning of dysphoric affect in France and in the Mediterranean tradition more generally (see Gaines 1982a, 1987; Gaines and Farmer 1986; and Good, Good and Moradi 1985, for fuller accounts of the patterning of dysphoric affect in this tradition).

All of these conditions (and others, such as *crise de foie*, the famous French "liver disease") are widely known and diagnosed in the popular arena and are diagnosed and treated in general and specialized medical practice, primarily the former. (There is a strong emphasis on general practice in France such that French physicians specialize far less frequently than in U.S.[4] The specialists' mentalities are considered narrow; the generalist is more knowing and wise.)

Sickness History

How might we explain French professional and lay ethnomedical entities that are absent from the medical nomenclature and nosology of American professional and lay ethnomedicine? From an empiricist standpoint, the two biomedicines focus upon and are derived from a unified biological theory (or economic reality for other sorts of empiricists) and must share a knowledge which reflects a putative external, biological reality. Since they appear not to, at least as regards this sickness domain, different levels of development might be suggested, i.e., one is more "developed" than another.

French medicine is much older than U.S. biomedicine. Indeed, aspects of American biomedicine are modeled on areas in French medicine, such as in the use of statistics (Cassedy 1984) and in the relating of research to clinical practice (Lesch 1984). Therefore, it would be appropriate to suggest that U.S. biomedicine is not yet sufficiently developed to identify these disorders. While some may see this as unlikely, one cannot help but notice the fact notice that U.S. medicine has indeed begun the construction of "diseases" whose sole symptom, not essence, is chronic tiredness, i.e., initial constructions of an "Epstein-Barr" viral infection and more recently, CFS (Chronic Fatigue Syndrome).

A macroeconomic political economic approach would likewise deny culture and explain differences in experience- and culture-distant terms by applying empty labels such as "core," "peripheral," or even "semiperipheral," despite the fact that such terms applied to such a developed country as France demonstrate their relativistic nature and, therefore, any lack of utility (see also Rabinow and Sullivan 1987 on this point). I suggest a more plausible and semantically rich cultural historical argument may be advanced; 1) there are important differences among biomedicines, and that 2) such differences derive in part from distinct historical experiences with various sickness events, i.e., sickness histories.

Sickness histories may relate to and involve a number of topics including: the conceptual development of nosological systems (e.g., Gaines 1992; Menninger 1963), the history of patient roles and experiences (e.g., Herzlich and Pierret 1985), the organization of medical and public health practices and methods (Brandt 1985; Cassedy 1984; Pernick 1985; Lesch

1984; Starr 1982; Weisz 1990), the development of illness and/or practice
conceptions and focal medical concerns (e.g., Foucault 1963; Kleinman and
Good 1985; Jackson 1985), systems of production and distribution of medical knowledge (Young 1980, 1981), systems of social knowledge, classification and communalism in medicine (Brandt 1978, 1985; Gaines 1982b,
1985a, 1986b, 1987, 1989, 1992; Pernick 1985).

In short, such histories would be interpretive histories of medical
knowledge, practice, and organization in their cultural contexts. Noting
that other writers have begun to show the role of theology and philosophy
in the shaping of the experience of dysphoric affect in the West (see Jackson
1985; Lutz 1985; Obeyesekere 1985), we may turn to a brief examination of
aspects of religious history in the West that bear on the French disorders.

Religion and Medical History in France

Historical material suggests that the three disorders are related and,
indeed, likely share a common origin. An examination of the psychiatric
history of the notions of *acedia, tristitia,* and *melancholie,* forms of what
Jackson (1985) calls "dejected states," provide an understanding of *spasmophilie, fatigué* and *triste/fatigué tout le temps.*

Jackson finds three forms of dejected states, acedia, melancholia, and
tristitia, all of which "belong to the history of religion, in particular to the
religious scheme of the cardinal sins in Christianity" (1985:44). The condition of acedia, a sin, developed out of the examination of the particular
experiences of members of the desert anchorite community near Alexandria
in the fourth century (A.D.). The isolation and inactivity produced mental
states which detracted from contemplation. The unusual mental states of
acedia soon acquired behavioral referents. Shifts in emphasis from one pole
(mental state) to the other (behavioral modes) have occurred through the
centuries. On the one hand, acedia was described as "carelessness,"
"weariness," "exhaustion," "negligence," (in contemplative duties) and, on
the other, as "apathy," "anguish," "sadness," and "low spirits" (Jackson
1985:45). Here, the two behavioral and affective poles are explicit.

The concern for acedia changed. Originally seen only negatively as a
sin, acedia acquired a positive meaning. This positive meaning derived
from the view that the conditions of sadness and weariness were a result of
one's "penitence for sin" and/or one's "desire for perfection" (p.48). These
notions spread widely in Christendom beyond the clergy to the laity
between A.D. 1200 and 1450, especially after the Lateran Council
(1215–16) decided on the need to extensively disseminate penitential literature, clerical manuals (for the newly required sermonizing), and catecheti-
cal handbooks (Jackson 1985:48; Wenzel 1960).

The penitential literature spread the new benevolent view of acedia and tristitia, a term used interchangeably with acedia. In this view acedia, because it was a condition that afflicted only the devout penitent, seems to have become thought of as a form of penance itself (Jackson 1985; Wenzel 1960); that is, dejection was the penance of the devout. Penance was seen "as medicine for the soul" (McNeill and Gamer 1938:44). The most common governing medical principle of the time held that "contraries cured contraries" (Jackson 1985; McNeill and Gamer 1938). (One is reminded here of homeopathy's dictum, "Like cures like.")

Jackson points out how acedia and tristitia gradually lost their theological affinities, and the positive and negative connotations became part of the culture area's secular/philosophical theories of emotions. They later appeared in the context of medicine. The component of positive sorrow "became more identified with the Christian tradition of the sufferer as an object for care, concern and cure" (1985:53–54). The conception developed further into melancholie as the Church lost its explanatory powers over human behavior and, subsequently, there developed a renewed interest in classical writers. This Renaissance brought forth melancholie as both a medical term for an illness (Menninger 1963) and as a popular term referring to sadness (Jackson 1985).

The popular term referring to sadness also developed an association with the term (from Aristotle) *melancholia* and was subsequently associated in Latin countries with the very bright and the gifted; melancholia and brilliance were seen as dispositional companions. It is possible to see this association as late as the last century in France. There, and then, one saw frequently the association of the intellectual and the experience of sadness and/or sad, wasting diseases such as tuberculosis. This was the romantic vision of the pale, wan (tubercular) artistic intellectual (e.g., see Sontag 1977).

This history, brief as it is, provides us with some understanding of the meaning of dejected states and dysphoria in French culture and history. The meaning of such states, their positive value, and their cultural significance, make us understand better the existence and elaboration of related sickness conditions in popular culture and in that culture's professional ethnomedicine. The ethnomedicine is an expression of that tradition.

Acedia and tristitia evidently are the source of fatigué and triste/fatigué tout le temps and probably spasmophilie, as well. Elsewhere in Latin America, one finds the folk disorder of sadness called tristitia. The two poles or faces of acedia are well-preserved in contemporary medical and popular discourse with the mental/affective face presenting as triste while the behavioral face appears as fatigué in the alternate names of the contemporary disorder, triste/fatigué tout le temps. Spasmophilie and fatigué may themselves represent these same two faces and suggest a dualism with many forms in French culture. As well, this dualism appears in other Latin and

Mediterranean countries because the history of acedia, and the other cultural forms of despair, is shared with them and with many U.S. ethnics.

Here we see the historical development of folk theories which later appear in a biomedicine. Other, less historical works have also shown the presence of what I have termed "folk theories" in U.S. professional ethnomedicine (e.g., Brandt 1978, 1985; Cassedy 1984; Gaines 1979) as well as other professional ethnomedicines in Germany (Maretzki and Seidler 1985; Maretzki, this volume; Townsend 1978; Verwey 1985), England (Helman 1985), Greece (Blue 1991, this volume), and Canada (Lock 1985; Katz 1985, n.d.). The impress of culture on the biomedicines of Asia generally also has been noted earlier (e.g., Lock 1980; Ohnuki-Tierney 1984; Reynolds 1979; Weisberg and Long 1984).

The disorders considered here are seen in France as biologically based disorders, though their etiology is psychosocial. In fact, we see a slightly different notion of human biology and its relation to thought and experience than found in the United States. States of the body, fatigué and spasmophilie, both express and embody culturally constructed existential conceptions. Multiple, diverse physical symptoms are to be understood as expressions of unhappiness, loss, and or disappointment. In this, the body is an expression of the mind; and this is not unusual (i.e., "somatization" in U.S. psychiatry), but rather normal, customary, and expected in lay and professional circles in Mediterranean (and New World Latin) lands. Finally, we note here that these disorders, along with *crise de foie*, appear to represent some of the 15 percent of French diagnoses that are *not* shared with other Western professional ethnomedicines (Helman 1990; Payer 1990).

Such differences have to do with an aspect of cultural history heretofore neglected, i.e., sickness history, which may be seen as the historical basis for thinking at the individual popular, folk, and professional medical levels in a particular culture. I suggest that cultures maintain continuity with their past in the medical domain by importing their particular repertoire of sickness histories into contemporary popular and professional (ethno)medicines. This historical process of continuity and importation is one means by which the demonstrable variation among the world's biomedicines is developed. Diseases, as elements of medical knowledge, may be seen in this way as products of sickness histories, not as products of current hypothesized material forces. A brief example from the U.S. will suffice to show the relevance of culture and sickness history for an understanding of biomedicines.

Sickness and Identity in America

In U.S. biomedicine, practitioners believe themselves to be focused on a universal, objective, external biology. In this biology, they find the source and locus of diseases, themselves objective, empirically evident, and universal (Mishler et al. 1981). However, if we explore the U.S. system of social classification, we will discover that much of the research and practice in biomedicine, including psychiatry, is not grounded in an objective, external natural biology but rather in a culturally constructed folk biology and folk genetics.

Systems of social identity are known to be based in culturally specific criteria of relevance. These distinctions are often articulated in terms of biology in the U.S., the "biology of race" (Blu 1980; Boas 1966; Domínguez 1977, 1986; Gaines 1980, 1986b). Here one finds the peculiar belief in, and social and economic institutions based upon, the existence of human "races," a form of social classification with virtually no empirical basis. Demonstrative of the lack of coherence of racial theories, one finds various classificatory schemes in use with varying criteria of differentiation including geography (e.g., "Asians," "Africans," "Europeans"), language (Hispanics), claimed skin color ("white," "red," "black," "brown," "yellow," etc.) and even religion ("Jews," "Christians," "Moslems").

Elsewhere, I have detailed the problematics of the notion of "race" in psychiatric clinical practice and medical research (e.g., Gaines 1980, 1982b, 1985a, 1986b, 1987), and therefore simply emphasize the obvious here, i.e., that such folk theories hold a prominent place in U.S. biomedicine, as do notions of gender. Theories of "race" and gender differences are both versions of a folk biological theory. Holders of such theories believe differences among the "races" or the sexes exist and are a result of biology rather than reflections, and the socially produced results of, their own prejudices. Apparently, these prejudices distort both cognition and perception, and should, therefore, logically find their way into psychiatric classifications, all things being equal (which they are not).

The deleterious effect on perception and cognition of racism is obvious, for example, in the common gross misrepresentation of biological reality encoded in the notion itself. For example, most Native Americans are biologically part European, in many cases largely so, and not infrequently, for southern Native Americans, part West African as well. And, virtually all U.S. blacks or "African-Americans" are biologically part European, and again in many cases largely so. And, again, quite commonly at least for southerners, they are also part Native American (Gaines 1985a, 1987, 1989; Hallowell 1976; Montagu 1962; Watts 1981). Examples of famous black Americans with known lineal antecedents as much or more from Europe and Native North America as from West Africa, include Charley Patton, the archetypical Delta bluesman, Muddy Waters, the 'father of electric blues,' Chuck Berry, the primary architect of rock 'n' roll, and entertainer Eartha Kitt, among tens of millions of others.

As well, among individuals who are considered "white" and trace their ancestry back to early settlers in the American South, it should be pointed out that such individuals have, as a virtual certainty, African (i.e., West African) ancestry and even more certainly have African-American relatives. (One family, the Hairstons, has recognized this fact and annually holds a family reunion which includes thousands of both "white" and "black" Hairston family members.) It is apparent that medical work considering biological differences among "blacks and whites" constitutes an U.S. cultural fiction in the context of an ostensibly empirical biomedical science.

While advocates of biological views claim that biology is the cause of homogeneity, evolutionary biologists, cognizant of the local nature of biology (and zoology or botany) resulting from local factors affecting reproduction, regard biology as the prime cause of *diversity* (Kleinman 1988; Rosenfield 1986; Watts 1981). As Rosenfield (1986:22) points out, "Qualities we associate with human beings and other animals are abstractions invented by us that miss the nature of the biological variation" (in Kleinman 1988:19). The construction of the science of biology in the last century has incorporated aspects of other fields and asserted itself. A self-evident, external reality which justified the delineation of a separate field of scientific endeavor was lacking; its contemporary presence as a separate discipline is then a constructed presence, *not* a reflection of a natural world (see Coleman 1987).

Research on the treatments of choice and treatment recommendations in U.S. biomedicine demonstrates that diagnostic and therapeutic choices are often made on the basis of patients' social identity, whether it is "race," class, or sex (see for example, Brandt 1985; Brill and Storrow 1960; Derogatis et al. 1971; Dorfman and Kliner 1962; Enright and Jaeckle 1963; Harding and O'Barr 1987; Lock 1985; Myers and Schaffer 1958). For example, we find that in the United States of the last century the use of anesthesia after its introduction was based on racial and gender stereotypes (Pernick 1985). Today, the determination of appropriate patients for heart bypass surgery and even postoperative pain medication is based on gender stereotypes (Tobin et al. 1987). The form of intervention in psychiatry, pharmacotherapy, or psychotherapy is likewise today largely dependent on stereotypic attributions of "racial" and sexual identity rather than on putatively empirical psychiatric signs, symptoms or diseases (e.g., Neighbors et al. 1989; and see MacKinnon and Michels 1971).

Social identity has implications for clinical care and medical research. In psychiatry "Blacks" and Hispanics are often seen as "not psychologically minded" or as belonging to that group of patients termed "psychologically unsophisticated" (MacKinnon and Michels 1971). Because of this classification, somatic, including pharmacological agents, are seen as treatments of choice. U.S. biomedicine's division of the social world into "races" is unique to it and expresses its cultural context. While other cultures have notions of "race," they are distinct from that found in the United States (e.g., Japan, South Africa, China). The U.S. version of folk biogenetics assumes behavioral, and/or biological homogeneity within categories and assumes the categories to be reflections of nature rather than culture. As a result, we find that pharmacological (e.g., Lin, Poland and Lesser 1986), epidemiological (e.g., Holden 1991; Sommervell et al. 1989; Vernon and Roberts 1982), as well as biomedical practice is conducted and interpreted in these putatively natural biological/genetic terms. Research in France on social classification, however, shows us that the social world there is divided according to very different, cultural criteria.

Social Classification in France: the Contrast

Research on French social classification in Strasbourg (1974, 1981–3),[5] the capital of Alsace, the most eastern province of France, revealed two distinct systems of classification, one French and the other Alsatian. The latter is, in fact, merely a variation of folk German theories of social classification, as Alsatian culture is one of German culture's (not the State of Germany) daughter cultures. (See Gaines [1978, 1980, 1985c] for detailed analyses of social classification, including religious identity in Alsace.)

French ethnic identity is symbolized by culture, primarily in the form of language competency. Thus, anyone, regardless of "race" can become a French ethnic, physical appearance is not germane. (Apparel can be, as it can indicate a rejection of French culture ("civilization") as one sees today among some Arabic speakers and historically among some Orthodox and Hassidic Jews. Such people are the targets of the right wing in France.) As a consequence, one does not find hyphenated French people; one is French or one is not. In my research I have met people who, in the U.S., would be called Vietnamese-, Greek-, Italian (i.e., Friulian)-, African-, Japanese-, Moroccan-, or Armenian-American(s). But, in France, they were all considered by self and others as French ethnics.

In contrast to the means of acquiring French identity, one can only be born an Alsatian (or German) ethnic. To claim an Alsatian identity, one must have a known lineal antecedent who was or is Alsatian. Hence, one cannot assume the identity regardless of language competence, religion, residence, marriage, or appearance; one simply cannot become Alsatian. Among Alsatians, we find a racial theory that states that people are what they are because of their "blood" (*blut*), which is inherited. Therefore, individuals who are seen as phenotypically different, but who in fact have Alsatian ancestry, may be rejected as Alsatian ethnics. Informants from other lands (India, Africa, Asia) tell me that in Alsace, "they are a bit racist," but do not say this of the rest of France. These facts suggest the cultural basis of affiliation and of biology and genetics as used by this group; they constitute an "ethnobiology" and an "ethnogenetics."

We see two theories of cultural belonging, one cultural and one biolog-ical. We note, however, that the biological conceptualization of the Alsa-tian, and its parent Germanic tradition, is a folk biology and a folk theory of genetics and inheritance. The notion of biology as the key to psychiatric differences is in fact of German origin and comes directly from Kraepelini-an German psychiatry (Gaines 1992; Young 1988), and today may be found in both medical and popular domains (Townsend 1978).

The social world of France is classified in ways which are not compara-ble with American social classification. As a result, the clinical practices and research found in America based upon American notions of "race" are pecu-liar to U.S. biomedicine (see Farmer, this volume). However, I do not sug-gest that the French neither make invidious distinctions nor hold communal-istic views. Rather, I suggest their criteria and categories are different.

Biology as Key Symbol

These brief observations suggest that particular forms of communal-ism play a large role in U.S. medical ideology, practice and education (Brown 1979). Biological notions such as "race" and gender differences in U.S. medicine have evolved with U.S. social history and as such are part of the sickness histories of the United States which are not shared with France. In the same biological vein, one notes that writers concerned with women as subjects and objects of medical practice in the U.S. have shown the falsity of the assumptions or the assertions of the neutrality of biomedical knowledge and practice as regards women, thereby demonstrating the sexist nature of biomedical theory and practice (see Barrett and Roberts 1980; Brandt 1985; Harding and O'Barr 1987; Lock 1985; Tobin et al. 1987).

We can but mention the development of slavery, immigration of vari-ous ethnic groups in this and the last century, and the suffrage, labor, and civil rights movements to bring to mind the social history of communalism in the U.S. Communalism is *intrinsic* to U.S. biomedicine because of its cul-ture's social history. It contributes to making U.S. biomedicine uniquely American, not in the sense of an evil empire set apart and opposed to soci-ety or to culture, but as an expression of that culture and its history. As a cultural medicine, it *may be criticized both from within and without* the cultural tradition by those it fails to serve and those it serves to fail.

In expressing culture history, biomedicine's key concept, biology, serves as a key symbol (Ortner 1974). As Ortner explains, key symbols serve to unite disparate yet related cultural elements and to summarize cen-tral themes of culture. The biological, then, appears in part as a product of culture history and is symbolic not of universal realities but of the particu-lar histories of France and the U.S. Biology as symbol is as much a reflec-tion of culture history as of nature (the symbolic character of which also may be shown) (see Gordon 1988).

Biology as key symbol provides a sense of *Selbsverstandnis* (self understanding) of biomedicine as a group and for its member individuals. It also seems to serve to establish self-esteem and social stature within and outside of medicine; biology is the focus of the subculture's work and the basis, and therefore validation, of its asserted scientific, value-neutral theory and praxis.

Biology serves, too, as the criterion of ranking in the status system; it appears that the greater the possibility and extent of somatic intervention, the higher the status within U.S. biomedicine (see Johnson 1985). The context of practice, hospital or not, is the chief, but not the only, criterion in the status system of France.

In relating biology to technology, we find that technology is the tool which allows greater access to and manipulation of the biology of the patient. Hence the "discourse of competence" among physicians is found to be related to reputed mastery over new technology and greater biological knowledge of one physician over another or others (DelVecchio Good 1985), or of one medical specialty over another (Johnson 1985).

Historically we see that U.S. biomedicine self-consciously allied and identified itself with the biological sciences and with (French) statistics in the nineteenth century in order to appear scientific (Cassedy 1984) after having moved away from the identity of medicine as art under the influence of Rush. The new pose allowed practitioners to assume a valued identity, that of modernists (i.e., scientists) who were involved in "progress." (The idea of progress in medicine is another important symbol deserving analysis.) There developed, then, a "cloak of scientistic competence," through which U.S. medicine began to emphasize research and relate it to clinical practice, again under French influence, only sometime after the Civil War (Lesch 1984).

Despite its scientistic pose, biomedicine did not eliminate its nonbiological nineteenth-century adversaries; it incorporated them. Aspects of hydropathy, hygiene, homeopathy, and Thompson's botanics became part of U.S. biomedicine as did the Rushian notion of medical heroics. (Then as now the results were sometimes detrimental to the patient, as for example, the fact that the physician's assumption of the role of hero was often fatal to patient. The role of hero can still be seen in contemporary surgery and internal medicine [see, for example, Hahn 1985; Katz 1985, n.d.].)

Biology serves to unite disparate cultural themes, such as "professionalism, competence," (both deriving from Lutheran theology), scientism, "progress and objectivity." It also serves to summarize them. It serves as the focus and validation of medical work and establishes group and self-identity. But there are, as noted here, local and contextual variants for the meaning of the key symbol. Its polysemous nature provides it with a resilience which allows it to endure in the face of important criticisms about the value and utility of the biological perspective in dealing with human suffering.

This symbolic potency is adopted by contemporary psychiatrists who view their work in biological terms. This stance has increasingly come to dominate psychiatry since the introduction of the major tranquillizers, i.e., antipsychotics, in the 1950s (Kleinman 1988; Johnson 1985; Lin, Poland, and Lesser 1986). Biological psychiatry, which treats of the biological and locates the nosological entities of its clinical interest in biology, is seen as the "new psychiatry" and as the means by which psychiatry will raise its status within medicine and become part of "mainstream" medicine. The criteria of evaluation are not necessarily efficacious practices. Again, we see the symbolic meaning and use of the biological.

Conclusions

The contextually variant meanings of biology and other symbols of biomedicine need further examination if we are to unravel their condensed, multivocal meanings. The present paper has sought to provide some tools for the interpretive analysis of biomedicines. The notion of sickness history, as a component of culture history, was advanced as a useful device in identifying and understanding differences in French and U.S. biomedicines. Aspects of the meaning of biology in the two systems were shown to derive from culture history, not current social forces or relations.

We have seen that biology, the body, in France is a mode and expression of experience (see Csordas, this volume). In the United States, it tends to serve, among other things, as the putatively empirical basis for social classification. On that basis, practices are generated. The French illnesses would be seen as illegitimate, as "only" psychosomatic illnesses and, doubtless, as malingering in the United States. Conversely, the "racial" system of social classification used by U.S. science and society would likewise be rejected in France. But, both are believed to be grounded in a biology and are therefore quite "natural," or so it is assumed.

The biomedicines, then, appear not to be monoparadigmatic, though they often strive to present themselves as such (Engel 1977; Mishler et al. 1981). In regard to the notion of biology as symbol rather than as an ultimate reality, it is important to note that other professional medicines exist which, while biologically based, articulate *distinct biologies*, e.g., the professional ethnomedicines of India, China, and Japan. The view presented here is that professional ethnomedicines are, to paraphrase Evans-Pritchard, *moral systems, not natural systems*. They represent "local biologies."

I have tried to offer a view of professional Western biomedicines as cultural garments woven not of a single fabric, but of many. The cloaks which cover biomedicines conceal, yet embody, express, and perpetuate the existence of distinct threads of vital histories of conflict and accommodation. It is suggested here that biomedicines in anthropological research should be taken less for their monoparadigmatic, idealized biological countenances and more for their multiparadigmatic cultural realities—realities created and grounded in local cultural knowledge and history.

Acknowledgments

I would like to thank Drs. Allan Young and Arthur Kleinman, and Lisa Mitchell and two anonymous reviewers for helpful comments on drafts of the present paper; thanks to Sue Wasserkrug for editorial assistance. Any problems which remain do so in spite of their best efforts.

Notes

1. The label "bourgeois medicine" has been advanced by Singer (1986). This label serves to convey the ideology of its users rather than anything about the object of study. It reflects a problematic view of biomedicine as universal, monolithic, distinct and set apart and opposed to society and produced by an economic system (also see Wright and Treacher 1982a on this point).

2. This research was conducted in Paris and Strasbourg in the summer of 1982 with Paul E. Farmer while we were both at Duke University. A Duke University Major Grant funded the research.

3. Psychiatrists queried include some at Duke Medical Center, 1983, and Case Western Reserve University School of Medicine, 1984–87.

4. As a result, through the 1970s, 61 percent of French physicians were general practitioners while only 39 percent were specialists. In the United States, we find a striking difference with only 21 percent of active physicians in general practice and 79 percent in specialties (USDHHS 1983:6). This difference is a reflection of the very different nature and context of medical practice in France and the United States. It also reflects a very different notion of intelligence in the two countries. It is also relevant to point out that many medical specialties in France and the United States are not comparable. There are, as well, very different social organizations of medicine in the two countries, different bases of hierarchy, hospital privileges, use of physicians as sources of help and the usual site of patient healer contacts (Baszanger 1985; Cabridain 1985; Du Pouvourville and Renaud 1985; Katz 1985, n.d.; Johnson 1985; USDHHS 1983). Other major differences include care of the elderly and use of pharmaceuticals (Gaines n.d.; Lenoire and Sandier 1976).

5. My original year-long study in Strasbourg (1974) was funded by an NIMH training grant. Subsequent visits (in the early 1980s) were funded by Duke University Major and Minor Grants.

References

Abu-Lughod, Lila
1986 Veiled Sentiments. Berkeley: University of California Press.
Ackerknecht, E. H.
1948 Hygiene in France, 1815–1848. Bulletin of the History of Medicine 22: 117–155.

American Psychiatric Association
1980 Diagnostic and Statistical Manual III (DSM-III). Washington, D.C.: American Psychiatric Association.
1987 Diagnostic and Statistical Manual III-Revised (DSM-III-R). Washington, D.C.: American Psychiatric Association.

Apple, Dorian
1960 How Laymen Define Illness. Journal of Health and Human Behavior 1:219–225.

Baer, Hans, Merrill Singer and John Johnson
1986 Toward a Critical Medical Anthropology. Social Science and Medicine 23:95–98.

Bailey, F. G., ed.
1971 Gifts and Poisons. New York: Schocken.

Barrett, M. and H. Roberts
1980 Doctors and Their Patients: the Social Control of Women in General Practice. In Women, Sexuality and Social Control. C. Smart and B. Smart (eds.). London: Routledge and Kegan Paul.

Baszanger, Isabelle
1985 Professional Socialization and Social Control: From Medical Students to General Practitioners. Noal Mellott, trans. Social Science and Medicine 20:133–143.

Becker, H., B. Geer, E. Hughes and A. Strauss
1961 The Boys in White; Student Culture in Medical School. Chicago: University of Chicago Press.

Blu, Karen
1980 The Lumbee Problem. Cambridge: Cambridge University Press.

Blue, Amy V.
1991 Culture, *Nevra* and Institution: The Making of Greek Professional Ethnopsychiatry. Unpublished Ph.D. Dissertation in Anthropology. Case Western Reserve University. Cleveland, Ohio.

Boas, Franz
1966 Race, Language, and Culture. New York: The Free Press (orig. 1940).

Bosk, Charles
1979 Forgive and Remember. Chicago: University of Chicago Press.

Brandt, Allan
1978 Racism and Research: The Case of the Tuskegee Syphilis Study. The Hastings Center Report, Dec.: 21–29.
1985 No Magic Bullet. Cambridge: Harvard University Press.

Brill, N. and H. Storrow
1960 Social Class and Psychiatric Treatment. Archives of General Psychiatry 3:340-345.

Brown, E. Richard
1979 Rockefeller Medicine Men. Berkeley: University of California Press.

Cabridain, Marie-Odile
1985 Managerial Procedures and Hospital Practices: A Case Study of the Development of a New Medical Discipline. Noal Mellott, trans. Social Science and Medicine 20(2):167–172.

Campbell, John
1964 Honour, Family and Patronage. Oxford: Oxford University Press.

Cassedy, James
1984 American Medicine and Statistical Thinking 1800–1860. Cambridge: Harvard University Press.

Coleman, William
1987 (1971) Biology in the Nineteenth Century. Cambridge: Cambridge University Press.

Cornelisen, Ann
1971 Women of the Shadows. Boston: Little, Brown and Company.

Crapanzano, Vincent
1973 The Hamadsha. Berkeley: University of California Press.

Davis, John
1977 People of the Mediterranean. London: Routledge and Kegan Paul.

Derogatis, L., et al.
1971 Neurotic Symptom Dimensions as Perceived by Psychiatrists and Patients of Various Social Classes. Archives of General Psychiatry 42:454–464.

Dodier, Nicolas
1985 Social Uses of Illness at the Workplace: Sick Care and Moral Evaluation. Noal Mellott, trans. Social Science and Medicine 20(2):123–128.

Domínguez, Virginia
1977 Social Classification in Creole Louisiana. American Ethnologist 4(4): 589–602.
1986 White By Definition. Rutgers: University of Rutgers Press.

Dorfman, D. and R. Kliner
1962 Race of Examiner and Patient in Psychiatric Diagnosis and Recommendations. Journal of Consulting Psychology 26:393.

Douglas, Mary
1979 Cultural Bias. London: Occasional Papers of the Royal Anthropological Institute.

Dugan, Anna Baziak
1988 *Compadrazgo* as a Protective Mechanism in Depression. In Women and Health. Patricia Whelehan and Contributors (eds.). Granby, MA: Bergin and Garvey.

Eickleman, Dale
1976 Moroccan Islam. Austin: University of Texas Press.

Eisenberg, Leon
1977 Disease and Illness: Distinctions Between Professional and Popular Ideas of Sickness. Culture, Medicine and Psychiatry 1(1):9–24.

Engel, George
1977 The Need for a New Medical Model: A Challenge for Biomedicine. Science
       196:129–135.

Enright, John and Walter Jaeckle
1963 Psychiatric Symptoms and Diagnosis in Two Subcultures. International Jour-
       nal of Social Psychiatry 9:12–17.

Frankenberg, Ronald
1980 Medical Anthropology and Development. Social Science and Medicine 14B
       (4):197–207.
1988 Gramsci, Culture and Medical Anthropology: Kundry and Parsifal? or Rat's
       Tail to Sea Serpent? Medical Anthropology Quarterly *(n.s.)* 2(4):324–337.

Freidson, Eliot
1961 The Patients' Views of Medical Practice. New York: Russell Sage.
1975 Profession of Medicine. New York: Dodd Mead.

Foster, George and Barbara Anderson
1978 Medical Anthropology. New York: John Wiley and Sons.

Foucault, Michel
1963 Naissance de la Clinique. Paris: Presses Universitaires de France.

Foulks, E., D. Freeman, F. Kaslow, and L. Madow
1977 The Italian Evil Eye. Journal of Operational Psychiatry 8:28–54.

Gaines, Atwood D.
1978 The Word and the Cross. Unpublished Ph.D. dissertation in Anthropology.
       University of California at Berkeley. Berkeley, California.
1979 Definitions and Diagnoses. Culture, Medicine and Psychiatry 3(4):381–418.
1980 'Race' and Culture as Cultural Systems: Ethnicity in Strasbourg. Presented
       at the American Anthropological Association Meeting. December, Washing-
       ton, D.C.
1982a Cultural Definitions, Behavior and the Person in American Psychiatry. In
       Cultural Conceptions of Mental Health and Therapy. A. Marsella and G.
       White (eds.). Dordrecht: D. Reidel.
1982b Knowledge and Practice: Anthropological Ideas and Psychiatric Practice. In
       Clinically Applied Anthropology. N. Chrisman and T. Maretzki (eds.). Dor-
       drecht: D. Reidel.
1985a Alcohol: Cultural Conceptions and Social Behavior Among Urban 'Blacks.'
       In The American Experience with Alcohol: Contrasting Cultural Perspec-
       tives. L. Bennett and G. Ames (eds.). New York: Plenum.
1985b The Once- and the Twice-Born: Self and Practice Among Psychiatrists and
       Christian Psychiatrists. In Physicians of Western Medicine. R. Hahn and A.
       Gaines (eds.). Dordrecht: D. Reidel.
1985c Faith, Fashion and Family. Anthropological Quarterly 58(2):47–62.
1986a Trauma: Cross-Cultural Issues. In Advances in Psychosomatic Medicine: Vol-
       ume 16; Psychosomatic Aspects of Trauma. L. Peterson and G. O'Shanick
       (eds.). Basel: Karger.
1986b Disease, Communalism and Medicine. Culture, Medicine and Psychiatry
       10(4):297–303.

1987 Cultures, Biologies and Dysphorias. Transcultural Psychiatric Research Review 24(1):31–57.
1989 Alzheimer's in the Context of "Black" (Southern) Culture. Health Matrix. 6(4):33–38.
1991 Cultural Constructivism: Sickness Histories and the Understanding of Ethnomedicines Beyond Critical Medical Anthropologies. In The Anthropologies of Medicine. B. Pfleiderer and G. Bibeau (eds.). Wiesbaden, Germany: Vieweg Verlag.
1992 From DSM-I to III-R: Voices of Self, Mastery and the Other: A Cultural Constructivist Reading of United States Psychiatric Classification. In The Cultural Construction of Psychiatric Classification. C. Nuckoles (ed.). Social Science and Medicine Special Issue/Section (In Press).
n.d. Physicians and Pharmacy in France. ms.

Gaines, Atwood D. and Paul E. Farmer
1986 Visible Saints: Social Cynosures and Dysphoria in the Mediterranean Tradition. Culture, Medicine and Psychiatry 10(4):295–330.

Gaines, Atwood D. and Robert A. Hahn, eds.
1982 Physicians of Western Medicine: Five Cultural Studies. Culture, Medicine and Psychiatry Special Issue 6(3).

Gaines, Atwood D. and Robert A. Hahn
1985 Among the Physicians: Encounter, Exchange and Transformation. In Physicians of Western Medicine: Anthropological Approaches to Theory and Practice. R. Hahn and A. Gaines (eds.). Dordrecht: D. Reidel.

Geertz, Clifford
1971 Islam Observed. Chicago: University of Chicago Press.
1973 The Interpretation of Cultures. New York: Basic Books.
1983 Local Knowledge. New York: Basic Books.

Gilmore, David
1982 Anthropology of the Mediterranean Area. In Annual Review of Anthropology. Palo Alto, California: Annual Review Press.

Good, Byron
1977 The Heart of What's the Matter: The Semantics of Illness in Iran. Culture, Medicine and Psychiatry 1(1):25–58.

Good, Byron and Mary-Jo D. Good
1982 Toward a Meaning-Centered Analysis of Popular Illness Categories: "Fright Illness" and "Heart Distress" in Iran. In Cultural Conceptions of Mental Health and Therapy. A. Marsella and G. White (eds.). Dordrecht: D. Reidel.

Good, Byron, Mary-Jo D. Good and Robert Moradi
1985 The Interpretation of Iranian Depressive Illness and Dysphoric Affect. In Culture and Depression. A. Kleinman and B. Good (eds.). Berkeley: University of California Press.

Good, Mary-Jo DelVecchio
1985 Discourses on Physician Competence. In Physicians of Western Medicine: Anthropological Approaches to Theory and Practice. Robert A. Hahn and Atwood D. Gaines (eds.). Dordrecht: D. Reidel.

Gordon, Deborah
1988 Tenacious Assumptions in Western Medicine. In Biomedicine Examined. Margaret Lock and Deborah Gordon (eds.). Dordrecht: Kluwer Academic Publishers.

Hahn, Robert
1985 A World of Internal Medicine: Portrait of an Internist. In Physicians of Western Medicine: Anthropological Approaches to Theory and Practice. R. Hahn and A. Gaines (eds.). Dordrecht: D. Reidel.

Hahn, Robert and Atwood Gaines, eds.
1985 Physicians of Western Medicine: Anthropological Approaches to Theory and Practice. Dordrecht: D. Reidel.

Hahn, Robert and Arthur Kleinman
1983 Biomedical Practice and Anthropological Theory. In Annual Review of Anthropology. Palo Alto: Annual Reviews, Inc.

Hallowell, A. I.
1976 American Indians, White and Black. In Contributions to Anthropology: Selected Papers of A. Irving Hallowell. A. I. Hallowell. Chicago: University of Chicago Press.

Harding, Sandra and Jean F. O'Barr, eds.
1987 Sex and Scientific Inquiry. Chicago: University of Chicago Press.

Helman, Cecil
1985 Disease and Pseudo-Disease: A Case History of Pseudo-Angina. In Physicians of Western Medicine: Anthropological Approaches to Theory and Practice. R. Hahn and A. Gaines (eds.). Dordrecht: D. Reidel.
1990 Culture, Health and Illness (2nd ed.). London: Wright.

Herzlich, Claudine and Janine Pierret
1985 The Social Construction of the Patient: Patients and Illnesses in Other Ages. Noal Mellott, trans. Social Science and Medicine 20:145–151.

Herzlich, Claudine
1973 Health and Illness. New York: Academic Press.

Holden, Constance
1991 New Center to Study Therapies and Ethnicity. Science 251:748.

Hughes, Charles
1968 Medical Care: Ethnomedicine. In International Encyclopedia of the Social Sciences. New York: Free Press.
1990 Ethnopsychiatry. In Medical Anthropology. Thomas Johnson and Carolyn Sargent (eds.). Westport, CT: Greenwood Press.

Jackson, Stanley
1985 Acedia the Sin and Its Relationship to Sorrow and Melancholia. In Culture and Depression. A. Kleinman and B. Good (eds.). Berkeley: University of California Press.

Johnson, Thomas
1985 Consultation Liaison Psychiatry. In Physicians of Western Medicine: Anthropological Approaches to Theory and Practice. R. Hahn and A. Gaines (eds.). Dordrecht: D. Reidel.

Katz, Pearl
1985 How Surgeons Make Decisions. In Physicians of Western Medicine: Anthropological Approaches to Theory and Practice. R. Hahn and A. Gaines (eds.). Dordrecht: D. Reidel.
n.d.   The Active Posture of Surgeons. ms.

Kleinman, Arthur
1980 Patients and Healers in the Context of Culture. Berkeley: University of California Press.
1986 Social Origins of Distress and Disease. New Haven: Yale University Press.
1988 Rethinking Psychiatry. New York: Free Press.

Kleinman, Arthur, Leon Eisenberg, and Byron Good
1978 Culture, Illness and Healing. Annals of Internal Medicine 88:251–258.

Kleinman, Arthur and Byron Good, eds.
1985 Culture and Depression. Berkeley: University of California Press.

Koos, E. L.
1954 The Health of Regionville: What People Thought and Did About It. New York: Columbia University Press.

Lee, Dorothy
1959 View of the Self in Greek Culture. In Freedom and Culture. D. Lee. Englewood Cliffs, New Jersey: Prentice-Hall.

Lenoire, C. and S. Sandier
1976 La Consommation Pharmaceutique en France et aux U.S.A. Paris: Centre de Recherches et de Documentation sur la Consommation (CRDC).

Lesch, John E.
1984 Science and Medicine in France. Cambridge, MA: Harvard University Press.

Leslie, Charles, ed.
1977 Asian Medical Systems. Berkeley: University of California Press.

Letourmy, Alain
1985 An Economic Approach to the Daily Activities of Private General Practitioners. Noal Mellott, trans. Social Science and Medicine 20(2):173–180.

Lin, K.-M., R. Poland and I. Lesser
1986 Ethnicity and Psychopharmacology. Culture, Medicine and Psychiatry 10(2):151–165.

Lock, Margaret
1980 East Asian Medicine in Urban Japan. Berkeley: University of California Press.
1985 Models and Practice in Medicine: Menopause as Syndrome or Life Transition? In Physicians of Western Medicine: Anthropological Approaches to Theory and Practice. R. Hahn and A. Gaines (eds.). Dordrecht: D. Reidel.

Lutz, Catherine
1985 Depression and the Translation of Emotional Worlds. In Depression and Culture. A. Kleinman and B. Good (eds.). Berkeley: University of California Press.

MacKinnon, Roger and Robert Michels
1971 The Psychiatric Interview in Clinical Practice. Philadelphia: W. B. Saunders.

Maretzki, Thomas
1985 Including the Physician in Healer-Centered Research: Retrospect and Prospect. In Physicians of Western Medicine: Anthropological Approaches to Theory and Practice. R. Hahn and A. Gaines (eds.). Dordrecht: D. Reidel.

Maretzki, Thomas and Eduard Seidler
1985 Biomedicine and Naturopathic Healing in West Germany: A History of a Stormy Relationship. Culture, Medicine and Psychiatry 9(4):383–427.

McNeill, J. and H. Gamer
1938 Medieval Handbooks of Penance. New York: Columbia University Press.

Menninger, Karl, Jr.
1963 The Vital Balance. New York: The Viking Press.

Merton, R., G. Reader and P. Kendall, eds.
1957 The Student-Physician. Cambridge, MA: Harvard University Press.

Mishler, Elliot, et al.
1981 Social Contexts of Health, Illness and Patient Care. Cambridge: Cambridge University Press.

Montagu, Ashley
1962 The Concept of Race. American Anthropologist 64:919–928.

Myers, Jerome and Leslie Schaffer
1958 Social Stratification and Psychiatric Practice: A Study of An Out Patient Clinic. In Patients, Physicians, and Illness. E.G. Jaco (ed.). Glencoe, IL: Free Press.

Navarro, Vincente
1976 Medicine Under Capitalism. New York: Prodist.

Neighbors, H., J. Jackson, L. Campbell and D. Williams
1989 The Influence of Racial Factors on Psychiatric Diagnosis. Community Mental Health Journal 25(4):301–310.

Obeyesekere, Gananath
1985 Depression, Buddhism and the Work of Culture in Sri Lanka. In Culture and Depression. Arthur Kleinman and Byron Good (eds.). Berkeley: University of California Press.

Ohnuki-Tierney, Emiko
1984 Health and Illness in Contemporary Japan. Cambridge: Cambridge University Press.

Ortner, Sherry
1974 On Key Symbols. American Anthropologist 75:1330–1346.

Parsons, Talcott
1951 The Social System. New York: Free Press.

Payer, Lynn
1988 Medicine and Culture. New York: Henry Holt.
1990 Borderline Cases: How Medical Practice Reflects National Culture. The Sciences 30(4):38ff.

Peristiany, John, ed.
1966 Honour and Shame: The Values of Mediterranean Society. London: Weidenfeld.

Pernick, Martin
1985 A Calculus of Suffering. New York: Columbia University Press.

Pitt-Rivers, Julian, ed.
1963 Mediterranean Countrymen. Paris: Mouton.

Pliskin, Karen
1987 Silent Boundaries. New Haven: Yale University Press.

Pouvourville, Gérard Du and Marc Renaud
1985 Hospital System Management in France and Canada. Social Science and Medicine 20(2):153–165.

Rabinow, Paul and William Sullivan, eds.
1979 Interpretive Social Science, A Reader. Berkeley: University of California Press.
1987 Interpretive Social Science: A Second Look. Berkeley: University of California Press.

Reynolds, David
1979 Morita Psychotherapy. Berkeley. University of California Press.

Rhodes, Lorna Amarasingham
1990 Biomedicine as a Cultural System. In Medical Anthropology. Thomas Johnson and Carolyn Sargent (eds.). Westport, CT: Greenwood Press.

Rosenfield, I.
1986 Neural Darwinism: A New Approach to Memory and Perception. New York Review of Books 33(15):21–27.

Rubel, Arthur
1977 The Epidemiology of a Folk Illness: *Susto* in Hispanic America. In Culture, Disease and Healing. David Landy (ed.). New York: Macmillan.

Scheper-Hughes, Nancy
1988 The Madness of Hunger: Sickness, Delirium, and Human Needs. Culture, Medicine and Psychiatry 12(4):429–458.

Singer, Merrill
1986 Developing a Critical Perspective in Medical Anthropology. Medical Anthropology Quarterly 17:128–129.

Sommervell, P.D. et al.
1989 The Prevalence of Major Depression in Black and White Adults in Five United States Communities. American Journal of Epidemiology 130(4):725–735.

Sontag, Susan
1977 Illness as Metaphor. New York: Vintage Books.

Starr, Paul
1982 The Social Transformation of American Medicine. New York: Basic Books.

Taussig, Michael
1980 Reification and the Consciousness of the Patient. Social Science and Medicine 14B:3–13.

Tobin, Jonathan, et al.
1987 Heart Bypass Surgery. The Washington Post. Quoted in San Francisco Chronicle. July 22, p.3.

Tousignant, Michel
1984 *Pena* in the Ecuadorian Sierra. Culture, Medicine and Psychiatry
      8(4):381–398.

Townsend, J. M.
1978 Cultural Conceptions and Mental Illness. Chicago: University of Chicago Press.

Turner, Victor
1975 Dramas, Fields and Metaphors. Ithaca: Cornell University Press.

United States Department of Health and Human Services (USDHHS)
1983 Comparison of Health Expenditures in France and the United States,
      1950–1978. NCHS, Hyattsville, M.D.: USDHHS Publication No. 83–1405.

Vernon, S. and R. Roberts
1982 Prevalence of Treated and Untreated Psychiatric Disorders in Three Ethnic
      Groups. Social Science and Medicine 16:1575–1582.

Verwey, Gerlof
1985 Psychiatry in An Anthropological and Biomedical Context. Dordrecht: D.
      Reidel.

Waitzkin, Howard
1979 Medicine: Superstructure and Micropolitics. Social Science and Medicine
      13A:601–609.

Watts, E.
1981 The Biological Race Concept and Diseases of Modern Man. In Biocultural
      Aspects of Disease. H. Rothschild (ed.). New York: Academic Press.

Weisberg, D. and S. O. Long, eds.
1984 Biomedicine in Asia: Transformations and Variations. Culture, Medicine and
      Psychiatry Special Issue 8(2).

Weisz, George
1990 Water Cures and Science: The French Academy of Medicine and Mineral
      Waters in the Nineteenth Century. Bulletin of the History of Medicine
      64:393–416.

Wenzel, S.
1960 The Sin of Sloth: Acedia in Medieval Thought and Literature. Chapel Hill:
      University of North Carolina Press.

Wright, Peter and Andrew Treacher, eds.
1982a The Problem of Medical Knowledge: Examining the Social Construction of
      Medicine. Edinburgh: University of Edinburgh Press.

Wright, Peter and Andrew Treacher
1982b Introduction. In The Problem of Medical Knowledge: Examining the Social
      Construction of Medicine. P. Wright and A. Treacher (eds.). Edinburgh:
      University of Edinburgh Press.

Wylie, Laurence
1957 Village in the Vaucluse. Cambridge: Harvard University Press.

Young, Allan
1980 An Anthropological Perspective on Medical Knowledge. Journal of Medicine
      and Philosophy 5:102–116.

1981   The Creation of Medical Knowledge: Some Problems of Interpretation. Social
       Science and Medicine 15B:379–386.
1982   The Anthropologies of Illness and Sickness. In Annual Review of Anthropolo-
       gy. Palo Alto: Annual Review Press.
1988   Reading DSM-III on PTSD. Paper presented at the Conference on Medical
       Anthropologies: Western European and North American Perspectives. Uni-
       versity of Hamburg. Hamburg, West Germany. December 4–8.
1990   Moral Conflicts in a Psychiatric Hospital Treating Combat-related Posttrau-
       matic Stress Disorder (PTSD). In Social Science Perspectives on Medical
       Ethics. George Weisz (ed.). Dordrecht: Kluwer Academic Publishers.

7

Too Close for Comfort: Schizophrenia and Emotional Overinvolvement Among *Mexicano* Families

Janis Hunter Jenkins

Alejandro and I have always gotten along well because we are very *afinados* ("in tune") with one another. In nearly all situations we don't even need to speak because we already know what the other is thinking. This is because we are exactly the same, in all things in life. It's very normal.

    (Opening interview statement from the mother of Alejandro)

I have to walk with her and keep my arm around her. If she leaves and goes outside, she would try to break away. (But) all day long I keep my arm around her.... Only God knows what I have been through!

    (Opening interview statement from the father of Gabriella)

Introduction

  At issue in the psychiatric and anthropological literature is the question of whether substantial differences exist in family members' responses to a relative with a major mental disorder. In this chapter, my principal interest is to highlight anthropological and clinical dimensions of individually variable (and sometimes deviant) constructions of family worlds within particular cultural contexts. Such differences have long been thought to be of therapeutic significance to the patient (Fromm-Reichman 1948; Bleuler 1978). In psychological and medical anthropology, however, fascination with such variations generally stems from a rather different interest, that is, in the existence of variations in representations of illness (e.g., response to "the problem" on the part of patients, family, and community) for their intrinsic interest as a dimension of culture (Farmer & Good 1990; Jenkins 1988a,b; Kleinman 1988).

  Only recently have the theoretical and empirical aspects of these two problems converged: cultural interpretations and representations of illness are an important domain of inquiry not only because they vary substantially across cultures but also because they mediate the very course of clinical illness (Karno et al. 1987; Jenkins 1988a,b, 1991b). The essential interrelation of cultural and clinical realities should help to dissuade those who would regard either illness representations or psychiatric symptomatology as discreet occasions of anthropological or psychiatric exotica, respectively.

A case in point is the study of "emotional overinvolvement" (EOI), developed over the past three decades as part of the "expressed emotion" (EE) research initiated by George Brown and his colleagues in England (Brown, Birley, and Wing 1972; Vaughn and Leff 1976). Studies of "expressed emotion" have revealed that certain features of the familial emotional climate are significantly associated with patterns of relapse for both schizophrenia and depression (Hooley, Orley, and Teasdale 1986; Karno, Jenkins, de la Selva et al. 1987; Vaughn and Leff 1976). In particular, patients who reside with relatives who are highly critical, hostile or emotionally overinvolved are likely to experience a relapse of symptomatology during the course of nine-month follow-up. It is perhaps the clinical relevance of these findings that has made expressed emotion the most thoroughly investigated psychosocial construct in psychiatric research. Indeed, studies of expressed emotion have been conducted internationally (North America, Europe, Asia, Australia, Africa) and applied to a full array of psychiatric and nonpsychiatric conditions (Jenkins and Karno 1992, n.d.).

Although the expressed emotion literature has made an empirically important contribution toward explicating particular features of the sociocultural milieu that may mediate the course and outcome of psychiatric disorder, several pressing issues require further examination. As Jenkins and Karno (1992, n.d.) have recently argued, principal among these is the elaboration of the nature and cultural meaning of the EE factors. Theoretical elucidation of expressed emotion necessarily entails interpretation of the specifically cultural dimensions of the construct: indigenous interpretations of the nature of the problem, the meaning of kin relations, the identification of cultural rule violations, and the ethnopsychology of emotion (Jenkins 1991b).

An underlying premise of the expressed emotion research is that emotion is an atmosphere that permeates interactive settings. This conceptualization is much in line with that of Harry Stack Sullivan's (1940) view of human interactive processes that construct symptom and sentiment. In contrast with a static, traditional psychoanalytic conception of feeling emerging from the intrapsychic constitution of individuals or, sociologically speaking, as symbolic strategies for negotiating social interaction, the paradigm of expressed emotion bridges intrapsychic and social symbolic processes. As I have argued elsewhere (Jenkins 1991b), "(t)o the extent that selves, self-esteem, persons and identity are dynamically constituted through the formative influence of kin interaction, social response to mental disorder does vary, and we must be concerned with how that variation may be important to the course of illness."

In this chapter I explore selected psychocultural dimensions of emotional overinvolvement. I pose the following questions: (1) What are the conceptual roots of EOI? (2) How commonly does emotional overinvolvement occur within families of persons with schizophrenia? (3) What are the common features of EOI? (4) Is emotional overinvolvement a culture-bound concept that applies only to British or Anglo-American families?

Conceptual Background of Emotional Overinvolvement

Emotional overinvolvement, as defined by Brown and colleagues (1978), is a construct which taps a variety of affective and behavioral features on the part of kin towards an ill relative: overconcern; unusually self-sacrificing and devoted behavior; extremely overprotective behavior; emotional displays; dramatization; and a lack of objectivity. In a retrospective account, Brown recalled that the inception of EE research in the late 1950s was an attempt to explore the relationships between the social environment and course of schizophrenia (Brown 1985). Brown's interest, however, was conceived in terms of a departure from psychiatric thinking of the time concerning the etiological relevance of psychopathological family factors. Brown was interested in the examination of everyday aspects of family life that could be important to the course and outcome of schizophrenia:

> I was skeptical about the published discussions of the role of family relationships in the etiology of schizophrenia. These dealt only with parents and emphasized enduring, deeply disturbed relationships. It was not that such relationships did not occur and might not at times be of some etiological significance. We had certainly come across a number of them in our visits, and they tended to be interviews that stood out in our memories. But such families were in fact uncommon, and it seemed most unlikely that they would provide a general explanation for what we were observing...it seemed important that the occasional presence of deeply disturbed or unusual relationships between parents and patients should not be allowed to dominate our thinking. If I had any hunch about what was going on, it was that it often involved something a good deal less fundamental, indeed, commonplace. (Brown 1985: 21–22)

Brown's sense that something "commonplace" held the greatest significance for social mediation of the course of psychiatric disorder proved justified. With or without the presence of a person who suffers from schizophrenia, criticism—the principal element of the EE construct—is indeed an everyday occurrence within families. More rarely, one observes families disturbed by high degrees of emotional overinvolvement. My own experience in this regard echoes that of Brown's: the observation of such families is striking, to say the least.

While there really is no concept in the family psychopathology literature that directly mirrors emotional overinvolvement, several related or parallel concepts have been developed. For example, the concepts of "enmeshment" (Minuchin 1974) and "symbiosis" (Goldenberg and Goldenberg 1980) are both used to convey an extremely close proximity and emotional intensity within families. An underlying assumption of concepts such as these is that the integrity of the self has been violated; the boundedness of the patient's self has been transgressed.

Aside from the conceptual domain they cover, concepts such as *enmeshment* and *symbiosis* differ from *emotional overinvolvement* in two important ways. First, the concept of EOI is an empirically derived, global measure that is based on specific types of evidence gathered within a research interview situation. Thus, EOI is not equivalent to more clinically obtained judgments made within specifically therapeutic situations. Second, and perhaps more important, these concepts differ substantially in how they have been applied: concepts such as enmeshment, marital skew and schism, and double bind, for that matter, have been formulated to account for presumed family etiological features of schizophrenia, whereas emotional overinvolvement has been confined to features that have been empirically associated with the course of illness. Contrast Brown's statement above about the presumed "normality" of most families of persons with schizophrenic illness with Lidz and Fleck's perspective (1960:323 emphasis added): "Our studies of the intrafamilial environment in which schizophrenic patients grow up follow the clinical observation that schizophrenic patients virtually always emerge from homes marked by serious parental strife or eccentricity."

Lidz and Fleck's (1960) investigation of sixteen middle and upper middle class families of persons with schizophrenia revealed several characteristic family features. These included an imperviousness to "other" and an inordinate intrusiveness between parents and their disturbed offspring. From the child's viewpoint, the essential parental figures were not objects from which she or he must become separated, but instead become embodied within her/his self and thereby continue to exert direction over one's life. Also typically present was a pronounced conflict between parents, manifest either as dominance ("marital skew") or hostility ("marital schism") (Lidz and Fleck 1960). According to Lidz and Fleck, a central problem for families such as these is the problem of control, especially control over incestuous proclivities of both parents and children.

As an etiological research tradition, this work has focused on a variety of presumed "schizophrenogenic" factors thought to be productive of psychosis (Fromm-Reichmann 1948). However, as I have summarized else-where (Jenkins 1991b), there are several problems with this line of research. First, because the relevant data are constructed from retrospec-tive instead of prospective accounts, the claim for the etiological impor-tance of family psychopathology has not yet been demonstrated empirically. Second, unlike operational outlines for emotional overinvolvement, the methodological definitions of key concepts from this early tradition in fami-ly psychopathology are often vague and applied with little analytic preci-sion. Third, this research paradigm can appropriately be critiqued on femi-nist grounds since the term *schizophrenogenic* has typically been applied to mothers for a disproportionately noxious influence they are alleged to exert. Finally, the general predominance of biogenetic and psychopharma-cological paradigms in current psychiatric research poses a challenge to family researchers interested in environmental factors.

Assessing Emotional Overinvolvement:
The Camberwell Family Interview

Expressed emotion is assessed through administration of the Camber-well Family Interview (CFI) to relatives who live with the patient. The CFI is a semistructured interview schedule of one and one-half to two hours duration. It is normally completed in the family home. The practice of interviewing in the home often serves to enhance researcher-respondent rapport and maximizes the possibility of obtaining relatives' emotional atti-tudes toward the problem. The CFI inquires into a variety of features of everyday family life. Principal strengths of this interview schedule are the qualitative, open-ended format and informant focus. The interviewer clear-ly conveys interest in obtaining detailed, specific reports of the relatives' own thoughts and feelings concerning their ill family member. Typically, the CFI yields rich narratives of daily events, activities, and interactions within the household. In particular, qualitative aspects of family interac-tions and relationships are probed, including reports of irritability, quar-reling, intimacy, and affection. Audiotaped interview materials on rela-tives' attitudes, feelings, and responses toward their ill family member are rated according to the principal expressed emotion scales: criticism, hostili-ty, and emotional overinvolvement (Vaughn and Leff 1976).

Emotional overinvolvement is rated on the basis of affective and behavioral features observed during the interview. Most notably these include unusually self-sacrificing and extremely overprotective behavior, dramatization, and emotional displays during the narration of events. While all of these features are considered together when rating emotional overin-volvement, greater emphasis is generally placed on self-sacrificing and over-protective behaviors. Such actions are interpreted as "unusually" or "overly" involved with reference to culturally expectable behaviors in the specific context of caretaking for a relative who suffers from schizophrenia.

The method for assessing the degree of EOI displayed by a relative calls for use of a six-point rating scale. Lower ratings (0–2) indicate an absence or low level of EOI, whereas a rating of 3 indicates a moderate degree of EOI. Ratings of 4 or 5 are applied only in those instances in which pronounced degrees of this factor are in evidence. Reliable use of the rating scales generally requires a training period of several months duration. High levels of inter-rater reliability among interviewers, as well as cultural adaptations of the EE rating scales, have been summarized elsewhere (Karno et al. 1987; Jenkins, Karno and de la Selva, n.d.).

Cultural Validity of the EOI Construct

In our longitudinal study of expressed emotion, clinical and anthropological evidence gathered during the pilot phase had suggested the cultural relevance of investigating emotional overinvolvement within Mexican-descent populations (Canino 1982; Ramirez and Arce 1982). Our approach to adaptation of the scale was anthropological, insofar as it identified the target behavior as unusual from an indigenous viewpoint. Thus, emotional overinvolvement was defined in accord with behaviors considered to be culturally unusual by Mexicans (or Mexican-Americans) themselves. This strategy was essential because analytic norms derived elsewhere (i.e., England) could not be expected to be of direct cultural relevance or meaning among a Mexican-descent population.

Mexican cultural orientations suggest to relatives that ideally they should display a high degree of involvement in kin affairs. This general cultural orientation certainly applies within the context of severe or serious illness. As we imagined, the particular nature and meaning of EOI among Mexican relatives was not the same as that observed among British or Anglo-American families (Leff and Vaughn 1985; Vaughn 1986). For instance, as interpreted in the British context, a particularly devoted relative might visit the hospital daily and bring along home-cooked food. Certainly this would not be similarly judged in the Mexican-descent context. In fact, regular and typically daily trips to the hospital may well be expected from female kin. The Mexican-descent mothers would underscore what for them was obvious: regular visits were necessary because this may have been their son or daughter's first experience of being away from family. They also voiced their worries about their son or daughter's vulnerability in a geographically (sometimes an adjacent county) and culturally (English-speaking American) distant hospital. Indeed, the substantive features of self-sacrificing and overprotective behaviors were culturally distinctive (see Leff and Vaughn 1985; Vaughn 1986, for comparisons).

Emotional Overinvolvement among Mexican-Descent Families

Seventy families were included in the study of expressed emotion among Mexican-descent families (Karno, Jenkins, de la Selva et al. 1987). In each of these families, one relative had recently been hospitalized for an acute schizophrenic episode according to the diagnostic criteria of the Present State Examination. The majority of these families were Catholic, first-generation, immigrant *Mexicanos* who were primarily or solely Spanish-speaking. The principal kin designations of the key relatives were as follows: 68 percent parents, 21 percent siblings, and 18 percent spouses. The sociodemographic characteristics of the sample have been more fully summarized elsewhere (Karno, Jenkins, de la Selva et al. 1987).

Of the 109 key relatives for whom the Camberwell Family Interview was administered, only eleven (or 11 percent) were rated "high" (scores of 4 or 5) on the scale for emotional overinvolvement. Nearly all of these relatives were female relatives, including seven mothers, two sisters, and one wife. With but one exception, this patient group was male. The predominant trend (in ten of eleven cases) was for this high EOI relationship to be a cross-sex phenomenon. The sole instance of high EOI for a male occurred for a father with his daughter. Interestingly, in this case (summarized below) the (single) father described himself as "both mother and father to my children."

How do the principal findings from the EE research paradigm articulate with assertions such as those made above by Lidz and Fleck, that all families of persons with schizophrenia can be characterized as "disturbed?" Cross-cultural studies of emotional overinvolvement among Indian (Wig et al. 1987), Mexican-descent (Karno et al. 1987), Anglo-American (Vaughn et al. 1984), and British (Brown, Birley and Wing 1972; Vaughn and Leff 1976) kin indicate relatively few relatives (0–21 percent) were considered high on this factor. These data contradict the general assertion that families of persons with schizophrenia can be characterized as pathologically disturbed. Moreover, in some societies (e.g., India), the entire concept of emotional overinvolvement may be of limited relevance. As applied to the Mexican-descent families, these data run counter to clinical and ethnographic characterizations of Latin American women (see Canino 1982) as "self-sacrificing" and "overprotective."

Characteristics of Emotional Overinvolvement

Having emphasized the relatively uncommon occurrence of high degrees of EOI in the sample of 109 Mexican-descent relatives, we now turn our attention to an examination of those eleven (or 11 percent) relatives who did display high levels of EOI. Interpretive analyses of this distinctive family phenomenon have not been advanced by expressed emotion researchers but are essential (1) to convey the often exotic features associated with it, and (2) to consider how it poses a situation of special vulnerability for persons coping with the day-to-day realities of schizophrenic illness.

Analysis of the specific group of relatives who scored high on EOI (scores of 4 or 5) reveals a coherent set of particular characteristics that differed from those of the other relatives (i.e., those considered "moderate" or "low" on this factor). Among high EOI Mexican-descent relatives, features of self-sacrificing and overprotective behaviors were culturally distinctive in form (see Leff and Vaughn 1985; Vaughn 1986, for additional comparative materials):

1. somatic complaints specifically in relation to their relative's illness (articulated as indigenous conditions of *nervios* (see Guarnaccia and Farias 1988; Jenkins 1988a and 1988b for further discussion of this indigenously defined condition);
2. suicidal thoughts or death wishes in relation to the relative's schizophrenic illness;
3. risking dangerous circumstances by enduring highly threatening or physically abusive behaviors;
4. reports of chronic and extreme suffering, fear, anxiety, and worry in relation to the illness;
5. major alterations in family activities and caretaking roles (i.e., cessation of family orientation and the adoption of a nearly exclusive dyadic relationship with the ill relative);
6. abandonment of employment or social activities to stay home and "guard" or "protect" the ill relative;
7. intrusive or vigilant behavior concerning the ill relative in the absence of circumstances (e.g., immanent danger) that would clearly require it;
8. highly emotional and dramatic narration of stories and events.

The above constellation of behaviors is culturally unusual, even in the face of serious family illness. Such was often the consensus of other household members (e.g., daughters, husbands). It was not uncommon for them to report that the high EOI relative had become overly embroiled in an intolerable situation, and that this had created considerable conflict within the family.

Typical statements by relatives considered high in EOI are "I am completely overwhelmed by this," or "I've devoted my whole life to looking after Jesus," even if there is evidence that Jesus does not need such caretaking. These kin would often report that their lives were filled with nothing but suffering. The cultural identification of such behaviors and attitudes as deviant is crucial to the cross-cultural validity of the concept. In this regard, it is noteworthy that other kin in the home did not reinforce these emotionally overinvolved orientations with comments such as "she's a saint" (see Gaines and Farmer 1986). Instead, these relative would make statements such as "that's too much" or "my mother's lost it." This cultural definition of emotional overinvolvement as strange or undesirable is the basis for use of the EOI concept in this particular setting. We turn now to the case materials to illustrate the particular nature of family relations characterized by high EOI.

Case Studies in Emotional Overinvolvement in *Mexicano* Families

1. The Mother of Alejandro

Alejandro Fuentes is twenty-three years old. He was born in Mexico but has been raised in the U.S. since the age of three. He lives with his parents and eight-year-old brother in a modest three-bedroom home near downtown Los Angeles. According to his mother and father, he first became ill at the age of seventeen, following a farewell party given by his friends and *novia* (fiancée) in honor of his imminent departure to serve in the U.S. Air Force. As was family custom, he telephoned his father at an appointed hour (10:30 P.M.) to be picked up at the party. When Sr. Fuentes arrived, however, Alejandro was nowhere in sight. After driving around for a short while, Sr. Fuentes found Alejandro wandering around confused and disoriented, making strange comments, and behaving in a bizarre fashion. Sr. Fuentes took his son to a local university psychiatric hospital the next morning, where he underwent one week of inpatient treatment. Since that time Alejandro has received outpatient therapy (consisting primarily of antipsychotic drugs) with apparently satisfactory results, but he was hospitalized twice again at three-year intervals, following psychotic decompensations in which he stopped eating and sleeping, had visual and auditory hallucinations, and was delusional (especially believing he had special powers to control others). For example, he cited his special powers involving a nuclear reactor (implanted in his head) and "travels" to the planet Venus.

Although Alejandro has suffered recurrent psychotic episodes, he generally functions well in periods prior to onset of such episodes. He worked in regular full-time jobs, socialized with his *novia* (fiancée) and friends, and participated in a local church group. The pattern has been that he may experience a recurrence of symptoms when he stops taking his medication or suffers a severe personal upset.

Sra. Fuentes is an attractive *Mexicana* who looks younger than her forty-seven years. She generally dresses casually at home, insisting upon relaxed, gracious living with family members. Her home is well maintained in a comfortable style, with family photographs adorning many of the walls and a music room (with piano and flute) just off the living room. When the research interviewers arrived, she insisted upon beginning with snacks and coffee. She then began to speak about herself and her interests as an artist and musician (flautist).

Sra. Fuentes' style of speaking is quite dramatic, shifting from a whisper to an emphatic, urgent tone of voice and then back again to a whisper. Moreover, while her customary style of speaking was dramatic she nonetheless conveyed even stronger affect when talking about Alejandro's illness, weeping several times during the course of the interview. She breathlessly described the onset of Alejandro's illness *"como una bomba...terrible... espantoso...durorosa...no te puede imaginar"* (like a bomb...terrible...terrifying...very difficult...you can't imagine). She reported chronic and disabling problems of *nervios* (nerves) in relation to Alejandro's illness. Worse still, she sometimes feels like dying or killing herself because, she asserts, she simply "cannot bear" the situation any longer.

Sra. Fuentes does not believe that Alejandro has full control over his behavior and places blame for his illness on others. During the course of the interview, she narrated stories of what she construes as mistreatment of Alejandro by his former fiancée (Marta) and friends. For example, she reports being concerned that he was not getting enough sleep due to Marta's late evening telephone calls. She also stated that she didn't know if he was eating properly because he did not come home for lunch and would often not eat dinner at home, preferring to go straight away to her (Marta's) house after work.

Alejandro's devotion to his fiancée was, in his mother's view, his psychic undoing. This was so, she claimed, because Alejandro was unwittingly being victimized by Marta's manipulations and abuse of him. She cited the following examples as evidence of her son's mistreatment. Although she could not be specific, she "knew" that Marta was seeing other men. Most telling for Sra. Fuentes, however, was her observation of an interaction between Marta and another woman friend in which they discussed engagement rings. Marta, congratulating her friend on her recent engagement, asked her friend to see her ring. Marta's casual comment, "It's just like mine, but the stone is bigger," provided, in Sra. Fuentes' estimation, unequivocal evidence that Marta did not appreciate Alejandro, that Marta was materialistic, and that her son was a fool. It was also likely evidence that Marta's family did not like Alejandro because he did not have a career and was therefore "not good enough" for her. Thus, from this seemingly minor incident Sra. Fuentes recited a litany of related problems that could only result in one outcome: her son needed to break off the engagement with Marta. When Alejandro did not agree and made no such moves to break his engagement, she told him how deeply hurt she was that *"no tenia la dignidad"* (he did not have the dignity) to break up with her.

Though she emphasized how much it hurt her personally, she also reported it hurt "us" (referring to her relationship with her son), going on to narrate the hurt it had caused her husband, too. In terms of her son's emotional frame of mind, she claimed to know that Alejandro also was deeply wounded, despite his verbal and behavioral evidence to the contrary. Her knowledge of her son's inner thoughts and feelings was extrapolated from those of her own, she explained, which were essentially the same. (See epigraph at beginning of this chapter for her narrative statement).

Nevertheless, a great source of consternation to Sra. Fuentes is behavior on the part of Alejandro indicating that he did not know what his mother's expectations were. For example, she reported that he sometimes behaved without regard to the "family rules" which she regarded as inviolate. These included not allowing friends or anyone "from the outside" to visit the home, not keeping any bedroom doors shut for privacy, not being "discourteous" through open disagreement, and not socializing with anyone of whom the family did not approve. Her family, she explained, does not socialize with many people to preserve the *agarre* (union) of the family. What was critical, from her viewpoint, was that Alejandro understand that preservation of family union means that he must conform and behave as a "true" family member, i.e., not to go against the rules or try to impose his own ideas. In Sra. Fuentes's view, it is her son's failure to embrace this "understanding" that has resulted in family chaos and turmoil.

The fact that Alejandro would socialize with friends (prior to his illness) brought his mother endless misery. She complained bitterly that she would have to watch for him "suspended...always looking over her shoulder, wondering what could be happening with Alejandro...it was horrible." Her constant vigils occurred within the context of Alejandro working full time and maintaining a busy social calendar, all activities he pursued through use of public transportation or the family car. During the periods in which Alejandro suffered an actively psychotic episode, he did not work or socialize as much as when he was well. Nevertheless, Sra. Fuentes did not distinguish between his symptomatic versus nonsymptomatic periods and reported that her behavior and feelings toward her son did not vary in relation to his illness. Although she has turned to her husband for support for her own illness (*nervios*) and suffering caused by Alejandro's sickness, her self-presentation sharply focused on the dyadic components of the mother-son relationship.

From this case summary, several features of this mother's behavior, attitude, and affective style are taken as criterial evidence for a high degree of EOI. In terms of reported behavior, her emotional response to the onset of her son's illness may have been somewhat exaggerated, evidenced in her comments that it was, "like a bomb...terrible...terrifying...difficult." Her marked concern for her son was reflected in unusually self-sacrificing behavior, including extreme, disabling problems associated with *nervios* and passive suicidal ideation. Instances of extremely overprotective behavior include prohibitions concerning socializing with friends (including not allowing any family friends into the home), and constant vigils ("suspended, looking over her shoulder") in wait for Alejandro to come home any time he was outside of the home.

These factors (e.g., prohibitions concerning friends, vigils) are evaluated as overprotective because nothing untoward had ever come to pass concerning Alejandro, and these behaviors therefore exist in the absence of circumstances that might justify or warrant them. For example, if every time Alejandro left the house trouble generally ensued upon his return, his mother's reaction might well be justified. This appears, however, not to have been the case. A similar logic applies to the family rule that no one be allowed to have their own bedroom door shut. Other examples of overprotective behaviors include this mother's admonition to break off her son's engagement despite the fact that, according to her own report, no conflict or trouble actually existed between her son and his fiancée. Her apparent telepathic knowledge of his hurt despite his statements and behavior to the contrary are also instances of overprotective (and perhaps intrusive) behavior. Finally, there are several behaviors that occurred within the context of the interview that are indicative of overconcern. These include the mother's crying several times during the course of the interview and extreme dramatization in the narration of events. Taken together, all of the foregoing evidence is used in a global judgment to conclude that this mother, relative to others interviewed and observed in the sample of 109 key relatives, scored high on the scale for emotional overinvolvement.

2. The Father of Gabriella

A different example of high emotional overinvolvement concerns 69-year-old Sr. Vasquez, father of eighteen-year-old Gabriella (see also Jenkins 1991b for a summary of this case). The family, consisting of Sr. Vasquez, Gabriella, and his four younger children, lives in East Los Angeles. Since the mother in this family is reported to have "abandoned" the family, Sr. Vasquez says he is "both mother and father to my children." The onset of Gabriella's illness is said to have occurred in her early teens. At this time, she was insomniac and would scream and cry from midnight until dawn. Her father repeatedly took her to be healed by *curanderos* (healers) in Mexico but their treatment apparently offered little relief. In the *curanderos*' view the problem was caused by "female trouble" triggered by the onset of menstruation.

A related factor, according to Sr. Vasquez, was that his daughter's troubles with *nervios* (nerves) were linked to his belief that Gabriella was *"fuerte de naturaleza"* (has a strong sexual/physical nature). Moreover, Gabriella's problems were compounded by having been exposed to a morally objectionable environment in which the mother is alleged to have entertained numerous visiting lovers. In Sr. Vasquez' view, his daughter's condition would improve greatly were she to marry and become sexually active. He complained that Gabriella has often tried to kiss him and cling to him in an inappropriate manner. This behavior, he claims, places him in the uncomfortable position of having to scold her and push her away. To be more specific, Sr. Vasquez reported that Gabriella has begged him to have sexual intercourse with her on numerous occasions, which he says he declined.

When she is actively ill, Gabriella experiences auditory hallucinations, irritability, insomnia, and violent-destructive behavior (e.g., breaking windows, hitting/shoving family members). Nevertheless, she was able to attend school and regularly socialize with friends and church members. Sr. Vasquez disapproved such activities, urging Gabriella to remain home where he could take care of her. Despite the fact that the father received regular household assistance from a neighborhood girl, he demanded that Gabriella remain at home to also provide him with help. He claimed such help was essential to him because his vision was significantly impaired (legally blind).

His principle method of caretaking involved keeping his arm around her throughout the day (*"todo el dia la traia del brazo"*). He reported that he always kept her company, assisting her in everything from dressing and eating to going to the toilet. (His reasoning for this vigilant watch, he asserted, was to guard against clogging up the toilet with sanitary napkins, which Gabriella is said to have done on one occasion.) Also significant was the fact that he slept with his daughter and, as during the day, kept his arms around her constantly. He explained this behavior as an important deterrent to her escaping the home and perhaps encountering some kind of trouble. According to Sr. Vasquez, no such trouble had in fact ever actually transpired. He forthrightly denied that he slept with her or sexually abused her. For him, sleeping with her was a form of protection. During the course of the interviews, he narrated his story in quite dramatic fashion, often exclaiming: *"Ay Dios," "valgame Dios!" "Es mi hija; yo la quiero. Me apuro por ella."* (God; give me a break, God; it's my daughter; I love her; I have suffered because of her). He complained he has suffered terribly because of her and the constant worry he feels creates great difficulty with his *nervios*. Nevertheless, Sr. Vasquez remains steadfast in trying to think of new ways to prevent her from leaving the home and providing her with protection. In short, the principle sources of evidence for a high degree of EOI in father's behavior and attitudes are (1) an unusual means of protection (or caretaking) by staying with her constantly, keeping his arm around her, helping her to eat and dress, and sleeping with her throughout the night; (2) reports of extreme self-sacrifice and suffering; and (3) a dramatic emotional style and lack of objectivity (i.e., Gabriella's behavior did not appear to warrant his overinvolved behavior).

Summary and Conclusions

High degrees of emotional overinvolvement among relatives, as described above in the case studies, are relatively rare among relatives interviewed in the expressed emotion studies. Only eleven (or 11 percent) of the 109 key relatives interviewed within the Mexican-descent study were so considered. As illustrated in the two case studies, the notion of emotional overinvolvement focuses primarily on overprotective and self-sacrificing behaviors. When such behaviors are noted, the behavioral portrait may appear to resemble somewhat those conveyed through other constructs in the family therapy literature, such as enmeshment or symbiosis (Minuchin 1974; Goldenberg and Goldenberg 1980). This assumes a culturally particular concept of the self as a bounded entity, but the criteria for EOI and related terms are that these boundaries have been abnormally transgressed. The main operational issue concerning EOI is that it is not related to, or explained by, the degree of psychopathology or behavioral disturbance (Jenkins 1991b). Rather, EOI is an index of a relative's subjective impression of the severity of burden engendered by the illness (see Noh and Turner 1987 for review of "family burden").

It may also be that social ecological features (such as household size and composition) are important to an understanding of emotional overinvolvement (Parker 1988). Certainly the degree to which EOI appears linked to gender-related sex roles is significant. With but one exception, all kin rated high are female and all patients male. The fact that when high degrees of EOI are present they are more often observed for women is not surprising given the cultural dimensions it taps (e.g., caretaking and affective attachments ideally relegated to women). The exception that proves the rule is that the (only) Mexican father (Sr. Vasquez, above) considered high on EOI was a single parent who portrayed his role as "both mother and father to my children." Observation of the cross-sex dynamic also makes it possible to hypothesize about a potentially sexualized component of EOI.

Toward a Psychocultural Conception of Emotional Overinvolvement

While the theory of emotion underlying the concept of emotional overinvolvement remains unelaborated in most empirical work in the expressed emotion paradigm, it is markedly distinct from the current trend in anthropology in which the elaboration of an ethnopsychology of emotion is looked for in the density of lexical elaboration (Lutz 1988) or in the degree to which emotions become "hypercognized" (Levy 1984). More relevant here are notions of emotional atmosphere (Bateson 1958) and the force of emotion (Geertz 1973). Harry Stack Sullivan (1940), in his writings defining the self-system as "all a person's characteristic, customary interpersonal devices for protecting himself against emotional distress and for seeking more emotional comfort," understood that emotional atmospheres are reciprocally created in the interpersonal space inhabited by related selves (Chapman 1976:95). Similarly, Sullivan defines a psychiatric disorder as any state in which a person shows inadequate or inappropriate performance in interpersonal relationships, encompassing everything from marital adjustments to psychoses (Chapman 1976:190ff.). Moreover, he implies that the definition of psychiatric disorders is to some extent influenced by changing social and cultural concepts about the kinds of behavior that are "adequate" or "appropriate." This definition therefore emphasizes that a person with a mental disorder must always be considered in the context of his or her broader interpersonal and social situation. I would argue that our understandings of these processes must dialectically incorporate the reciprocal relationship between kin interpretations of schizophrenic illness, on the one hand, and the perceived impact or burden of the illness on kin, on the other.

This theory also implies the presence of emotion as a destructive force within and between the self-systems of any interpersonal situation (Jenkins 1991b). Only recently, as in the luminary work of Michelle Rosaldo (1984), has the important issue of the "cultural force" of emotion received much attention in anthropology. According to Renato Rosaldo (1989:2), the notion of force here does not refer to emotion as cultural abstraction or ideal. In this sense, emotional overinvolvement can be considered a destructive force among kin and a failure to preserve culturally appropriate boundaries among self-systems. The force of emotional overinvolvement stems from the breakdown of the self-systematic capacity for emotional protection. In other words, it is dependent upon the nature of the self. Knowledge of cultural representations of the self underlie the cross-cultural validity of the EOI concept, because the requisite violation of boundaries entails a cultural psychology of a people (Shweder 1990) that is premised upon the notion of a bounded self.

To more fully consider this issue cross-culturally, we must posit the likelihood that no culture exists in which the self is completely without boundaries in some minimal sense (see Jenkins 1991b). In recent years, the clinical presentation of refugees and victims of torture (Jenkins 1990, 1991a) from all parts of the world suggests that trauma is inevitably an event for the self whether that self is "sociocentric or egocentric" (Shweder and Bourne 1982) or "indexical or referential" (Gaines 1982). Moreover, the universality of an incest taboo suggests the existence of such kin boundaries, and, as we have seen, some cases of emotional overinvolvement certainly exist on (or possibly over) the threshold of incest. The question of whether specific cultures seem to have the type of self requisite to this psychocultural dynamic must be addressed prior to the more complex search for cross-cultural variations in emotional overinvolvement.

Acknowledgments

This research was supported by the National Institute of Mental Health (NIMH) Research Grant MH 33502 (Marvin Karno, M.D., principal investigator) and by the National Alliance for the Study of Schizophrenia and Depression (NARSAD) Young Investigator Award (1988–1990) to me as a research fellow at Harvard Medical School. I wish to thank Thomas J. Csordas, Atwood Gaines, Marvin Karno, and Arthur Kleinman for their comments.

References

Bateson, G.
1958 Naven. Stanford, California: Stanford University Press.

Bleuler, M.
1978 The Schizophrenic Disorders: Long-Term Patient and Family Studies. New Haven and London: Yale University Press.

Brown, G.
1985 The Discovery of Expressed Emotion: Induction or Deduction? In Expressed Emotion in Families. J. Leff and C. Vaughn (eds.). New York, Guilford Press.

Brown, G., J. Birley and J. Wing
1972 Influence of Family Life on the Course of Schizophrenic Disorders: a Replication. British Journal of Psychiatry 121:241–258.

Brown, G, D. Quinton, M. Rutter, et al.
1978 Camberwell Family Interview: Notes on the Rating of Expressed Emotion. Unpublished manuscript.

Canino, G.
1982 The Hispanic Woman: Sociocultural Influences on Diagnoses and Treatment. In Mental Health and Hispanic Americans: Clinical Perspectives. R. Becerra, M. Karno and J. Escobar (eds.). New York: Grune and Stratton.

Chapman, A.
1976 Harry Stack Sullivan: His Life and His Work. New York: G. P. Putnam's Sons.

Farmer, P. and B. Good
1990 Illness Representations in Medical Anthropology: A Critical Review and a Case Study of the Representation of AIDS in Haïti. In The Mental Representation of Health and Illness. J. A. Skelton and Robert P. Croyle (eds.). A Volume in the Series Contributions to Psychology and Medicine. New York: Springer-Verlag .

Fromm-Reichman, F.
1948 Notes on the Development of Treatment of Schizophrenia by Psychoanalytic Psychotherapy. Psychiatry 11:263–273.

Gaines, A.
1982 Cultural Definitions, Behavior and the Person in American Psychiatry. In Cultural Conceptions of Mental Health and Therapy. Anthony Marsella and Geoffrey White (eds.). Dordrecht: D. Reidel.

Gaines, A. and P. Farmer
1986 Visible Saints: Social Cynosures and Dysphoria in the Mediterranean Tradition. Culture, Medicine and Psychiatry 10(4):295–330.

Geertz, C.
1973 Interpretation of Cultures. New York: Basic Books.
1984 "From the Native's Point of View": On the Nature of Anthropological Understanding. In Culture Theory: Essays on Mind, Self, and Emotion. R. Shweder and R. LeVine (eds.). Cambridge: Cambridge University Press.

Goldenberg, I. and H. Goldenberg
1980 Family Therapy: An Overview. Monterey, California: Brooks/Cole Publishing Co.

Guarnaccia, P. and P. Farias
1988 The Social Meanings of *nervios*: a Case Study of a Central American Woman. Social Science and Medicine 26:1223–1232.

Hooley J., J. Orley and J. Teasdale
1986 Levels of Expressed Emotion and Relapse in Depressed Patients. British Journal of Psychiatry 148:642–647.

Jenkins, J. H.
1988a Conceptions of Schizophrenia as a Problem of Nerves: a Cross-Cultural Comparison of Mexican-Americans and Anglo-Americans. Social Science and Medicine 26(12):1233–1244.
1988b Ethnopsychiatric Interpretations of Schizophrenic Illness: The Problem of *Nervios* Within Mexican-American Families. Culture, Medicine, and Psychiatry 12(3):303–331.
1990 Neither Here Nor There: Depression and Trauma Among Salvadoran Refugees in North America. Paper presented at McGill University Medical School to the Groupe Interuniversitaire de Recherche en Anthropologie Medical et en Ethnopsychiatrie (GIRAME). Montréal, Québec, Canada.
1991a The State Construction of Affect: Passion and Politics Among Salvadoran Refugees. Culture, Medicine and Psychiatry 15(2):139–165.
1991b Anthropology, Expressed Emotion, and Schizophrenia (The 1990 Stirling Award Essay). Ethos 19:387–431.

Jenkins, J., A. Kleinman and B. Good
1990 Cross-Cultural Aspects of Depression. In Advances in Mood Disorders: Theory and Research, Volume I. Psychosocial Aspects. J. Becker and A. Kleinman (eds.). Los Angeles: Earlbaum Press.

Jenkins, J. H. and M. Karno
n.d. Inside the Black Box Called "Expressed Emotion:" A Theoretical Analysis of the Construct in Psychiatric Research. (Ms. submitted for publication.)
1992 The Meaning of Expressed Emotion. American Journal of Psychiatry 149(1):9–21.

Jenkins, J. H., M. Karno and A. de la Selva
n.d. Expressed Emotion Profiles and Schizophrenic Illness Among Mexican-descent Families. (Ms. submitted for publication.)

Karno, M, J. Jenkins, A. de la Selva, et al.
1987 Expressed Emotion and Schizophrenic Outcome Among Mexican-American Families. Journal of Nervous and Mental Disorders 175:143–151.

Karno, M., et al.
1987 Lifetime Prevalence of Specific Psychiatric Disorders Among Mexican American and Non-Hispanic Whites in Los Angeles. Archives of General Psychiatry 44:695–701.

Kleinman, A.
1988 Rethinking Psychiatry. New York: Free Press.

Leff, J. and C. Vaughn
1985 Expressed Emotion in Families: Its Significance for Mental Illness. New York: Guilford Press.

Levy, R.
1984 Emotion, Knowing, and Culture. In Culture Theory: Essays on Mind, Self, and Emotion. R. Shweder and R. LeVine (eds). Cambridge: Cambridge University Press.

Lidz, T. and Fleck, S.
1960 Schizophrenia, Human Integration, and the Role of the Family. In The Etiology of Schizophrenia. D. Jackson (ed.). New York: Basic Books.

Lutz, C.
1988 Unnatural Emotions: Everyday Sentiments on a Micronesian Atoll and their Challenge to Western Theory. Chicago: University of Chicago Press.

Minuchin, S.
1974 Families and Family Therapy. Cambridge, MA: Harvard University Press.

Noh, S. and R. Turner
1987 Living with Psychiatric Patients: Implications for the Mental Health of Family Members. Social Science and Medicine 25:263–71.

Parker, G., P. Johnston and L. Hayward
1988 Parental 'Expressed Emotion' as a Predictor of Schizophrenic Relapse. Archives of General Psychiatry 45:806–813.

Ramirez, D, and C. Arce
1982 The Contemporary Chicano Family. In Explorations in Chicano Psychology. A. Baron (ed.). New York: Praeger Press.

Rosaldo, M.
1984 Toward an Anthropology of Self and Feeling. In Culture Theory: Essays on Mind, Self, and Emotion. R. Shweder and R. LeVine (eds.). Cambridge: Cambridge University Press.

Rosaldo, R.
1989 Culture and Truth: The Remaking of Social Analysis. Boston: Beacon Press.

Shweder, R.
1990 Cultural Psychology—What is it? In Cultural Psychology: Essays on Comparative Human Development. J. Stigler, R. Shweder and G. Herdt (eds.). Cambridge: Cambridge University Press.

Shweder, R. and E. Bourne
1984 (1982) Does the Concept of the Person Vary Cross-Culturally? In Culture Theory: Essays on Mind, Self, and Emotion. Cambridge University Press.

Sullivan, H. S.
1940 Conceptions of Modern Psychiatry. New York: Norton and Company.

Vaughn, C.
1986 Patterns of Emotional Response in the Families of Schizophrenic Patients. In Treatment of Schizophrenia. M. Goldstein, I. Hand and K. Hahlweg (eds.). New York: Springer-Verlag.

Vaughn, C. and J. Leff
1976 The Influence of Family and Social Factors on the Course of Psychiatric Illness. British Journal of Psychiatry 129:125–137.

Vaughn, C., K. Snyder, S. Jones, W. Freeman and I. Falloon
1984 Family Factors in Schizophrenic Relapse: A California Replication of the British Research on Expressed Emotion. Archives of General Psychiatry 41:1169–1177.

Wig, N., D. Menon, H. Bedi, et al.
1987 Expressed Emotion and Schizophrenia in North India II. Distribution of Expressed Emotion Components Among Relatives of Schizophrenic Patients in Aarhus and Chandigarh. British Journal of Psychiatry 151:160–165.

Professional Ethnopsychiatric Ideologies and Institutions

8

Professional Ethnopsychiatry in South Africa: The Question of Relativism[1]

Leslie Swartz

Introduction

This chapter deals with the production of ethnopsychiatric knowledge in South Africa in the light of aspects of *apartheid* ideology and practice.[2] I shall argue that the concept of relativism is used in a distorted manner by the South African state as a means of legitimating its continuing power, and that this has far-reaching consequences for South African ethnopsychiatric theory and practice.

I introduce my argument by a brief consideration of the concepts of complementarism and relativism in ethnopsychiatric theory. I go on to show that allowing for the multiplicity of visions implied by these positions, the South African state's pseudorelativist discourse is in fact very constraining and coercive. Some key responses to this on the part of South African anthropologists opposed to the state strategy are presented, and form part of the context for the discussion of the production of psychiatric knowledge in South Africa that follows. Some case examples illustrate the realisation of these same issues in clinical practice. I shall argue that pragmatic attitudes towards practice in an unjust society may be seen, paradoxically, as perpetuating injustice. The concluding section of this chapter emphasizes the need to explore ideologies hidden within apparently rational, dispassionate approaches to the theory and practice of psychiatry.

Complementarism and Relativism in Ethnopsychiatric Theory

Devereux's Complementarism

Devereux's *Ethnopsychoanalysis* (1978) puts forth the thesis that complementarism is a necessary basis for the understanding of human behaviour. According to Devereux, complementarism is not a theory but a methodological generalization (p. 18) stating, essentially, that a multitude of theoretical perspectives on the same human activity will yield a more complete understanding than will a single perspective. The best-known intellectual precursor of Devereux's complementarism principle is Bohr's concept of complementarity from physics which, in fact, Devereux applies.

Bohr's concept attempts to deal with a central problem of quantum physics: the observation that phenomena respond to the process of their measurement. Bohr was certainly not the first to grapple with the relationship between observer and observed, but others used different ways to deal with the problem. For example, in his *The Logic of Modern Physics* (1932), Bridgman attempted to some extent to excise the problem of the observer-observed relationship from science by advancing his system of operationalism.

According to this method, objects and concepts are defined empirically by the operations it takes to measure them. This procedure of operational definition yields a recipe for defining concepts from one perspective only. Furthermore, the operations involved in any single definition are, generally speaking, replicable by any number of observers. Operationalism yields a series of empirical concepts which are ostensibly atheoretical and exist apart from any individual's assumptions: these concepts exist only in the recordable, infinitely replicable procedures which define and contain them.

Bohr, by contrast, confronted the observer-observed relationship by accepting that a phenomenon that is being observed is different from the same phenomenon when it is not being observed. Hence, different perspectives will yield different approximations to the thing out there which is ultimately not fully knowable because it is being studied. A single method of observation becomes impossible. In Anglo-American psychiatry the operationalist paradigm has enjoyed considerable power, the strongest product of which is possibly the DSM-III (1980) and its revision, the DSM-III-R (1987).

Devereux's support of complementarity can be seen as a fundamental response to a dominant ideology, an attempt to restore the observer to a central place in the study of human behaviour. Furthermore, Devereux's insistence on the validity of both psychological and sociological modes of explanation (or of both psychoanalysis and anthropology) seriously challenges the idea of a single truth in any science.

However, Devereux does not go so far as to suggest that any theory or perspective has value. Complementarism requires that the methods or theories used are valid (1978:18). Much of his work is concerned with searching for theories which have more utility than others. In his discussions of the phenomena he studies, furthermore, Devereux does not shrink from placing a value on what he sees. Hence he is prepared to commit himself to a notion of normality which is not contained simply by the particular context in which it appears but is defined as well by structural criteria which are relatively context-independent (1980:3–71). Devereux's concern then, is the realization or surface manifestation of structures in particular contexts.

Cultural Relativism

In a chapter in a book devoted to cultural factors in mental health and therapy, Shweder and Bourne (1982) contrast relativism with universalism and evolutionism as paradigms of understanding. They define these terms in the following way:

> Universalists are committed to the view that intellectual diversity is more apparent than real, that exotic idea systems, alien at first blush, are really more like our own than they initially appear.
>
> Evolutionists are committed to the view that alien idea systems not only are truly different from our own, but are different in a special way; *viz.*, other people's systems of ideas are really incipient and less adequate stages in the development of our own understandings.
>
> Relativists, in contrast, are committed to the view that alien idea systems, while fundamentally different from our own, display an internal coherency which, on the one hand, can be understood but, on the other hand, cannot be judged. (Shweder and Bourne 1982:98)

They argue that universalism is an approach which will (a) emphasize likenesses and overlook specific differences...and/or (b) examine only a subset of the evidence (p.98). This by now fairly standard attack on universalism (see Kleinman 1977) argues that an essentially trivial grid will be placed on data, and no adequate context for the data will be provided. In the field of ethnopsychiatry the perspective provides a somewhat superficial catalog of disorder which does not adequately address issues of sociogenesis (see, for example, Leff 1981).

Evolutionism, as Shweder and Bourne refer to it, is a view which attributes to some groups deficits in cognitive skills, intellectual motivation, pertinent information and linguistic tools (p.107). It is beyond the scope of this chapter to enter into discussion of Shweder and Bourne's treatment of the authors whom they describe as evolutionist, but the important point for this chapter is that they make a strong case to demonstrate that the concept of deficit tends not to be useful in cultural anthropology. Littlewood and Lipsedge (1982) have shown that evolutionism of the type to which Shweder and Bourne refer, i.e., a crude progressivism, or what Shweder (1984) elsewhere terms developmentalism, has a long and ignominious history in Western psychiatry. There is a particular affinity between evolutionism and psychiatry in that they both deal with human deficits, whether cognitive, emotional, or cultural, and evolutionism has been attractive even to psychiatrists of considerable sophistication. In linking the mental lives of savages with those of neurotics in the context of a theory which uses regression as a central concept, for example, Freud (1950), regardless of whatever else he was doing, was adding indirectly to the discourse of evolutionism.

The key feature which distinguishes relativism from either evolutionism or universalism is the way that it uses context. Nothing is explicable without context, and different contexts (including linguistic ones) nurture phenomena which cease to be directly comparable. Things are not essentially the same (universalism) or at different stages of development (evolutionism); they are radically and essentially different. The relativist view of the world is fundamentally more fragmented than either of the others but, it is argued, more accurate.

Different though relativism may be from universalism and evolutionism, however, relativism and universalism are equally attractive to liberal ideology, though at different levels. As Gellner (1985) puts it:

> Liberalism, tolerance, pluralism, incline many to find pleasure in the idea of a multiplicity of men and visions; but the equally reputable and enlightened desire for objectivity and universality leads to a desire that at least the world and truth be but one, and not many. (The tolerant endorsement of human diversity becomes very tangled if one realises that very many past and alien visions have themselves in turn been internally exclusive, intolerant and ethnocentric; so that if we, in our tolerant way, endorse them, we thereby also endorse or encourage intolerance at second hand. This might be called the dilemma of the liberal intellectual.) (p.83–4)

Psychiatry, being essentially a liberal enterprise (see Ingleby 1981), finds itself precisely in the dilemma to which Gellner refers. Part of the difficulty with psychiatric relativism is that the actual practice of psychiatry cannot be radically relativistic. Unlike the author of a descriptive (as opposed to prescriptive) grammar, for example, the mental health practitioner cannot simply observe and celebrate diversity; it is the job of the practitioner to intervene. Partly (though not entirely) because of this reality, Devereux (1980) refuses to abandon some universalist tenets. He recognizes the need for many perspectives (hence, his reliance on complementarism) but refuses to abandon his conception of normality. Hence, his statement that from a psychiatric viewpoint the valid criteria for normality are absolute (1980:5) is not a contradiction of complementarism but simply a statement of what Devereux sees as a fundamental aspect of psychiatry. In the end, psychiatry depends on a criterion of normality which can be adapted to context but which preexists examination of any particular culture.

Regardless of whether the distinction between normal and abnormal is seen as categorical or very unclear, and regardless of where the blame for abnormality is located, psychiatry as a practice always works on the principle that there are more or less desirable ways of living. Even if it is argued that different practitioners may have different criteria for what is desirable and that these criteria are themselves culturally determined, it is a universal necessity for practice to have criteria.

In concluding an essay designed, as he puts it, to destroy a fear (Geertz 1984: 263) about cultural relativism, Geertz (1984: 276) writes:

> The objection to an anti-relativism approach is not that it rejects an it's-all-how-you-look-at-it approach to knowledge or a when-in-Rome approach to morality, but that it imagines that they can only be defeated by placing morality beyond culture and knowledge beyond both. This, speaking of things which must needs be so, is no longer possible. If we wanted home truths, we should have stayed at home.

This quotation raises certain questions about the relationship between professional ethnopsychiatric practice and relativism. In discussing the different points of view in the field, Kleinman (1988:33) contrasts the extreme relativism of some antipsychiatry anthropologists with the universalistic fundamentalism of some card-carrying biological psychiatrists, calling both positions outrageously ideological. Clearly, the card-carrying biological psychiatrists, wherever they may go, stay at home with the home truths of biological psychiatry, and the antipsychiatry anthropologists are indeed in some danger of a when-in-Rome approach. Questions about relativism as a theoretical perspective inevitably become translated into questions about the nature of psychiatric practice, which is one form of social practice.

It is of course arguable that the distinction between theory and practice is often a false one and that any social or scientific practice is informed by theories implicit or explicit. Though these statements may be true, it is important to note that theories as they are used in practice are often modified and subtly changed, whether consciously or unconsciously. A distinction needs to be made between theory as it is conceived and theory in use, or theory as an item of cultural currency. A central question that needs to be raised in this regard is this: when theorists attempt to behave in a relativist way, do they behave in such a manner consistently? Is the tolerance associated with relativism likely to be applied equally to Afrikaners as it is to Blacks,[3] for example, or is tolerance, ironically, reserved for those who might in evolutionist discourse be termed primitives? These are clearly not questions about relativism in itself, but questions of this type become crucial in any analysis attempting to examine South African ethnopsychiatric knowledge and practice.

The Language of 'Relativism' in South Africa: A Strategy for Domination

A current major ideological task of the South African state is to create a vision of reality which will allow maintenance or entrenchment of power imbalances while at the same time giving the appearance of liberalization. Domination and oppression must be cast into other, more acceptable terms. Resistance also needs to be recast in order that it can be seen as an inappropriate response to state policy. In discussing the rhetoric of the South African state particularly since 1978, Posel (1984) argues,

> The new reformist language currently prominent within the South African state upholds...a standard of technocratic rationality, recognisable in two guises: in the call for realistic and pragmatic government, and in the powers assigned to experts in administering objective solutions to national problems. (p. 2)

The language of cultural relativism as used by the South African state depends on calls for recognition of cultural diversity not simply on moral grounds, but on practical grounds as well. Hence, it becomes the duty of the South African state to protect separate group identities (so that the cultures will not be swamped by others), but even more fundamentally it is also incumbent upon the state to recognize the facts of these identities purely in pragmatic terms. Posel points out that the state has increasingly presented cultural diversity as a fact which no pragmatist can afford to ignore. Hence, cultural diversity/multinationalism/ethnicity is presented as value-free, preexisting any policy. The state becomes bound by rules of common sense to respond to the facts, and its *apartheid* policy (or whatever its new guise) is seen as the only hardheaded, logical response to these facts. Thus a climate is created in which to deny the state's version of cultural relativism is to deny reality. Opponents of South African policy can then be cast as people who are out of touch with reality, or sentimental dreamers.

Posel's identification of the technicist cast to South African reformist language is particularly relevant to the present discussion. Ethnopsychiatry is a field dominated by experts of the type required by state strategy to provide objective solutions. The entire mental health enterprise, expertise in which is designated scientific, becomes an arena in which the dominance of the state ideology can be reproduced and confirmed scientifically. It may even be argued, as is implied in Littlewood and Lipsedge's (1982) work, that psychiatry in particular is an area where ideological reproduction is crucial. This is because of the association between 'primitives' and 'madness' as well as the social regulatory function of mental health practice. Scientific though psychiatry, clinical psychology and similar helping professions may be, they are however applied disciplines. They have to rely for their givens on common sense (i.e., ideologically influenced cultural knowledge) or more basic social sciences. Social anthropologists opposed to state policies have considered at some length issues concerning the nature of categories of culture in South Africa. Some issues concerning their response now will be considered.

Redefining Culture in South Africa: The Problem

A recent South African textbook aimed chiefly at undergraduate students and "interested general readers" states in its introduction, different races and ethnic groups, unique cultures and traditions, do not exist in any ultimate sense in South Africa, and are real only to the extent that they are the product of a particular worldview. (Sharp 1988:1)

The author of this introduction goes on to describe this view as "a heresy" (Sharp 1988:1), and much of the book amounts to a defence of this heretical position. The authors set themselves the task of laying bare what they term the changing discourse of domination (Sharp 1988:6) in South Africa, and they show how terms such as "race," "culture," "tribe," "tradition," and "community" have been used at different times to legitimate the interests of those who hold power in South Africa (cf. Posel 1984).

Heresy is a strong word to describe what may be termed a social constructionist[4] approach to the understanding of the production of ideas about groups. Its theological connotations are particularly apposite in the context of the history of the use of religion and the Dutch Reformed Church in particular as a basis for legitimation of *apartheid* ideology. The strength of the word *heresy* accurately reflects the intensity of feeling about the construction of groups that is the cornerstone of apartheid policy. At the time of writing this chapter, for example, it is still mandatory for each South African to be classified along racial lines. Though just recently dissolved officially, still, regardless of whether this classification seems relevant to persons thus classified, it determines where they may live, go to school, and whether they may vote in the House of Assembly, the whites-only house of parliament in which *de facto* the country's executive power is vested. It is not possible in South Africa to claim that groups of people are different from each other without at some level recalling, consciously or unconsciously, a major basis for justification of oppressive practices. In the same introductory textbook, Thornton writes that ideas about the existence of separate cultures,

have been used to justify repressive and brutal forms of government by arguing that, like an organism, a culture or nation must defend itself against internal, as well as external, enemies. If the initial premise that cultures are owned by nations is accepted, the activities of repressive state bureaucracies may be justified as a form of political hygiene. (1988:19)

In a lucid exposition which recalls many of the issues of debate in contemporary culture theory (Shweder and LeVine 1984), Thornton (1988) demonstrates the fact that many of the boundaries around cultures in South Africa (and elsewhere) have in fact been imposed on people within specific historical contexts. Thornton argues instead that modern anthropology should regard culture as a resource which can be used in social relations rather than as a static entity which defines people from the outside, and should in addition recognise the fact that culture changes. An important implication of his work is that to define people from the outside as belonging to a specific cultural group is to engage in a political act which has particular ramifications in South Africa.

These ramifications have been evident in various trends in the production of knowledge about culture in South Africa. Sharp (1981) has traced the history of the discipline known as *Volkekunde* (cultural anthropology), which is taught and applied in Afrikaans medium universities, which have been created by the South African government for nonwhites, and in various state organizations such as the Defence Force. *Volkekunde*, Sharp argues, assigns primacy to culture as a mode of explaining South Africa's diversity, and many of its strengths and weaknesses, and culture is taken as the basis on which all knowledge is to be built. As Sharp shows, the *Volkekunde* argument has been used repeatedly to provide scientific support for apartheid or separate development policies.[5] In this article and in a companion one (Sharp 1980) he demonstrates that the assumption of the primacy of culture is used as an analytical tool not only within *Volkekunde* but also in social anthropology—even among people critical of *apartheid* and similar policies.

In the face of an articulate attack on the production of ideas about cultural difference in the service of the current system of domination, it is tempting to opt for an approach which deemphasizes difference and emphasizes similarity. Kottler (1988) argues that this is indeed the position taken by the contributors to the Boonzaier and Sharp (1988) text mentioned. For example, Thornton (1988:18) states:

> In the marketplace and workplace, listening to music or watching television, at homes and in churches, people in fact experience the same desires, profess the same religions, follow the same leaders, and eat the same cornflakes, notwithstanding their multicultural condition!

Thornton makes four assertions here about what people in fact do:

1. They experience the same desires.
2. They profess the same religions.
3. They follow the same leaders.
4. They eat the same cornflakes.

An important feature of these statements for the purposes of this chapter is that all of them are easily translated into empirically testable questions (e.g., Do people coming from different cultures eat the same cornflakes?) except for the first. How does one know that people experience the same desires? In terms of the way that knowledge is divided in contemporary academic life, this becomes a difficult psychological, psychiatric, or (perhaps most appropriately) psychoanalytic question, not open to easy empirical investigation. As Kottler (1988) notes, the psychological dimension is ignored by the similarities position in South Africa. Yet this is a key dimension for ethnopsychiatry.

Kottler (1988) points out further that adhering to the similarities position is not the only way theorists can express dissatisfaction with state strategies.[6] Proponents of what she terms the differences position are not automatically in favour of government policy:

> It is irrelevant if the Government is telling Zulu people that they are bounded by their own special culture which is peculiar to them. They know who they are essentially, so that at one level can indeed be Zulu, yet at a deeper level are Africans with a worldview or orientation common to Africans in general; while in a more external sense they are also South Africans. (Ngubane [1988:11–12] as quoted by Kottler [1988:8])

Ngubane is suggesting that, in the face of dominant state ideology, it is more fundamentally heretical to note the importance of differences in a manner contrary to the way the state does, than to emphasize similarities rather than differences. This view, Ngubane would argue, is not one imposed from the outside but part of the cultural heritage of different South African groups (see Ngubane 1977), and is essential in the understanding of the psychology of black South Africans.

The Production of Psychiatric Knowledge in South Africa

Ethnopsychiatric knowledge in South Africa is caught between a variety of positions which may influence it: the pseudorelativism of state policy, the similarities counterattack, and the differences counter-counter-position.[7] I have demonstrated elsewhere the central position of state policy in providing a context for this knowledge (Swartz 1986, 1987). Given the nature of South African society, one might argue that psychiatric knowledge produced in this country is part of a broad conspiracy against Blacks (see Lambley 1980). I believe this view is inherently simplistic and extremely unfortunate. Psychiatric knowledge in South Africa, as in other countries, has a primarily pragmatic motivation (Swartz and Foster 1984). The aim of much South African research is to create knowledge which will contribute to the understanding and treatment of mental illness in black people.

I make this point not simply because I wish to protect myself from counterattack by some South African colleagues but because I believe that conspiracy theories in general are not useful. Though conspiracy theories have a popular history in psychiatry (Laing and Esterson 1964; Szasz 1971) they are often based on the belief that evil intent is at the basis of work which either is in itself racist or oppressive in orientation or comes to be used for oppressive purposes. This belief is reductive in that it locates ideology in individual motives and fails to take account of the extent to which ideology determines what is sayable, what cannot be said or seen, and what becomes common sense.

In trying to establish a framework for understanding production of psychiatric knowledge in South Africa, I shall draw on Said's (1978) discussion of Orientalism. In the introduction to his argument, Said identifies a number of meanings for the term. According to Said, the most obvious definition of Orientalism is as an academic field. It can also be defined as "a style of thought based upon an ontological and epistemological distinction made between the Orient and (most of the time) the Occident"(p.2).

Most importantly for Said's purposes, however, and for this discussion, Orientalism can be seen as a discourse in Foucault's sense:

> My contention is that without examining Orientalism as a discourse one cannot possibly understand the enormously systematic discipline by which European culture was able to manage—and even produce—the Orient politically, sociologically, militarily, ideologically, scientifically and imaginatively during the post-enlightenment period. Because of Orientalism the Orient was not (and is not) a free subject of thought or action. This is not to say that Orientalism unilaterally determines what can be said about the Orient, but that it is the whole network of interests inevitably brought to bear on (and therefore always involved in) any occasion when that peculiar entity the Orient is in question. (p. 3)

South African psychiatry, like Orientalism, can be seen as an academic discipline but also as part of a cultural discourse which creates its object. Ethnopsychiatry in particular creates its object of study and constellates it as part of a particular kind of discourse. The fundamental notion of this discourse is that of otherness. I use this term in contradistinction to that of difference in that I take difference to be relatively more value-neutral and otherness more closely associated with the forms of cultural reproduction I discuss below. The notion of otherness is one which serves to perpetuate divisions and also to define the not-other. By defining the other or the bizarre, South Africans writing in the field of ethnopsychiatry are simultaneously defining both themselves and their own culture.

Writing in the *South African Journal of Ethnology*, a journal with a strong *volkekunde* flavour, De Villiers makes the following series of statements:

> In Xhosa tradition illness is regarded as a type of misfortune..., consequently ideas about causes of illness are closely associated with ideas about causes of misfortune in general. (1985:48)
>
> Available information allows for a distinction between supernatural and natural causation. This distinction is made in relation to cultural considerations of the target population and it is not verbally expressed, possibly only existing in a subconscious awareness among the people who identify a particular cause, but not the type of causation.

While supernatural and natural causes are mutually exclusive, factors such as deterioration in a patient's condition may lead to reinterpretation of the cause, so that a natural cause is rejected for a supernatural one. (p. 52)

These quotes place themselves as much by what they omit as what they say. They imply that supernatural causation is the "province" of Xhosas, that the link between illness and misfortune is unique to this group (or groups of this "type"). Even physicians in the biomedical tradition do in fact have a range of ways of responding to illness, not all of them neatly fitting into a "natural" pigeonhole (Hahn and Gaines 1985). De Villiers does not address this issue, but by implication disallows an examination of similarities between her subjects and Westerners. The second quotation also makes an implicit link between irrationality and "Xhosa culture" by focusing on what she terms the "subconscious." One wonders how many groups *consciously* choose explanatory models!

De Villiers's treatment of the natural/supernatural distinction is but one of many South African examples (Swartz 1985a, 1986, 1987; Swartz and Foster 1984). It is not an accident that the work which is challenging the implicit models in South African work is also critical about its own assumptions and theoretical base. Mills (1985) begins to challenge dominant South African models; Heap (1985) very clearly relegates the ideology of 'otherness' to a back seat in her discussion of health and illness in Lesotho. The 'relativism' which is apparently value-free in South African work can quite easily be seen as an example of knowledge determined by ideological climate. To focus on similarities rather than differences, one must first take on a series of South African cultural assumptions, to deconstruct, as it were, one's own position as a reproducer of ideology.

Producing Otherness in a Universalist Context

The discourse of otherness appears in other contexts besides the relativist or pseudorelativist work in South Africa. Much of conventional South African ethnopsychiatry—particularly that produced by proponents of ostensibly universalist (largely British) biomedical theory and practice—is intent on finding similarities between groups but remains locked within the discourse of otherness. Studies of this type often focus on similarities between psychiatric syndromes amongst various groups. I shall use an example to illustrate the problems with this position.

Using the Present State Examination (PSE) (Wing et al. 1974), Teggin et al. (1985) investigated the symptoms of schizophrenia in white, coloured, and Black psychiatric inpatients. Their study revealed great similarities in prevalence of syndromes. They conclude that this study provides qualified evidence for similarity in the psychiatric manifestations of schizophrenic patients from diverse cultural and social groups (p. 885).

How does this universalist conclusion (in the sense attacked by Kleinman [1977] as the old transcultural psychiatry) contribute to the discourse of otherness? Let us consider the manner in which the authors deal with the supposedly observed difference. "Blacks" were found to have significantly more olfactory hallucinations than were the other groups:

> Significantly more black patients were rated on the syndrome of olfactory hallucinations, which supports the findings...that these symptoms occur with relatively high frequency among Kenyan patients. (Teggin et al. 1985:686)

This statement lays bare some of the assumptions behind the approach. The authors do not explain how a finding in Cape Town, South Africa, can support a finding in Kenya, on a completely different population. No discussion is given as to why Kenyans and Black South Africans are comparable groups. Whether they are in fact comparable or not is beyond the scope of this chapter; reading the article in question, however, one might conclude that what unites Kenyans and Black South Africans is that both groups are black. To explain the differences observed, the authors are drawing on the otherness of *all Blacks*, regardless of how diverse the groups may be. If I am correct in my assumptions, then the authors of the article can be seen to be producing "blackness" as a concept, in the same way that Said speaks of the production of the Orient through the discourse of Orientalism. This otherness or blackness (replete with racist overtones, regardless of the intention of the authors) provides the background for any similarities seen.

The knowledge created by work of this kind is fundamentally decontextualized, its concepts (such as culture and mental illness) reified. Material reality is nothing more than a modifying factor, and the implicit dimension along which people are measured is that of otherness—a dimension which clearly elaborates aspects of South African state ideology.

Clinical Practice and the Search for Appropriate Models of Explanation

I have consistently argued thus far that South Africans in the field of ethnopsychiatry find themselves embedded within a particular dominant discourse, or at very least within the kinds of oppositional responses the discourse invites. By saying this I do not imply that South Africans are passive bearers of ideology. Nor do I accept that the majority of mental health professionals are out to do anything other than what they perceive to be the best for their patients. Nowhere are the difficulties of being a South African mental health professional more clear than in the field of actual clinical practice, where the demand to do one's best in structurally less-than-ideal circumstances is strongest. I shall illustrate the problems by means of case examples.

Case 1: Ms. A

Ms. A was a coloured woman[8] of very dark complexion (i.e., she looks Black), in her mid-thirties at the time of referral. She was divorced with one son and she lived with her parents and son in a house in a small city some 800 kilometers from Cape Town. She was referred to a large psychiatric hospital in Cape Town after the only psychiatric services (all outpatient) in her city felt they could no longer cope with her. Her presenting problem was that she would often find herself lying on the sidewalk with her legs apart and her panties beside her. She never had any recollection of how she had got into this state, and she thought that perhaps other people had taken her panties off her after knocking her out. Some indication of how she negotiated her sick role could be gleaned from the fact that she was taking eighteen different psychotropic drugs a day, dispensed by various different practitioners. On admission she was taken off all medication, with no apparent change in her behaviour. I was responsible for the management of the case.

During the first history-taking session, Ms. A, though apparently unaware of doing so, fondled my ankle with her bare foot. She spoke under pressure, and it was very difficult to keep her talking on the topic at hand (though she was by no means thought-disordered). I got the impression that the more rigidly I tried to keep to the standard (British-model) history taking format, the more irritated she became that I did not want to hear what she wanted to say. At the end of this unsuccessful interview, Ms. A asked me if I would give her twenty cents because she wanted to use the public telephone. I declined, and she went off to the dining hall for the evening meal. I was told the following morning that she had stood on a table there and claimed that she had just been raped. She had then lain on the floor. After this event, Ms. A settled well on the ward, and she was later discharged asymptomatic. Unfortunately, I am unaware of her follow-up details.

DISCUSSION

How does one interpret Ms. A's behaviour? Her arrival at the hospital caused considerable interest amongst the clinical staff. More junior members were encouraged to come to the ward and talk to Ms. A as, it was said, classic Freudian hysteria is now very rare in the Western world but is still seen in Africa in people "who are not white." I do not wish to enter into any discussion here of whether this statement is empirically true or not, but I do want to point out the implicit evolutionism—Ms. A and her ilk are 'curiosities,' bearers of an illness of the past.[9]

Clinically, this view of the patient seems to do little more than to distance the patient from the professionals. It provides a context in that it alludes to history, but in such a reified manner that it is not particularly useful. The discourse of otherness reinforces the divisions in South African society and more firmly defines the clinicians as culturally different from people of Ms. A's social stratum.

There were, however, other, less reductive ways of looking at the case of Ms. A. Her interaction with me, though clearly hysterical in a classical sense, also occurred within a particular context. I am a white South African; she is coloured. A stereotypical relationship (though in reality not the most common) between white and coloured South Africans is that of begging. The coloured person begs; the white either agrees or disagrees to give money.

In my role as a clinician I was attempting as far as possible to divorce myself from all preconceptions or cultural stereotypes that I might have, but this woman was reminding me that South African social factors do not stop at the hospital gates. She was forcing me to confront the ambiguity of my attempts at clinical neutrality. She was in a very real sense raped by me, both by my insistence on a mode of clinical procedure which did not adequately receive her view of herself, and by my white maleness. This white maleness in South African society offers the promise (the reality) of power which cannot be hers. Her request for money can be seen both as a demand that she be paid for allowing me the pleasure of my exercise of power (as a prostitute might be paid) and as an attempt to receive part of that power for herself. Part of why she saw herself as raped, I suspect, was that she was not paid.

This discussion is not designed to imply either that Ms. A was an innocent victim of my evil machinations or that she had consciously created an illness in order to expose contradictions in South African ethnopsychiatry. What I am suggesting, however, is that the case of Ms. A demonstrates the usefulness of focusing on the common cultural context encapsulating both clinician and patient. Goldstein's comment, "it takes two to make a diagnosis—a patient with a set of symptoms and a physician who gives them the label he deems appropriate" (1982:211), can be expanded to other aspects of the clinical encounter. Issues of power, class and colour existed for both me and Ms. A—they were not hers alone, and my behaviour was determined to some extent by my own emotional reactions to them. Our encounter crystallized for me much about my own position as a white South African whose concern for his patients is inextricably confounded with his own social position. Ms. A and I are equally part of a particular South African "culture."

A final question in this case is, Why hysteria? The essentially evolutionist reduction of hysteria to a relic of the Western past is not satisfactory. I cannot deal fully with this question here but will sketch some of the parameters for what I see as a more adequate contextual understanding. I must reiterate that this woman is classified coloured. She speaks English and Afrikaans at home. She does not belong to those groups in which, some would argue, spirit possession can be culturally acceptable (see for example Ngubane [1977]; Swartz [1986] gives an overview of some aspects of spirit possession in South Africa). The cultural explanation (in the sense used in South African state discourse), therefore, cannot be applied. An understanding of the matrix of Ms. A's familial and social relationships is necessary in this case. This includes some understanding of the woman's position within power relationships in South Africa. Foucault (1978) has suggested that the 'hysterization of women's bodies' (p.104), as he calls it, has been, since the eighteenth century, a feature involved in the harnessing of sexuality within a structure of power.[10]

> Sexuality must not be thought of as a kind of natural given which power tries to hold in check, or as an obscure domain which knowledge tries gradually to uncover. It is the name that can be given to a historical construct: not a furtive reality that is difficult to grasp, but a great surface network in which the stimulation of bodies, the intensification of pleasures, the incitement to discourse, the formation of special knowledges, the strengthening of controls and resistances, are linked to one another, in accordance with a few major strategies of knowledge and power. (1978:105–106)

This woman's "perverse pleasure" (p.105)—her hysteria—can be understood not only as a psychological problem but also as her contribution to an historically specific discourse. In his discussion of culture-bound syndromes in Malaya, Lee (1981) uses Turner's concepts of structure and anti-structure to argue that these syndromes are not pathological but: 'an integral part of Malay cultural reality' (1981:245). What I am arguing here with respect to Ms. A's hysteria is not that it is either normal or culturally acceptable (this is clearly not the case) but that it does have a function similar to that alluded to by Lee. It helps to reproduce the South African discourse of otherness precisely by presenting a picture of madness which is, apparently, so antiquated. Hysteria is a form of madness of the Western past (whether this is empirically true is irrelevant here—I am talking at the level of ideological production), and women like Ms. A reemphasize the Romantic association between darkness of skin and "the primitive." Ms. A, through the theatrical language of her condition, was informing me and other clinicians of how we had captured our own sexuality within what Foucault would call an appropriate domain. She was confirming us in our positions while at the same time reinforcing the image of otherness as crystallized within herself.

I do not pretend to have a complete explanation of Ms. A's behaviour. I do wish to suggest, however, that her symptoms and our reactions to them played some part in furthering our function (as clinicians) of reproducing South African power discourse. Our technicist response to her, such as the prescription of eighteen kinds of psychotropic drugs and attempts to take a formal history from a woman whose story was not formal, reproduced aspects of the language of legitimation in South Africa.

I do not think that clinically we served her badly at the hospital, and I also do not suggest that her being a South African mysteriously caused her to be an hysteric. Her case does illustrate, however, the way in which symptoms and response to them are elaborated within a particular ideological context and not simply in the context of many neatly separate cultures all having different norms, values, and so on. The ideological context to which I refer is not one which can be escaped by anyone, least of all by those who seek to enter what has been termed the "cosmology" or "worldview" of black people (Hammond-Tooke [1975]; Schweitzer [1983]). Mental health practice is inevitably involved in the reproduction of ideologies. Ms. A's case serves as an illustration of how both patients and clinicians are involved in the process.

Case 2: Mr. B

Mr. B was a Xhosa-speaking man in his late forties, a school principal in a rural area. Prior to admission he had been behaving increasingly bizarrely and had become verbally aggressive. His behaviour fitted the typical picture of frontal lobe syndrome, which was confirmed on examination and later treated.

It is not surprising in view of Mr. B's condition that he was difficult to manage during his time on the ward prior to the completion of his diagnostic assessment. The particular ward to which Mr. B was assigned had compulsory group meetings three times a week. He was extremely disruptive in these, complaining that nobody understood him. His command of English was excellent, but his Afrikaans (the home language of most of the other patients on the ward, all of whom were classified coloured) was poor. Most patients used Afrikaans in group meetings, much to Mr. B's annoyance. From the time of his second group meeting and until he was transferred to another ward, he spoke only Xhosa during group meetings, though he spoke English at other times. Nobody else on the ward (staff or patients) could understand Xhosa.

DISCUSSION

Mr. B's behaviour was clearly neither culturally determined nor culturally acceptable. However, the manner in which he expressed his dissatisfaction with the hospital exposed contradictions within the system. Like other such institutions in South Africa, the hospital was racially segregated. The form of segregation, however, did not follow the cultural lines as put forward in official government policy. Whites were placed in one section of the hospital, and all other patients in another. As it happens all the patients on Mr. B's particular ward were, except for Mr. B himself, coloured. All the staff were white or coloured. No special arrangements were made for Mr.

B's cultural needs. His choice to speak Xhosa in group meetings, which were ostensibly designed to facilitate patients' hospital adjustment, demonstrated clearly how the system was capable of making very little true provision for his needs. In multilingual societies clinical staff often are ignorant of their patients' home language (see, for example, Marcos et al. 1973), and clearly this is not an ideal situation anywhere. But the South African state claims that its policies are designed to give privileged place to what it terms 'cultural' matters, and furthermore by legislation it defines Black language groups as cultural groups. Mr. B, whatever else he was expressing with his clearly disturbed behaviour, was making an accurate attack on the dishonesty of the system which defined him in one way but made no positive provision for him in the light of this definition.[11] He also exposed some of the inadequacies of the rhetoric of South African ethnopsychiatry in that it claims to require knowledge of cultural factors but was in this case unable to cope with them adequately. As staff we were effectively silenced by Mr. B, and this took away our ability to provide a genuinely containing environment for him.

The cases of Ms. A and Mr. B both demonstrate how the model of separate, bounded cultures as used in South Africa can be of limited clinical value. In both cases there was a need to establish a model of understanding which incorporated both the clinician and the other culture patient. Recognition of this second type of model, however, is potentially subversive of the socially constituted clinician-patient relationship in that it emphasizes their similarities rather than differences. It also indirectly raises questions of appropriate clinical practice, which are considered in the following section.

Criticism and the Question of Professional Responsibility

The question of how to function as a clinician in a society which is not conducive to optimal mental health for all has been addressed by a number of authors, notably those espousing radical politics (Kovel 1981; Turkle 1978). In South Africa, which is regarded by many as a prerevolutionary society, the issue often becomes recast informally as, "what do we do until the revolution comes?" For purposes of this discussion I shall avoid the substantive question of what can be expected to happen to patterns of mental illness when (if?) the revolution does come. I shall focus instead on the debates about the present. Responding to a radical critique on South African industrial psychology by Nzimande (1985), Coldwell (1985) makes the implicit point that psychologists have to operate in the present and cannot simply wait for the future to arrive. Few could argue with this assertion, though some would say that to attempt to operate honestly as a clinician in *apartheid* society is to attempt the impossible. Leaving aside this view, the debate becomes one of the pragmatic aspects of practice under less than ideal, repressive conditions.

The issue of pragmatism, however, immediately recalls the technicist language of facing reality that has been shown earlier to be part of South African state strategy (Posel 1984). Thus Gillis (1977, 1978), for example, who has taken upon himself the unenviable task of defending South African psychiatry to the outside world, speaks of the realities of the situation in a manner which is not dissimilar to that used by the state. Given his chosen task, I doubt that he could have done otherwise, but the challenge he implicitly poses to critics of South African ethnopsychiatry is precisely this: it is all very well to carp and to make political statements, but for the welfare of our patients we have to adapt to the realities of the situation. Those who simply carp achieve nothing.

This is not a viewpoint to be dismissed lightly. Overburdened staff in mental institutions have only so much time and energy, and many have chosen to dedicate themselves as far as possible to the welfare of their patients within current social constraints. Politically speaking, to make the best of an unacceptable situation makes no sense at all; many feel that from the viewpoint of clinical ethics there is no choice. I do not question the motivation and dedication of many proponents of this position, but it can become counterproductive if it is presented preemptively as the *only* course of action. To argue that agreeing on the maximum benefit of one's individual patients is the only ethical way to proceed is to subscribe to a view which is politically naïve. As we have seen earlier, the knowledge produced this way is likely to reproduce dominant ideology willy-nilly and hence to entrench it. Clinicians who have no time for what may be termed armchair criticism may well contribute to that which they find unacceptable.

This does not imply that all critics of the function of the mental health professions within the South African state system are not practising clinicians. However, I have not seen any radical critique of the discourse of South African ethnopsychiatry from persons whose chief employment is within state health services. I am sure that it is not by accident that recent discussion of the role of mental health practice in the South African discourse has come from people employed largely in nonclinical university teaching positions (Dawes 1985; Psychology in Society 1983; Swartz 1985a; Swartz and Foster 1984). This fact can lead to a false and unfortunate split between practitioners within state services and critics of structures defining those services. It may be the case, indeed, that in order to function adequately within the state system one cannot question too much and too radically (even leaving aside issues of formal and informal censorship of such criticism). Hence the role of critic has to be split off and handed to those not similarly involved. The possibility of acrimony between groups on the issue of professional responsibility is, however, great in a polarized society.

This discussion may appear to be only tangentially related to the central question of the manufacture of 'cultural difference' with which this paper has been concerned. However, it highlights very centrally the fact that divisions within South African society do not necessarily coincide with those legislated by state policy. Even within professional groups, important differences which may well influence psychiatric practice exist. These positions are to greater or lesser degrees cast within the mould of or in response to dominant discourse.

Conclusions and Implications

This chapter has traced some issues in the production of a culturally constructed (Gaines 1988) language of pseudorelativism in South Africa and its relationship to conditions in South African ethnopsychiatry. I have demonstrated that the language of relativism plays a particular role within South African state strategy, in its academic disciplines in general and in psychiatry in particular. I have illustrated some ways in which relativism can be used to reproduce certain stereotypical pictures of mental illness. These images in turn reinforce the reality of images generated by the state. Case examples have illustrated how these issues are realized in clinical practice, and some of the questions and debates surrounding responsible clinical practice have been discussed.

Working in an unequal society like South Africa demonstrates the importance of taking account of power relationships. Knowledge, expression of distress, healing practices are not all qualities of human essence which alters in appearance in certain contexts but remains essentially the same. When exploring issues of knowledge the question of value is not one that can be swept aside. Not all knowledge is equal.

The pseudorelativist approach of the South African state does indeed take context into account, but only context of a particular kind. Context is reified into a cultural essence inherent within the patient—a product of belief in the primacy of racial categories. Other contexts which are deserving of more attention include the material context and the context of the clinical encounter.

Prejudice and discrimination which masquerade as relativism can be seen to be part of a discourse of domination, as Said's study of Orientalism shows, and, as I believe, is seen in South African ethnopsychiatry. The questions of power and resistance cannot legitimately be divorced from clinical practice. There is the constant reality that in defining patients clinicians are simultaneously defining themselves and their own position. Pure knowledge of a patient's real state of mind (i.e., divorced from this context) cannot be obtained. The task of building a South African psychiatry which takes adequate account of the different realities of patients—a psychiatry which Ngubane (in Kottler [1988]) would perhaps support—is severely impeded by the fact that 'difference' in this country almost invariably implies domination. Adequate knowledge of a range of social practices, however, remains essential.

Rychlak (1982) has suggested that psychotherapy operates in an "as if" mode—thus the therapist proceeds as if theories were empirically true and as if interpretation referred necessarily to objective reality while recognizing that we are not actually dealing in facts. Clinical practice anywhere demands this 'as if' approach, particularly in South Africa. There is a constant danger that unhelpful constructions will simply be reproduced through clinical practice. The more a group of people operates uncritically within a certain mode, the more reality the images of that mode appear to attain.

The truism that every science creates its own object applies well to South African ethnopsychiatry. Clinicians are socialized in a context in which differences between bounded cultural entities are presented as real and unproblematic. The rational, responsible clinical attitude towards these differences may be simply to acknowledge the differences but refuse to make value judgements. What at first glance may appear to be a different-but-equal model of psychopathology, however, may be a method of obscuring power imbalances. These imbalances, I would argue, need to be explored and exposed.

Notes

1. I am grateful to Atwood Gaines, Marion Heap, Tracey Miller, and Michelle Slone for their comments on drafts of this chapter. Financial assistance of the Mellon Foundation Grant is acknowledged with thanks. The opinions expressed in this chapter are my responsibility alone.

2. *Apartheid* has for some time not been the official policy of the South African régime, but the term provides a convenient shorthand for policies which, despite changing discourses of legitimation (Posel 1984), maintain racial difference as fundamental, and the protection of white power as central.

3. In this article I use the terms laid down by the South African Population Registration Act, as amended. These are white, coloured, Indian, and Black. This does not imply that I accept the validity of these categories. The term "coloured" presents particular difficulties: according to the South African Population Registration Act, 'coloured' is simply a ragbag category including all people who are not white and who are not Black. For a discussion of this see Swartz (1985a). Where I use the term "black" (i.e., without capitalization), it is a generic term, distinct from official usage, for all South Africans without franchise for the South African House of Assembly (i.e., coloured, Black and Indian people as defined by the Population Registration Act).

4. Gaines (1988:2) argues that the term "constructionism" has negative connotations: "the term *constructionism* suggests coming to the study of lay and professional medicine, or any other domain of culture, with preconceived ideas. Such ideas constrain, limit and block understanding(s)." He suggests that the approach

he develops as "cultural constructivism" is more useful in the medical anthropological arena than social constructionism. The negative connotations he sees as implicit in the term "constructionist" are important in the text in question.

5. Other notions have, of course, been used (or misused) as well in the service of state ideology, including those of "justice," "fairness," and even "democracy"!

6. It should be noted that proponents of what Kottler (1988) terms the "similarities" position do not set themselves up purely to produce knowledge questioning the South African state. Thornton (1988), like other contributors to the Boonzaier and Sharp (1988) volume, questions a range of received truths held by people from a wide variety of political perspectives.

7. I do not suggest here that these three positions are historically distinct or even that they follow the order in which I have presented them. The schematization of state policy's—"similarities," "differences"' is, however, useful here as it illustrates some of the complexity of ideological forces impinging on ethnopsychiatric practice.

8. "Coloured," as I have noted before, is very much a ragbag category for people who fit in neither the "white" nor the "Black" pigeonholes (see Swartz 1985a). The category includes people of so-called "mixed race," and "Cape Malay" people, but excludes "Indians." Those classified 'coloured' in South Africa range in appearance from people indistinguishable from "whites" to those indistinguishable from "Blacks."

9. This is in all probability a gross oversimplification of the epidemiology of hysteria, but the fact that it was "common knowledge" in the institution in question is an interesting piece of information in itself.

10. I have argued elsewhere that *anorexia nervosa* can fruitfully be understood under this rubric (Swartz 1985b).

11. Since the time of Mr. B's stay, a large psychiatric hospital chiefly for coloured patients has opened. Black patients alone are now treated on the formerly Black/coloured side of the older institution. This has led to a greater awareness of the particular needs (including linguistic) of Black patients. It is, however, interesting that in discussion of current moves to integrate all psychiatric facilities by race, concern is being expressed by some about the problem of white and Black patients' not being able to communicate with each other, or feeling "culturally alienated"' from each other. I had no knowledge of this type of talk, which applies equally to communication gaps between coloureds and Blacks, when they were together for many years in the same wards.

References

American Psychiatric Association
1980 Diagnostic and Statistical Manual of Mental Disorders, Third Edition (DSM-III). Washington, D.C.: American Psychiatric Association.
1987 Diagnostic and Statistical Manual of Mental Disorders, Third Edition, Revised (DSM-III-R). Washington, D.C.: American Psychiatric Association.

Boonzaier, Emile and John Sharp (eds.)
1988 South African Keywords: Uses and Abuses of Political Concepts. Cape Town, South Africa: David Philip.

Bridgman, Percy W.
1932 The Logic of Modern Physics. New York: Macmillan.

Coldwell, D. A. L.
1985 Reply to Nzimande. Psychology in Society 3:43–48.

Dawes, Andrew R. L.
1985 Politics and Mental Health: the Position of Clinical Psychology in South Africa. South African Journal of Psychology 15:55–61.

De Villiers, Stephne
1985 (Consideration of) Illness Causation Among Some Xhosa-Speaking People. South African Journal of Ethnology 8:45–52.

Devereux, George
1978 Ethnopsychoanalysis. Psychoanalysis and Anthropology as Complementary Frames of Reference. Berkeley: University of California Press.
1980 Basic Problems of Ethnopsychiatry. Chicago: University of Chicago Press.

Foucault, Michel.
1978 The History of Sexuality. Volume I: An Introduction. Robert Hurley, trans. New York: Random House.

Freud, Sigmund
1950 Totem and Taboo. James Strachey, trans. London: Routledge and Kegan Paul.

Gaines, Atwood D.
1988 Cultural Constructivism: Sickness History and the Understanding of Ethnomedicines Beyond Critical Medical Anthropologies. Paper presented at the Conference, Medical Anthropologies: Western European and North American Perspectives. December. University of Hamburg. Hamburg, West Germany. Also 1991. In Anthropologies of Medicine. B. Pfleiderer and G. Bibeau (eds.). Wiesbaden: Vieweg Verlag.

Geertz, Clifford
1984 Anti-Anti-Relativism. American Anthropologist 86:263–278.

Gellner, Ernest
1985 Relativism and the Social Sciences. Cambridge: Cambridge University Press.

Gillis, Lynn S.
1977 Mental Health Care in South Africa. The Lancet, October 29:920–921.
1978 Mental Health Care in South Africa. The Lancet, April 8:767.

Goldstein, Jan
1982 The Hysteria Diagnosis and the Politics of Anticlericalism in Late Nineteenth-Century France. Journal of Modern History 54:209–239.

Hahn Robert A. and Atwood D. Gaines, eds.
1985 Physicians of Western Medicine. Anthropological Approaches to Theory and Practice. Dordrecht, Holland: D. Reidel.

Hammond-Tooke, W. D.
1975 African World-View and its Relevance for Psychiatry. Psychologia Africana 16:25–32.

Heap, Marion
1985 Health and Disease in two Villages in South Eastern Lesotho: A Social Anthropological Perspective. Unpublished Masters of Social Science thesis. University of Cape Town.

Ingleby, David
1981 Understanding 'Mental Illness.' In Critical Psychiatry. David Ingleby (ed.). Harmondsworth: Penguin.

Kleinman, Arthur
1977 Depression, Somatization and the 'New Cross-Cultural Psychiatry.' Social Science and Medicine. 11:3–10.
1988 Rethinking Psychiatry: From Cultural Category to Personal Experience. New York: The Free Press.

Kottler, Amanda
1988 South Africa: Psychology's Dilemma of Multiple Discourses. Ms. Department of Psychology, University of Cape Town.

Kovel, Joel
1981 The Age of Desire. Reflections of a Radical Psychoanalyst. New York: Pantheon Books.

Laing, Ronald D. and Aaron Esterson
1964 Sanity, Madness and the Family. London: Tavistock Publications.

Lambley, Peter
1980 The Psychology of Apartheid. London: Secker and Warburg.

Lee, Raymond
1981 Structure and Anti-Structure in the Culture-Bound Syndromes: the Malay Case. Culture, Medicine and Psychiatry 5:233–248.

Leff, Julian
1981 Psychiatry Around the Globe: A Transcultural View. New York: Marcel Dekker.

Littlewood, Roland and Maurice Lipsedge
1982 Aliens and Alienists. Ethnic Minorities and Psychiatry. Harmondsworth: Penguin.

Marcos, L. R., M. Alpert, L. Urcuyo and M. Kesselman
1973 The Effect of Interview Language on Evaluation of Psychopathology in Spanish-American Patients. American Journal of Psychiatry 130:549–553.

Mills, Janet J.
1985 The Possession State *Intwaso:* An Anthropological Re-appraisal. South African Journal of Sociology 16:9–13.

Murray, Colin
1981 Families Divided: The Impact of Migrant Labour in Lesotho. Johannesburg: Ravan Press.

Ngubane, Harriet
1977 Body and Mind in Zulu Medicine. An Ethnography of Health and Disease in Nyuswa-Zulu Thought and Practice. London: Academic Press.
1988 Reshaping Social Anthropology. Paper presented at the University of Durban-Westville, August.

Nzimande, Bonginkosi
1985   Industrial Psychology and the Study of Black Workers in South Africa: A
       Review and Critique. Psychology in Society 2:54–91.

Posel, Deborah
1984   Language, Legitimation and Control: The South African State after 1978.
       Social Dynamics 10:1–16.

Psychology in Society Editorial Staff
1983   Editorial. Psychology in Society 1:1–20.

Rychlak, Joseph
1982   Some Psychotherapeutic Implications of Logical Phenomenology. Psychother-
       apy: Theory, Research and Practice 19:259–265.

Said, Edward W.
1978   Orientalism. London: Routledge and Kegan Paul.

Schweitzer, Robert D.
1983   A Phenomenological Explication of Dream Interpretation among Rural and
       Urban People. Unpublished Ph.D. Dissertation. Rhodes University, South
       Africa.

Sharp, John
1980   Can We Study Ethnicity? A Critique of the Fields of Study in S. African
       Anthropology. Social Dynamics 6:1–16.
1981   The Roots and Development of Volkekunde in South Africa. Journal of
       Southern African Studies 8:16–36.
1988   Introduction: Constructing Social Reality. In South African Keywords: Uses
       and Abuses of Political Concepts. Emile Boonzaier and John Sharp (eds.).
       Cape Town, South Africa: David Philip.

Shweder, Richard A.
1984   Anthropology's Romantic Rebellion Against the Enlightenment, or There's
       More to Thinking Than Reason and Evidence. In Culture Theory: Essays on
       Mind, Self and Emotion. Richard A. Shweder and Robert A. Le Vine (eds).
       Cambridge: Cambridge University Press.

Shweder, Richard A. and Edmund J. Bourne
1982   Does the Concept of the Person Vary? In Cultural Conceptions of Mental
       Health and Therapy. Anthony J. Marsella and Geoffrey M. White (eds.).
       Dordrecht, Holland: D. Reidel.

Shweder, Richard A., and Robert A. LeVine, eds.
1984   Culture Theory: Essays on Mind, Self and Emotion. Cambridge: Cambridge
       University Press.

Swartz, Leslie
1985a Issues for Cross-Cultural Psychiatric Research in South Africa. Culture,
       Medicine and Psychiatry 9(1):59–74.
1985b Is Thin a Feminist Issue? Women's Studies International Forum 8:429–437.
1986   Transcultural Psychiatry in South Africa Part I. Transcultural Psychiatric
       Research Review 23:273–303.
1987   Transcultural Psychiatry in South Africa. Part II. Transcultural Psychiatric
       Research Review 24:5–30.

Swartz, Leslie and Don Foster
1984 Images of Culture and Mental Illness: South African Psychiatric Approaches. Social Dynamics 10:17–25.

Szasz, Thomas
1971 The Manufacture of Madness. London: Routledge and Kegan Paul.

Teggin, Anthony F., Ronith Elk, Oved Ben-Arie and Lynn S. Gillis
1985 A Comparison of Catego Class 'S' Schizophrenia in Three Ethnic Groups: Psychiatric Manifestations. British Journal of Psychiatry 147:683–687.

Thornton, Robert
1988 Culture: A Contemporary Definition. In South African Keywords: Uses and Abuses of Political Concepts. Emile Boonzaier and John Sharp (eds.). Cape Town, South Africa: David Philip.

Turkle, Sherry
1978 Psychoanalytic Politics. Freud's French Revolution. New York: Basic Books.

Wing, J. K. et al.
1974 Measurement and Classification of Psychiatric Symptoms. London: Cambridge University Press.

9

The Birth of the *Klinik*:* A Cultural History of Haitian Professional Psychiatry

Paul Farmer

To the memory of Marie-Thérèse "Ti Tap" Joseph,
who is sorely missed.

Introduction

The Republic of Haïti, long saddled with a reputation as an impoverished and backward outpost of exoticism, has few professional psychiatrists. This fact, like so many others concerning Haïti, conceals far more than it reveals, for it suggests a provincialism that is not borne out by ethnography. Many anthropologists would be startled by the fluency with which Haitian psychiatrists discuss the social construction of illness categories, the myriad ways in which culture shapes psychopathology, and other topics that are, in most settings, the province of medical anthropologists alone. Interviews with Haitian psychiatrists reveal them to be on far more familiar terms with anthropological concepts than, for example, their North American and French counterparts.[1]

In this regard, Haitian psychiatrists resemble other intellectuals from that country. Often drawn to European and American academic fashions and frequently trained in the "First World," they are nonetheless aware that the categories and disciplinary boundaries of metropolitan knowledge are socially constructed. In other words, the content and contours of this knowledge are the products of historically and culturally peculiar preoccupations and bound indissociably to certain linguistic categories. To cite Louis Mars, the *doyen* of Haitian psychiatry: "By deepening (our understanding) of the relationship between *culture* and *personality* in the Haitian setting, we came to understand the flimsiness of the French categories that we were using so uncritically, mechanically imposing Western concepts on Haitian reality" (Mars 1966:8).

---

*Haitian patois for "Clinic."

For most of this century, the imposition of Western concepts on Haitian reality has been regarded with profound ambivalence by the very people who employ these concepts. Haitian intellectuals are caught on the horns of their own contradictions, both internal ones and those stemming from their country's position in a larger cultural and economic system. These contradictions are reflected in the fact that the majority of Haitian psychiatrists now practice in North America. They are reflected in the confusing and contradictory conventional wisdom about things Haitian. The country is the hemisphere's "poorest," we are told; Haïti, land of painters and poets, has the richest cultural traditions in the Americas. Haïti is the most illiterate of American states; its intellectuals have produced more books per capita than those of any other New World nation, with the exception of the United States.[2] Haïti's mentally ill are the subject of abuse and cruelty; the burden of stigma is lighter in Haïti than many other places, and the mentally ill are the beneficiaries of humane therapeutic alternatives that evolved in the absence of biomedical care.

Any revealing study of Haitian professional psychiatry requires not only an historical approach that would sketch the development of the specialty in Haïti, but also an understanding of the contradictions that continue to mark the careers of psychiatrists, as well as the illness experiences of their patients. An account with explanatory power must be fully alive to political economy and, especially, to history.

Madness and the Burdens of History

The Republic of Haïti is Latin America's oldest independent nation. In 1791, in the confusion that reigned after the collapse of the French *ancien régime*, a slave revolt began in the colony of Saint-Domingue, the "Pearl of the Antilles" and the source of more than two-thirds of all French colonial wealth. Under slave and mulatto leadership, the revolt took on the dimensions of a veritable war of liberation. Although Napoléon dispatched an enormous armada to reconquer the territory, the French could not match the combined effect of tropical diseases and the slaves' desperate determination. In November 1803, Napoléon's troops surrendered to the former slaves, and the independence of Haïti was proclaimed.

Despite the importance of Saint-Domingue to the French economy, investments in health-care infrastructure had been negligible. On the eve of the Revolution, there were a few miserable military hospitals. The white minority was treated at home. The black majority received care in plantation sick bays, or not at all. From the detailed testimony of the colony's most careful observer, we may surmise that the mentally ill also lacked care. Shortly before the Revolution, Moreau de Saint-Mery (1984:1034–1035) wrote of "madmen severely locked-up in jail or poorly kept by their masters," and deplored the absence, in Port-au-Prince, of "a place to receive the most unfortunate of all beings, those who, while not sunk to the level of brutes are nonetheless deprived of the Creator's greatest gift to man."

Regarding the conditions a decade later, at the close of the war of independence, Bordes (1979:16–17) offers the following summary: virtually all of the island's doctors and surgeons had fled. The majority of hospitals and other institutions had been destroyed; only the military hospitals in Port-au-Prince and Cap Haïticn (formerly Cap Français) remained. The towns were in shambles, without sewers or latrines. What little care could be delivered was offered by orderlies who had worked in hospitals, or by midwives, herbalists, and bonesetters. Bordes writes of a

> host of technically unprepared health workers in the presence of a pop-
> ulation newly liberated from slavery, living for the most part in primi-
> tive huts, without water or latrines, and undermined and decimated by
> the infectious diseases against which they were so poorly protected.
> Oppressive legacy from our former masters, thirsty for profits, and lit-
> tle interested in the living conditions and health of the indigenous popu-
> lation.[3]

This oppressive legacy continues to mark the course of a nation born too soon, a nation whose Enlightenment ideals swam, and often drowned, in a sea of racism and proslavery sentiment. For Haïti was quite literally an island of radical anthropology, the sole voice of racial equality in the Americas. These geopolitical arrangements were darkly mirrored in academic circles. Haïti's elite emulated European fashions in literature and science, but were confronted with prejudices that they could not comfortably accept; members of this elite represented, after all, the world's self-proclaimed "Black Republic." The struggle to counter the dominant, racist models of human capacity may well be the chief reason that anthropological concepts have played such an important role in Haitian academic, literary, and political discourse.[4] Such concepts have played a key role in the evolution of a properly Haitian psychiatry, although not until this century. During the nineteenth century, it seems clear that the role of biomedicine in treating mental affliction was minor.

The Nineteenth Century: Dominance of the "Folk" Sector

In his history of the first 100-odd years of Haitian medicine, Ary Bordes says almost nothing about the care of the mentally ill. His omission might merely reflect a consensus that cut across many classes: mental illness was beyond the scope of physicians and other "secular" healers. The scant literature on mental health in nineteenth-century Haïti presents a somewhat monolithic picture. It suggests that the vast majority of the population believed that mental problems were of "supernatural" origin and not amenable to treatment by physicians; however, the universality of any one etiologic theory is dubious. In addition, no professional psychiatrists were practicing in the country during that period. It is not surprising, therefore, that, during the nineteenth century, the treatment of mental illness in Haïti was almost exclusively in the hands of "folk" practitioners or in the popular sector.

Writing of twentieth-century problems and using contemporary census data, Kline (1960:4–5) poses a question also relevant to nineteenth-century Haïti. Noting that psychoses tend to have a worldwide incidence of between three to seven per one thousand population, he estimates between twelve thousand and twenty-one thousand psychotics in Haïti. Aware that the professional sector is not involved in the care of these persons, he asks: "Does the extended family system care for psychotics in such a way that they do not need hospitalization? Does it reject them and, if so, where are they? Dead, perhaps? Are psychotics able to function with at least partial productivity in the extended family system?"

Kline's questions were somewhat rhetorical, as he believes that psychosis in rural Haïti was treated in the folk sector. The study of Haitian professional psychiatry thus requires consideration of the therapeutic systems that preceded, are classed with, and occasionally complemented the newer professional psychiatry. In this chapter, "popular sector" refers to family-based and social nexus-based therapy, as well as self-care. The term "folk practitioners" is used to describe a heterogeneous groups of nonprofessional or nonbureaucratized healers. In Haïti, this group might subsume voodoo priests and priestesses (*houngan* and *mambo*), herbalists (*dokte fey*), Catholic priests, and Protestant pastors. Although the research presented here has been largely within the professional sector of health care, it also is necessary to examine the far larger popular and folk sectors. These spheres often overlap so much that such terms are useful only with considerable caution. (See Kleinman [1980] for the model of the local healthcare system.)

We know little about the home-care afforded the mentally ill. Bijoux (1982) reports that those who could, confined their family members or sent them, in the manner of lepers, to a small island off the northern shores of Haïti. Writing of an unspecified "past," Douyon (1965:61) says that "mental problems constituted a shame for the family. If they did not wander like shadows throughout the house, unnoticed, non-persons, these patients were relegated to a room, off-limits to visitors." Further, we do not know which units of analysis—household or extended family or community—are appropriate to a discussion of care in the popular sector.

There is, however, a vast literature on voodoo, and interviews with Haitian psychiatrists indicate that psychiatric interventions are most often compared with this religious system. Voodoo looms large in virtually every study of, or commentary on, mental disorder in Haïti. Mars (1966:7) suggests that the bulk of "ethnopsychological works in Haïti have stemmed from the study of voodoo possession crisis and from research on mental illness." Although the psychotherapeutic nature of voodoo has not been the subject of a major investigation, many researchers have provided impressionistic accounts of its role in treating the nation's mentally ill. Given the synchronic nature of these studies, we are obliged to suspend temporarily our historical approach, even though voodoo clearly is changing, and twentieth-century analyses have only limited relevance as regards the role of voodoo in earlier periods.[5]

A few of these studies offer comparisons between Haitian and cosmopolitan therapies. Kiev (1961:260) asks whether "the Voodoo priests' functions could meet minimal criteria for what could be considered psychotherapy." In this and subsequent publications, he describes "native theories of psychiatric illness." He concludes that there are striking similarities between modern psychiatry and the therapeutic system afforded by voodoo; between psychiatrist and voodoo priest: "The *hungan* can diagnose a number of syndromes suggestive of depression, the schizophrenias, hysteria, paranoia, and mental deficiency" (Kiev 1961:475). Kiev presents a brief case study of the treatment, by a voodoo priest, of a woman with a history of mania. Some of his research examines emic constructions. He notes, for example, that possession "is explained in much the same way as *folie*—the *loa* supplants the soul of the possessed and takes control of his mind and body" (Kiev 1961:471–472).

Just as it is possible to exaggerate opposition, so too is it possible to exaggerate similarities. In tracing the commonalities between the two systems, Kiev relies heavily on categories borrowed from North American psychiatry. In fact, he refers to voodoo as "native psychiatry." The fact that voodoo healing takes place in a highly ritualized, group setting, while therapy is most often a dyadic relationship, is significant. Some Haitian observers have highlighted differences, rather than similarities, between the two therapeutic systems. A brief essay by one of Haïti's most prominent psychiatrists, Dr. Legrand Bijoux, deals with the "psychiatric aspects of voodoo." In a historical overview written in 1982, Bijoux suggests that some agitated patients were severely beaten and tortured in "voodoo exorcism ceremonies." A more thorough examination of voodoo exorcism reveals an altogether tame ritual, and underlines the need of many to see voodoo as "barbaric" (see Trouillot 1983, Hurbon 1987, Métraux 1972).

Many conclusions have been drawn from such anecdotal research. One is that the chief determinant of choice of practitioner is the perceived etiology of the illness.[6] Other factors, such as perceived severity and course, cost of treatment, and access to various alternatives, usually are not considered in these studies, but are of primary importance in this poor and agrarian nation (see Coreil 1983). Further, there is significant ideological and religious heterogeneity among the peasants and urban poor. Many of these papers perpetuate an assumption of cultural uniformity among Haitians. Voodoo is depicted as providing the ideological background for one and all. Haitians who profess other faiths are either dishonest or repressing.

Research in Haitian villages suggests that explanatory models of illness are much more complex. These facile oppositions between natural/supernatural and, let us say, psychiatric/nonpsychiatric, are not often so neat. Illnesses classes as "natural" may be referred to as "God's illness" (*maladi bondye*), but they are also caused by microbes, stress, and ill fortune, to name only a few oft-cited factors.[7] Conflicting beliefs about etiology may be simultaneously entertained by the sufferer, within the family, and by the larger group of consociates who play some role in managing illness. A number of factors other than ideas about causation enter into the unfolding negotiations that result in help-seeking. For most Haitians, choice of practitioner is constrained by economic considerations, religious affiliation, sex, and age, all independently of etiologic belief.

Finally, the larger sociopolitical milieu has often loomed large as regards any question regarding voodoo. Access to this therapeutic system has often been constrained by law. During the American occupation, for example, voodoo was outlawed and its practitioners persecuted. The largely French Catholic clergy later joined forces with the mulatto elite and initiated the ignorant and equally unsuccessful "antisuperstition campaign." There have been more indigenous attempts, also without success, to extirpate voodoo. More recently, the flight of Jean-Claude Duvalier (whose father, at least, was seen as an ally of voodoo), has led to the expression of much antivoodoo sentiment. In 1986, several *houngan* were murdered, and scores of temples were destroyed. This violence illustrates the marked cultural and religious heterogeneity of Haïti, and calls into question the pat conclusions of Kiev (1961) and many others who divide Haïti into two internally homogeneous groups: the small, wealthy elite, and the large, poor majority. We turn again to this subject below, in a detailed examination of the practice and ideology of Haitian psychiatrists.

Early Twentieth-Century Attempts to Medicalize Mental Illness

Given the cultural heterogeneity of the Haitian people, it is not surprising to learn that some representatives of "official" medicine had long tried to counter mental illness with pharmacologic treatments. According to one report, "stimulants" and "tranquilizers" were used as deemed appropriate (Bijoux 1982). From the beginning of this century, wealthy Haitians could send their mentally ill family members abroad, especially to Cuba, for treatment. Today, several Miami psychiatrists treat Haitians currently living in Haïti. But, then as now, the number of families able to afford such treatment was tiny.

Such therapeutic interventions may have been far from typical during the first decades of the century. It is hard to assess with certainty popular attitudes toward the mentally ill. In the same article that states, "there is...not the same type of stigma attached to mental illness as in certain other parts of the world," Kline and Mars (1960:48–49) observe that "as a rule (disturbed patients) were manacled inside their huts." As in Europe, the great majority of seriously agitated or violent cases often were subjected to draconian measures of restraint: straitjackets, manacles, or solitary confinement in dungeons. Those who "lost their minds" without becoming violent or in some other way dangerous, wandered the streets, exposed, reportedly, to ridicule and physical abuse (Bijoux 1982).

The first decade of the century brought delayed waves of French fashions: herbal treatments, "talk therapy," hypnotism, and pharmacologic agents. Improvement in medicalized care for the mentally ill was, at best, tenuous. The entire country was, in fact, unstable. By the turn of the century, Haitian sovereignty, ever fragile, was violated in almost continuous fashion. Haitian waters were invaded regularly by the representatives of most of the world's imperial powers. Between 1849 and 1914, the United States sent warships to Haïti's shores no less than twenty-four times, usually on the pretext of protecting the property or rights of a U.S. citizen. Germany also had significant interests in Haïti, and the North Americans were increasingly skittish about European, especially German, influence in the famous "back yard" of the United States. In 1915, the Marines disembarked, and the long and hated American occupation of Haïti began.[8]

As despised as the occupation was, notes one Haitian historian, the majority of North American physicians dispatched to Port-au-Prince came to command "the respect and the gratitude of the population" (Corvington 1984:177). A significant change in the treatment accorded the mentally ill occurred in 1929, when the American-directed public health department turned its attention on "wandering madmen." An empty military barracks was commandeered for the confinement of violent or otherwise bothersome mentally ill patients. At Beudet, the mentally ill, "received care which, although insufficient, had nonetheless previously been denied them" (Corvington 1987:179).

Called "Camp de Beudet" by the Haitians, and dubbed "Camp General Russell" by the North American of the same name, the new asylum was situated about two kilometers from the town of Croix de Bouquets, a market town in the Cul-de-Sac Plain. The internees, it seems, did not receive specialized care; there was no doctor at Beudet. Instead, nurses from the occupying forces were their keepers. One of these, a man named Rieser, is remembered as having demonstrated a great deal of good will toward his wards and doing much to improve the lamentable conditions at Beudet.[9]

The American occupation of Haïti affected the training and interests of psychiatrists, as well as the care accorded the mentally ill. There was a sudden efflorescence of fascination with folklore. Throughout the nineteenth century, there had been marked interest in anthropology. This peculiar vocation stemmed from the rejection, by literate Haitians, of European and U.S. "scientific" racism. During that century, Haïti may well have been the world's chief source of explicitly antiracist literature. In literary efforts, the Haitian elite's self-ascribed task was to show to a sceptical Europe and North America that "the black race" was every bit as capable as they of "civilization" and "refinement." The majority of the nation's writers produced works that were largely derivative of whatever was in style in Paris.

Both of these traits of the nineteenth-century Haitian elite—widespread interest in countering the anthropology of the day and an uncritical enthusiasm for continental literary fashions—came into play in the intense debate sparked by the invasion of the United States Marines. The introduction of North American racism, which tended to class people as black or white, upset a carefully calibrated dynamic, forcing issues of race, ethnicity, and cultural identity. The Haitian intellectuals, born to privilege, took great offense that mere foot soldiers from North America would dare to consider themselves superior to members of the Créole elite. The response to the "indiscriminate" racism of the occupying forces was a literary and political movement known as *indigènisme*. If the occupation was the stimulus for the movement, then the remarkable Jean Price-Mars was its guiding force. Price-Mars, an anthropologist-sociologist trained in medicine, deplored the Haitian elite's "cultural bovaryism," and insisted that they acknowledge their Haitianism. Within a few years after the 1927 publication of Price-Mars' influential book of essays, *Ainsi Parla l'Oncle*, literary and political discourse was ethno-this and ethno-that:

> Dès lors, les écrivains commencerent a se referer avec orgueil a leur couleur noire, considerée jusqu'alors comme une tare; ils reconnurent l'heritage de l'Afrique ancestrale et proclamerent avec joie leur negritude. Aux dieux de vaudou qui avaient été relegués dans les hounforts et traités avec mépris, on reconnut alors droit de citer. "L'assoor" remplace la flute occidentale. (Castro 1988:167)[10]

Although the effects of this vogue were seen most clearly in *les belles lettres*, the trend paved the way for the advent of Haitian ethnopsychiatry. The desire to understand human behavior in scientific terms led Dorsainvil (1931) to discuss trance and other dissociative states in voodoo as pathologic, and he proposed neuropsychiatric explanations of such phenomena. Price-Mars countered prevailing prejudices by asking, "Is voodoo possession a form of hysteria?" It most certainly is not, he concluded, and his work led to a heightened awareness of the effects of culture on behavior, and threw into doubt any firm line between the normal and the abnormal. In fact, the eminent French anthropologist Roger Bastide credits Price-Mars with the succinct statement of this central problematic:

> Dr. Price-Mars was thus the first to open the way to the modern theory of the cultural or sociological normalcy of possession, and that is (because), in examining and analyzing (possession), he refused to cloak himself in class prejudices and to accept the biased viewpoint of the elite. (Bastide 1956:200)

1936: The Advent of Cosmopolitan Medicine

The United States, now uncontested in its quest for control of Haïti, withdrew its Marines in 1934. At least one of the North American nurses remained at Beudet, however, to care for his charges. But despite the good intentions of a few expatriate nurses, the care there remained purely custodial until 1936. That year marked the return of Dr. Louis Mars, the first Haitian physician to receive specialty training in psychiatry. When he reached his homeland, he reported, quite naturally, to the sole institution concerning itself with the mentally ill. His impressions of Camp de Beudet remain vivid, as a recent commentary would suggest:

> What a frightful reality it was! The quarantine of the mentally ill like the plague-stricken of the Middle Ages, in Europe; their physical and mental deprivation: no beds, no medication, no supplies, no trained personnel. Decrepit chambers from which rose screams, calls, lamentation. These men, these women, these children: nonpersons.

By then, this twenty-bed facility housed 250 patients.[11] The building was indeed decrepit, and becoming more so, with holes in the roof and little in the way of maintenance. There was little in the way of medication, for that matter: the total *monthly* budget for Beudet was no more than $20. Malaria, avitaminosis, and malnutrition were rampant (Kline and Mars 1960).

"The history of (Haitian) medicine," notes Bordes (1979:v), "is largely the history of institutions and of individuals. Little doctrine and few important works." So it was with psychiatry. In his brief history, Bijoux (1982) speaks of two periods: "before 1936, or before the return of Louis Mars, and after 1936, or after the return of Louis Mars." Mars' initial shock at Beudet spurred him to action. He initiated the nation's first serious campaign to improve the lot of the mentally ill. In the first decades after the end of the Occupation, Mars stood alone in his attempt to inform the Haitian elite about mental illness. In the context of the present account, Mars' tireless energy to improve care for the mentally ill is not as striking as his second vocation, anthropology. Louis Mars, physician-anthropologist, was the son of another physician-anthropologist, Jean Price-Mars.

Louis Mars later became, with Roger Bastide and Georges Devereux, one of the founders of Europe's first school of ethnopsychiatry.[12] The psychiatrist's "intellectual activism" followed the example of his father. Mars *fils* approached political, religious, and other leaders to accomplish what Bijoux has termed the "systematic medicalization" of the care offered at Beudet. Emblematic of this change: the "camp" became the "asylum" after the occupation ended. Dr. Mars made repeated attempts to educate the literate minority through newspaper articles, seminars, and speeches to different clubs and organizations in Port-au-Prince. In 1941, he established the Ligue Nationale d'Hygiène Mentale. His work was reinforced by the activism of several others, including Jean Price-Mars, who in the same year founded the Institut d'Ethnologie. Dr. Louis Mars was honored with a post in psychology and began to teach at the institute.[13]

In 1946, a 133-page booklet entitled "La Lutte Contre La Folie" (The Struggle Against Mental Illness—ed.), intended for nonprofessionals, was published. Mars lobbied successfully for the introduction of psychiatry into the curriculum and vocabulary of students of medicine and nursing. He continued to teach anthropology, and his interest in the discipline seemed to deepen. In 1946, Louis Mars was named Director of the Institut d'Ethnologie, which became formally affiliated with the Université d'Haïti.

Despite the fact that he located pathology within individuals, rather than in the sociopolitical sphere, Mars occasionally engendered the ill will of those in power. His work, he recently noted, was "not without danger." The Haitian authorities "threatened with imprisonment those who attacked it by describing the sordid misery of the insane, the Asylum's total lack of equipment, the enormous difficulties that confronted the students and volunteers who brought their help to these unfortunate persons." In 1941, Mars secured international funding for a psychiatric hospital, but the project was blocked by the Haitian government. Mars persisted, and in 1948 he was able to lay the cornerstone of the new edifice. "Shortly thereafter," he notes, "the work stopped. The funds had disappeared."

It took another decade of commitment for Mars to build an enduring resource for mentally ill Haitians. The Centre de Neurologie et Psychiatrie Mars et Kline was built and organized through the combined efforts of Mars, the Haitian government, the late Nathan Kline (a U.S. psychiatrist), three pharmaceutical companies, and sectors of the Haitian public. The establishment of the clinic, the explicit goal of which was to "make available to the public the advances of modern psychiatry," constituted an important milestone in the evolution of professional psychiatry in Haïti.

What, precisely, were those advances of modern psychiatry? For Mars, the chief advance was the advent of effective antipsychotic medications. As the institution's name suggests, Mars wished to incorporate neurology, again emphasizing the material foundations of psychiatry. But there were other reasons for pharmocologic interventions. Those involved in building the Center knew that thousands of psychotic Haitians were entirely unattended by physicians. Long hospitalizations were out of the question. Above all, perhaps, was the unexpressed fear that the new facility might come to resemble Beudet. The goal was thus to provide, during very brief stays, medications to individuals experiencing acute psychotic breaks. Therefore, its prime movers refer to the center as "the first deliberately and consciously drug-centered treatment program" (Kline and Mars 1960:50–51), and they advance it as a model for other countries. The influence of Dr. Mars would have been even greater had he not been banished during the reign of another physician-anthropologist, François Duvalier. After two decades in exile, Mars has recently returned to his country, where he continues to write and teach.

Haitian Professional Psychiatry: The Current State of Affairs

What professional-sector psychiatric care is currently available in Haïti, and to whom is it available? Given the expressed desire to "make available to the public the advances of modern psychiatry," what has happened to this cultural system, elaborated, after all, in radically different settings? If indigenization denotes the process by which a therapeutic system is altered following its export to a new cultural setting (Kleinman 1980), how has professional psychiatry been *indigenized*? In an attempt to answer these questions, I interviewed practitioners of what might be called "Haitian ethnopsychiatry." I counted nine such psychiatrists in Haïti.

Before briefly examining the experiences and ideology of a rather remarkable psychiatrist, I will sketch the status of professional psychiatry in Haïti. The specialty is still an urban commodity. However, it is no longer available solely to the wealthy and to the acutely psychotic. There are several psychiatric facilities in Port-au-Prince and the surrounding area: the Centre de Neurologie et Psychiatrie Mars et Kline, which opened in February of 1959, saw almost forty thousand patients in the first twenty years of operation. Its main objectives remain the diagnosis and treatment of acute cases requiring short-term hospitalization and long-term follow-up. Both the services and the treatment regimens are heavily subsidized and are intended for people from a broad spectrum of economic backgrounds. Still, there remains a silent minority of those unable to seek care there. An inability to purchase expensive medications is often responsible for termination of care in the professional sector.[14]

The Asile de Beudet is now the Hôpital Défilée de Beudet, and it continues to house and care for some relatively stable, chronic patients. It is still a grim and depressing place. Although improvements have been made, it remains overcrowded, understaffed, and grossly undersupplied. In 1979, the Clinique d'Hygiène Mentale of the Faculté des Sciences Humaines opened to offer services to certain patients with "behavioral disorders." There are several private psychiatric clinics, all in the capital, of which four offer inpatient care. Dr. Legrand Bijoux reports seeing, in twenty years of private practice, more than five thousand patients: some sixteen hundred children and adolescents, and thirty-four hundred adults.

Psychiatry is now part of the formal curriculum at the national medical school. Theoretical courses are taught by a psychiatrist, and clinical clerkships are offered at the Centre Mars et Kline. Psychiatric nursing is taught at the nation's three nursing schools, again through theoretical courses and clinical rotations at the Centre. Versions of the discipline are taught at the Faculté d'Ethnologie and the Faculté des Sciences Humaines, where anthropologists, sociologists, psychologists, social workers, and mass-communications technicians are trained. Students of practical nursing at l'École Nationale d'Infirmières Auxiliares de Port-au-Prince receive some theoretical instruction and also visit the Centre Mars et Kline. Similar instruction is planned for the rural auxiliary nursing schools, although many of these efforts have been hampered by the social unrest of recent years.

The term *la vulgarisation* refers to attempts by the practitioners of professional psychiatry to disseminate their ideology in the popular and folk sectors. A kind of planned indigenization, *vulgarisation* is accomplished through the publication of books written for nonprofessionals, newspaper and magazine articles, conferences, and addresses of the sort initiated by Louis Mars, and continues by his students and successors. Haïti has low rates of literacy; regular radio programs are broadcast in Haitian Creole by Dr. Jeanne Philippe. At the time of this writing, seven psychiatrists now practice in Port-au-Prince and contribute to educational and *vulgarisation* services.

What have been the results of *vulgarisation*? One Haitian psychiatrist makes bold claims for the campaign that was initiated by Louis Mars:

> The past 30 years have been marked by a remarkable evolution in the popular conception of mental illness. It has gone from the idea of behavioral troubles as the result of a curse or a spell cast on an individual or a family (concept of supernatural illness) to (the idea) of a natural illness affecting the brain. (Bijoux 1982:19)

The process of indigenization is not one that is fully amenable to conscious control. The impact of the psychiatrists' campaign is far less palpable in rural Haïti, where long-standing ways of configuring mental disorder continue to shape the contours of illness realities. Although the version of reality advanced by the physicians have not replaced the more indigenous understandings, some of the categories and treatment modalities of psychiatry have been incorporated into rural Haitian responses to madness. Anthropologists have demonstrated that new illness categories and ideas about them are often "adopted" by older interpretive frameworks. "As new medical terms become known in a society," notes Good (1977:54), "they find their way into existing semantic networks. Thus, while new explanatory models may be introduced, it is clear that changes in medical rationality seldom follow quickly."

Thanks in large part to the contributions of Price-Mars and Mars, psychiatrists in Haïti have never been hostile to voodoo. They have, however, competed with *houngans* and other adepts for patients, and voodoo remains the therapeutic system with which professional psychiatrists compare their own services. Some psychiatrists, aware of the importance of indigenous models and familiar with the ethnography of their country, have attempted to co-opt popular discourses on mental illness and the explanatory models embedded in them. Dr. Bijoux, for example, declares that he will welcome the day when all voodoo priests declare to their mentally ill clients: "Your supernatural problems are resolved; your spiritual uneasiness dissolved. The rest of your treatment must be offered by a mental-health technician" (Bijoux 1982:19).

Theory and Practice in Haitian Ethnopsychiatry

As noted at the outset, a number of Haitian psychiatrists have demonstrated striking familiarity with concepts more native to anthropology than to medicine. Although Dr. Mars was familiar with the reigning concepts of cultural anthropology and clearly appreciated the role of culture in shaping psychopathology, he was in no sense a radical relativist. It was the brain— not some immaterial "mind"—that was altered in madness. His intent was to medicalize not only the treatment of mental illness, but also his compatriots' beliefs about its etiology. Because Mars believed the etiologies of mental illness to be fundamentally organic, the obvious remedies were pharmacologic:

> The concept of mental illness as a form of medical disease is virtually unknown in Haïti, not only among the potential patient population but among the population in general. When the first few patients treated with drugs showed rapid improvement, a spokesman for a group of natives asked one of us (Dr. Mars) if he was an houngan, i.e., a voodoo priest, because the voodoo priests are supposed to be the only people skillful enough to cure such ailments. (Kline and Mars 1960:48)

The "organicist" position may have been overstated because it was perceived to be a politically expedient one, although it failed to shield Mars from the political currents that have swept through (and occasionally swept away) all professions in Haïti. For Mars clearly suggested that the role of culture could be quite determinant in psychopathology.

In North American psychiatry, concepts such as 'person' and 'self' are rarely problematic. Yet unexamined folk notions of personhood exert determinant effects on diagnosis and treatment of mental disorder, as Gaines (1979, 1985) has demonstrated in a number of studies. Writing of North American psychiatry, he notes:

> The key conception of person *organizes* cultural knowledge which gives rise to the explanatory model of patient and healer. That is, a nonmedically focused notion, that of person, lies behind and organizes patients' and healer' thinking about sickness episodes. Put another way, we may say that a cultural or folk theory underlies and gives shape to cultural knowledge and direction to cultural thinking about sickness. (Gaines 1985:230–231)

In his work with psychiatrists in such diverse setting as California, Hawaii, and "Bible Belt" North Carolina, Gaines has found that psychiatrists' conceptions of person are most often implicit or "unconscious." Not so among the Haitian ethnopsychiatrists who, unprompted, will hold forth at great length about the significance of these constructs to the experience of mental illness. Haitian psychiatrists demonstrate a heightened awareness of anthropological concepts. Highly elaborate commentary on "the notion of person" serves as an example of the effects of such sophisticated theory on the practice of Haitian psychiatry. Appreciation of the cultural construction of the notion of person or self—which is not the same as the widely shared appreciation of the process of socialization into individual personhood— seems to lead Haitian psychiatrists to a relativism rare outside of anthropology or philosophy. For example, Dr. Jeanne Philippe, citing barriers to the indigenization of psychotherapy, offered the following observations:

> In Haïti, in general, people are very reticent. They don't like to answer question.... There is always an aura of mystery, of suspicion. Certainly, this is extreme right now (1986), but we have always had this in Haïti. Perhaps it is not surprising, then, that the most common mental illness in Haïti is paranoia, paranoid reactions. Nor is this surprising, at least to me, as mental illness is, in my opinion, the exaggeration of the cultural temperament. In this way, culture shapes psychopathology, and helps to determine the sorts of problems one seems most often.

When pressed as to the lineaments of this cultural temperament, Dr. Philippe turned directly to the concept of the person. A chief source of dissonance between Western psychiatric theory and Haitian ethnopsychology was, she said, differing notions of the person, of the individual:

> Even in the middle classes, there is a tendency to live in and for the group. To use the expression of Dr. Louis Mars, this renders the Haitian idea of the individual very "diffuse." There isn't really an individual distinct from the group, or distinct, even, from the universe. And thus can one be harmed: there are so many strands linking one to the social and material world.[15]

If personality is socially and culturally constructed, as many Haitian psychiatrists insist, then it stands to reason that nosologies and etiologic theories elaborated in radically different settings will have limited applicability in Haïti. The difficulties confronted by Dr. Philippe in attempting to apply her Canadian psychiatric training in a Haitian setting will not surprise anthropologists, but her response to these difficulties are thoroughly Haitian:

> Right away, I found it impossible to apply what I had just learned. I knew there was an anthropology department (at the state university), and so I enrolled. And I learned anthropology. I completed my master's degree there. Since then, I have never received or treated a patient without taking into account all relevant aspects of his or her social, economic, religious background. I seek the full cultural complex.

Seeking the full cultural complex later led Philippe to the Institut des Hautes Études of the University of Paris, where she completed her doctorate in anthropology. Her advisors there were Roger Bastide and George Devereux.[16] This intellectual genealogy serves as another reminder that the high level of awareness of such implicit categories is due not to the recent resurgence of anthropological interest in self, but is rather a recognizable bend in the stream of French anthropology. Devereux was a student of Marcel Mauss, who offered, as the 1938 Huxley Memorial Lecture, an analysis of the notion of person.[17] Lévi-Strauss (1950:xxii) notes the relevance of Mauss's theory to any critical understanding of the boundary between normal and abnormal:

> The very notion of *mental illness* is to be questioned. For if, as Mauss suggests, the mental and the social merge together, then it would be absurd, in instances in which social and psychological are in direct contact, to apply to one of these two orders a notion (like illness) that has no meaning without the other.

Conclusions

Recent anthropological study of biomedicine has shown that Western medicine, including psychiatry, is an enormously varied *potpourri* of ideology and practice (see Hahn and Gaines 1985). But most social scientists interested in biomedicine have worked in industrialized countries in North America, Europe, and Asia. Impressionistic accounts of cosmopolitan medicine in "Third World" settings have tended to be dour assessments. Stories about the medical bourgeoisie or the misapplication of Western medical knowledge in non-Western settings are intended to shock—or amuse. Biomedicine in the Third World is seen as a parody of the profession as practiced in the industrialized countries.

This disparaging cliché does not hold true among Haitian psychiatrists, whose engagement with both North American and French professional psychiatry has tended to be critical and reflexive. At least three reasons explain this awareness. One of these is unique to Haïti but reflects the experience of physicians from Africa, Asia, and Latin America who have sought psychiatric training in the Northern Hemisphere. Social construction of psychiatric theories and nosologies is much more apparent to one who does not share the cultural knowledge (such as the notion of person, or the boundary of normal/abnormal) underpinning the psychiatric orthodoxies of the moment. Dr. Philippe expressed this idea when she said that she "found it impossible to apply what I had just learned."

A second major reason is peculiarly Haitian and reflects the role of antiracist anthropological discourse in the world's first "Black Republic." The birth of the first large black elite in the periphery of the European capitalist system meant that Haitian intellectuals depended on European readings of the world—the were often schooled in Paris—but were required to challenge those readings as ethnocentric and socially constructed. In Haïti more than any other setting, the social construction of categories is taken as a given. The majority of Haitian psychiatrists would agree with Dr. Legrand Bijoux: "All good psychiatry must draw on sociology and anthropology." Such a dictum would occur to few North American or French psychiatrists. Similarly heightened sensibilities are of much more recent vintage in sub-Saharan Africa and the rest of the Caribbean.[18]

The third reason for the heightened awareness of anthropological issues among Haitian psychiatrists also is related to history and political economy. In a small country with an extremely low literacy rate and little upward mobility, the literati becomes a sort of intellectual jack-of-all-trades, hence the profusion of hyphens among the small elite of physician-anthropologist-statesmen, poet-senators, novelist-engineers, etc. The specialization that has for decades characterized cosmopolitan medicine is less common in Haïti.

What barriers to the indigenization of an exogenous therapeutic system might one encounter in Haïti? Three main types of barriers—cultural, political, and economic—are easily discerned. These are not, of course, discrete categories. The cultural barriers are not difficult to elucidate and include widely held models of illness that took shape in contexts in which medical response to mental disorder was simply not an option. Although its Haitian practitioners may be ahead of their North American or French counterparts, professional psychiatry has not yet come to terms with a number of behaviors that are clearly not abnormal in local context (e.g., possession and trance during voodoo ceremonies, "bad blood" in response to emotional shocks). Rural Haitian notions of self are frankly inconsonant with those held in professional psychiatry, and etiologic beliefs may lead the mentally ill away from doctors and toward those better able to "manipulate the spirit," as more than one Haitian psychiatrist would have it.

If the models of behavior and normalcy elaborated in the First World are readily seen, by Haitian psychiatrists, as culture-bound and needing "deconstruction" before they have applicability in Haïti, how were they indigenized following their export to a new cultural setting? The most common response to this question, when posed to Haitian psychiatrists, has been "by tailoring concepts to Haitian culture." Some mentioned "anchoring these concepts in Haitian reality," and still others, such as Philippe, "sought the full cultural complex." All psychiatrists interviewed felt it their professional duty to be informed about the religious affiliations of their patients, but interviews suggested that this interest ran the gamut from respect and affirmation of the patient's beliefs to the somewhat disingenuous attempt to co-opt the explanatory models of voodoo.[19]

Sociopolitical barriers are also in place: a climate of fear does not foster the interchange so central to many versions of psychotherapy.[20] Further, a publishing, or "vulgarizing," psychiatrist runs political risks by underlining the *social* causes of mental illness. This was underlined in a review of Jeanne Philippe's *Classes Sociales et Maladies Mentales en Haïti*:

> To posit the existence of sociogenesis, as does the very title of the work, is to distinguish it from two other approaches: psychogenesis leads to the elaboration of often unverifiable hypotheses; biologism...leads to no attempts to modify the environment. (Thébaud, in Philippe 1985:iv)

Shortly after the publication of the third edition of her study of the sociogenesis of mental illness, Philippe decided to pull copies from circulation to avoid the ire of a collapsing dictatorship that was suddenly attempting to silence criticism.

Psychotherapies have been, historically, largely middle-class enterprises. The near absence of such a class in Haïti—an issue of political economy—erects both logistic and cultural barriers to the indigenization of these systems. That economic barriers help to erect or maintain cultural and political ones will surprise no one who has worked in a poor, rural, and agrarian society. There are enormous problems of access to care in Haïti, a country of more than six million with only seven psychiatrists now seeing nonprivate patients at least part-time.[21] There also are the barriers of urban/rural bias: the country is largely rural, but every psychiatrist practices in urban Haïti. If a peasant with mental disorder does make it to the clinics of Port-au-Prince, continuity of care is threatened: medications are costly, and regular follow-up is necessary. For example, a patient living in a village in the Central Plateau may be less than fifty miles from the Centre Mars et Kline, but it takes no less than five hours on public transportation to cover this distance. Add to this the hours of waiting in the clinic, and it is clear that a simple follow-up appointment requires an overnight stay in Port-au-Prince, an unhospitable and somewhat dangerous city.

In summary, Haitian psychiatrists have come a long way in "tailoring psychiatric concepts to Haitian culture." From French and North American clinical settings, they have ushered in the *klinik*, a properly Haitian version of clinical psychiatry. But much remains to be done before the majority of Haitians with mental illness have access to psychiatric care. Even then, the contributions of such efforts may be negligible next to the forces that keep Haïti poor. These forces contribute to pathology of every description. One of the people who encouraged me to write this chapter was a brilliant young woman, Marie-Thérèse, from a poor family from the Plateau Central, diagnosed by psychiatrists at the Centre Mars et Kline as having manic-depressive disorder. For years, she struggled with keeping appointments and purchasing expensive medications, only to die of infectious complications of childbirth. "You see," her mother said, "she died not from being crazy. It's this country that killed her."

Notes

1. My assessment is based on impressions, rather than serious comparative research. But I have worked with psychiatrists in France, and my training in medicine has included significant exposure to North American psychiatry.

2. Such, at least, is the opinion of Edmund Wilson, *The Nation*, October 14, 1950, p. 341.

3. Paragraphing altered. Translations in this paper are my own except as noted.

4. A brief historical account of Haïti's role in larger economic systems is found in Farmer (1988a). The Haitian elite lost this struggle, perhaps in part because many of its members believed themselves congenitally superior to the authentic heirs of the Haitian Revolution: the peasants.

5. See Hurbon (1987), Métraux (1972), and Trouillot (1983) for historical perspectives on Haitian voodoo.

6. For example, Kiev makes much of the indigenous distinction between "supernatural" and "natural" illness causation, asserting that "supernatural illnesses can be treated only by *hungans* and *mambos*" (1961:261).

7. The goal of this essay is not to review these complexities, but illness in Haïti and among Haitians has been discussed by many anthropologists including Bastien (1987), Coreil (1983), Courlander (1960), Farmer (1988b), Herskovits 1975), Hurbon (1987), Laguerre (1987), Métraux (1972), Murray (1976), Philippe (1985), and Weidman (1978).

8. For an excellent account of the years leading up to the Occupation, see Plumer (1988); for an important account of the era, see Castro (1988).

9. Beudet remained, however, a frightful place. That it was used for political

purposes as well as therapeutic ones is suggested by Castro (1988:205), who notes that President Stenio Vincent sent one of his rivals to the asylum in 1935, "sous prétexte qu'il était devenu fou." ("Under the pretext that he had gone mad"—ed.)

10. "Since then, writers have referred with pride to their black color which was earlier considered a defect; they rediscovered the heritage of ancestral Africa and proclaimed their negritude with joy. As for the voodoo gods, who had been relegated to the [social outcastes] and treated with contempt, one rediscovered the right to refer to them. The [indigenous] *l'assoor* replaced the Western/European flute" (ed.).

11. Kline and Mars (1960:49) note, "an amazing factor was the stability of the population at approximately 250 persons. This was achieved by virtue of the fact that the 15 admissions a month were exactly balanced by an average of five discharges, five escapes, and five deaths."

12. Indeed, Devereux credits the Haitian physician with coining the term "ethnopsychiatry." (see chapter 1—ed.)

13. The Institute (l'Institut d'Ethnologie) is not to be confused with the Bureau d'Ethnologie, founded the same year by another intellectual giant, Jacques Roumain. The Institute was devoted to teaching; the Bureau was a research center, and soon included a museum.

14. For example, in the village in which I have for some years conducted research, the two persons believed locally to have mental disorders have been treated by healers in both the professional and folk sectors. Long-term pharmacotherapy has been a failure due to the high cost of antipsychotics, and also the difficulty of maintaining contact with a psychiatrist in far-off Port-au-Prince. Psychotherapy has not been attempted.

15. For the reader familiar with the ethnography of Haïti, this may sound odd. Many students of Haitian culture have characterized rural Haïti as less communal than other Latin American cultures. Yet this seeming paradox may be resolved by agreeing with Dr. Philippe who argues that Haïti is sociocentric, but the unit of social nexus is smaller and more kin-determined, perhaps, than in other countries in the region.

16. The latter wrote the preface to the third edition of her thesis, in which he recalls, "Dr. Philippe arrived in Paris with her files and notes in order, her thesis topic already chosen; her project was grounded in sensible methodology, and (was) feasible."

17. Reprinted as "Une categorie de l'esprit humain: la notion de personne, celle de 'moi'," in Mauss (1950: 331–362). ("A Category of the Human Mind: the Notion of the Person, that of the 'Self'")

18. See, for example, Fisher's excellent (1985) study of mental illness on Barbados.

19. The much-touted cooperation between the professional and folk healers may be more important on paper than in reality. There are, in any case, no formal arrangements obtaining between voodoo priests and the practitioners of psychiatry.

20. For an idea of the dimensions and mechanisms of this fear, see the excellent journalistic account by Wilentz (1989).

21. There are, it is said, more Haitian psychiatrists practicing in the city of Montréal than in the entire Republic of Haïti.

References

d'Ans, André-Marcel
1985 Remy Bastien et l'Ethnologie Haïtienne. Introduction. In Le Paysan Haïtien et sa Famille. R. Bastien. Paris: Karthala.

Bastide, Roger
1956 Le Dr. J. Price-Mars et le Vodou. In Témoignages sur la Vie et l'Oeuvre de Dr. Jean Price-Mars. Port-au-Prince: Imprimerie de l'État.

Bastien, Rémy
1987 Maladies en Haïti. Paris: Dunod.

Bijoux, Le Grand
1982 La Vie en Haïti. Haïti: Farmer Publishing.

Bordes, Ary
1979 Évolution des Sciences de la Santé et de l'Hygiène Publique en Haïti. Tome 1. Port-au Prince: Centre d'Hygiène Familiale.

Castro, George
1988 In Haïti. Boston: Farmer Publishing.

Coreil, Jeannine
1983 Parallel Structures in Professional and Folk Health Care: A Model Applied to Rural Haïti. Culture, Medicine and Psychiatry 7:131–151.

Corvington, Georges
1984 Port-au-Prince au Cours des Ans: La Capitale d'Haïti sous l'Occupation 1915–1922. Port-au-Prince: Imprimerie Henri Deschamps.
1987 Port-au-Prince au Cours des Ans: La Capitale d'Haïti sous l'Occupation 1922–1934. Port-au-Prince: Imprimerie Henri Deschamps.

Courlander, Harold
1960 The Drum and the Hoe: Life and Lore of the Haitian People. Berkeley: University of California Press.

Dorsainvil, J. C.
1931 Vodou et Névrose. Port-au-Prince: La Presse.

Douyon, Lamarck
1965 Les Maladies Mentales et Nous, Haïtiens. Revue de la Faculté d'Ethnologie 10:61–65.

Farmer, Paul
1988a Blood, Sweat, and Baseballs: Haïti in the West Atlantic System. Dialectical Anthropology 13:83–99.
1988b Bad Blood, Spoiled Milk: Bodily Fluids as Moral Barometers in Rural Haïti. American Ethnologist 15(1):62–83.

Fisher, Lawrence
1985 Colonial Madness: Mental Health in the Barbadian Social Order. New Brunswick, NJ: Rutgers University Press.

Gaines, Atwood D.
1979 Definitions and Diagnoses: Cultural Implications of Psychiatric Help-Seeking and Psychiatrists' Definitions of the Situation in Psychiatric Emergencies. Culture, Medicine, and Psychiatry 3(4):381–418.
1985 The Once- and the Twice-Born: Self and Practice Among Psychiatrists and Christian Psychiatrists. In Physicians of Western Medicine, Robert Hahn and Atwood Gaines (eds.). Dordrecht: D Reidel.

Good, Byron
1977 The Heart of What's the Matter: The Semantics of Illness in Iran. Culture, Medicine and Psychiatry 1(1):25–58.

Hahn, Robert and Atwood Gaines, eds.
1985 Physicians of Western Medicine: Anthropological Approaches to Theory and Practice. Dordrecht: D. Reidel.

Herskovits, Melville
1975 Life in a Haitian Valley. New York: Farrar, Strauss and Giroux.

Hurbon, Laennec
1987 Le Barbaire Imaginaire. Port-au-Prince: Deschamps.

Kiev, Ari
1961 Folk Psychiatry in Haïti. The Journal of Nervous and Mental Disease 132(3):260–265.

Kleinman, Arthur
1980 Patients and Healers in the Context of Culture. Berkeley: University of California Press.

Kline, Nathan
1960 Comments During Roundtable Discussion. In Psychiatry in Underdeveloped Countries. Nathan Kline (ed.). Washington, D.C.: American Psychiatric Association.

Kline, Nathan and Louis Mars
1960 The Haïti Psychiatric Institute: Centre de Psychiatrie. Psychiatry in the Underdeveloped Countries. Nathan Kline (ed.). Washington, D.C.: American Psychiatric Association.

Laguerre, Michel
1987 Afro-Caribbean Folk Medicine. South Hadley, MA: Bergin and Garvey.

Lévi-Strauss, Claude
1950 Introduction. In Anthropologie et Sociologie. Marcel Mauss. Paris: Presses Universitaires de France.

Mars, Louis
1946 La Lutte Contre la Folie: Port-au-Prince: Imprimerie de l'État.
1947 La Crise de Possession. Port-au-Prince: Imprimerie de l'État.
1956 L'Institut d'Ethnologie. In Témoignages sur la Vie et l'Oeuvre de Dr. Jean Price-Mars. Port-au-Prince: Imprimerie de l'État.
1966 Témoignages I: Essai Ethnopsychologique. Madrid: Taller

Mauss, Marcel
1950 Anthropologie et Sociologie. Paris: Presses Universitaires de France.

Métraux, Alfred
1972 [1959] Haitian Voodoo. Hugo Charteris, trans. New York: Schocken.

Murray, Gerald
1976 Women in Perdition: Ritual and Fertility Control in Haïti. In Culture, Natality, and Family Planning. J. Marshall and S. Polgar (eds.). Chapel Hill: University of North Carolina.

Philippe, Jeanne, ed.
1985a Les Causes des Maladies Mentales en Haïti (2ème ed.). Port-au-Prince: Éditions Fardin.
1985b Classes Sociales et Maladies Mentales en Haïti (3ème ed). Port-au-Prince: Éditions Fardin.

Pluchon, Pierre
1987 Vaudou, Sorciers, Empoisionneurs: de Saint-Domingus à Haïti. Paris: Karthala.

Plumer, John
1988 Mental Problems in Haïti. Boston: Farmer Publications.

Saint-Mery, Moreau de
1984 La Santé en Haïti. Port-au-Prince: Éditions Fardin.

Thébaud, Elder
1985 (1979) Notes de Lecture: Classes Sociales et Maladies Mentales en Haïti. In Classes Sociales et Maladie Mentales en Haïti (3ème ed.). Jeanne Philippe (ed.). Port-au-Prince: Éditions Fardin.

Trouillot, Henock
1983 Introduction à une Histoire du Vaudou. Port-au-Prince: Éditions Fardin.

Wilentz, Amy
1989 The Rainy Season. New York: Simon and Schuster.

Weidman, Hazel
1978 The Miami Health Ecology Project Report. Volume 1. Miami: University of Miami.

10

Psychiatrist and Patient in Japan: An Analysis of Interactions in an Outpatient Clinic*

Naoki Nomura

Introduction

The problems of communication in medical settings have been recognized in the United States since the 1950s, particularly in the setting of psychiatric institutions. Working in mental hospitals requires both attention and a great deal of sensitivity to people's expressive behavior. The latter is a consequence of the nature of patients' presenting illnesses. Several classic studies have illustrated the complexity of social interaction in psychiatric hospitals. Stanton and Schwartz (1954) documented in detail the working relationships developed among the staff, the psychiatrists, and the patients in order to create a better therapeutic ward environment.

William Caudill's classic work (1958) demonstrated how the events taking place in various parts of the hospital are in fact interrelated and form parts of an ongoing institutional social system. Erving Goffman (1961) critically examined the social situations of the patients and the staff in the mental hospital and explained the "total institutional" processes through which the patient's self is degraded, humiliated, and made to conform to institutional exigencies. Aside from these comprehensive works on entire institutions, there are many other studies concerned with aspects of the medical consultative process—interaction between patients and medical practitioners (e.g., Pendleton and Hasler 1983).

A number of studies have appeared which take account of cultural factors in psychiatrist-patient relations. In the case of Japan, Caudill and Doi attempted to characterize Japanese patterns of patienthood and doctor-patient relationship in mental hospitals (Caudill 1961; Doi 1962; Caudill and Doi 1963). According to their observations, Japanese psychiatric hospitals have a "family-like" atmosphere. Unlike American institutions, those in

*This chapter was substantially reorganized and rewritten by the editor and edited by Sue Wasserkrug, with the permission of the author.

Japan encourage mutual dependency (as an actively mutual relationship, also unlike America) in all relationships including that between psychiatrist and patient. They observed that patients frequently would say to their doctors, "I am completely in your hands." In so doing, patients indicate that they want to be cared for and are, in effect, asking to be allowed to take a dependent position vis-à-vis the doctor. The physician (generally) accepts and even fosters this desire of the patient (Caudill and Doi 1963; see also Nomura 1987a).

Through his cross-cultural survey on Japanese and American patienthood in mental institutions, Yamamoto (1972) confirms the observation that the Japanese patient conceives of her- or himself as a child in a family and appears to be very concerned with developing and maintaining strong ties of benevolent paternalism with both the doctor(s) and the nurses (see also Nomura 1987 a,b).

In the United States, however, the psychiatrist-patient relationship appears more contractual and less affectively charged. Western patient-physician relations are not seen in terms of a kinship idiom (e.g., Hahn and Gaines 1985; Lock and Gordon 1988). The U.S. patient might verbalize, "As long as my doctor knows his business, it does not matter whether he likes me personally or not." In contrast, the Japanese patients do not usually judge or evaluate the ability or the talent of their doctors. Rather, they seek simply to put themselves into their hands (Yamamoto 1972).

Munakata (1986) has investigated some characteristics of mental health care in contemporary Japan. Some of his findings are relevant here. He found: (a) The average length of stay in a mental hospital in Japan is one of the longest in the world; (b) mental hospitals in Japan are usually privately owned (86 percent), whereas in the United States almost the reverse is true (8 percent); (c) Japanese mental hospitals are relatively small, the average size being 250 beds; and (d) hospitalization for mental illness costs considerably less for the patient in Japan than it does in the United States.

One of the key sociocultural factors, according to Munakata (1986), is that in Japan (as well as in China and Korea) the primary care responsibility for the sick, the handicapped, and the elderly falls to their families and relatives. This responsibility has been put into statutory form in those countries, suggesting the cultural source of law. Under Japan's present Mental Health Act, a part of which was somewhat revised in 1988, family members still make the final decision regarding admission and discharge of the patient. When families are unable to offer care at home, they send their sick member(s) to the hospital, often telling them to remain and consider it (the hospital) their "home." The patients, for their part, may resign themselves to hospital life, feeling that they must not trouble their families and relatives by insisting on returning home, even though they may wish to do so.

These sociocultural and psychological factors reported by researchers are useful points of departure when we consider psychiatrist-patient interaction in Japan. This study, however, focuses on an aspect neglected by earlier studies: the psychiatrist-patient interaction in an outpatient psychiatric clinic setting. I focus on meetings between a doctor and patients in the outpatient clinic of a mental hospital. The analyses of interactions demonstrate cultural as well as interactional factors imbedded in verbal and nonverbal exchanges between the doctor and his patients.

Setting

The Hospital

My work was conducted during 1984–1985 in a small, private mental hospital, here called Hiraoka Hospital, in central Japan. At the time of my fieldwork, about 150 patients were hospitalized there. This figure was slightly below the average number of patients for such hospitals. The hospital had three main patient wards: the locked, the unlocked, and the elderly's ward. Eighty to ninety percent of patients in the locked and unlocked wards were diagnosed as schizophrenic. Throughout the course of the year, I was fortunate to be permitted to participate as an anthropologist in almost every aspect of hospital life. The scenes, presented as cases in this paper, are excerpted from my larger ethnographic study (see Nomura 1987a).

Staffing and Social Organization

There were four psychiatrists and twenty-eight nurses, including student nurses and attendants in the hospital. The hospital had four full-time psychiatrists (three males and one female). Except for the day when she/he was in charge of the outpatient clinic, the psychiatrist's day at the hospital began at 10 a.m. S/he would first come into the doctors' room (*ikyoku*) where there were desks for all except the psychiatrist who was serving as the director of services. Upon arrival, the psychiatrist would call the wards and ask if there had been any change(s) in his or her patients. The conditions of the patients were reported by the nurse on duty. At this point, the doctor might give orders for medication or make suggestions to resolve some problem of the patient's. S/he sometimes had to go to the ward and see a patient if immediate attention was needed. Each psychiatrist was responsible for thirty to forty patients scattered among the three wards.

The psychiatrist's everyday schedule was more flexible than that of the nurses'. The psychiatrist was freed from day-to-day involvement with the patients. After calling the wards, the psychiatrist would sit down and write orders, look at the examination results, or discuss patient problems with the nurse, either on the phone or in person. The psychiatrist often met the patients in person in the therapy room. Such meetings were usually requested in advance by the patient. These meetings were called *mensetsu* ("interviews").

Mensetsu were held, generally, for every new patient and whenever a patient had some troubles with other patients or with relatives. The psychiatrist's role was, by turns, often like that of a counselor or a parent figure. Sometimes it was like that of an active therapist.

Each psychiatrist was obliged to work with outpatients at least once a week. The outpatient clinic, located inside the main building, was open six days a week. When seeing outpatients, the psychiatrist's day began at 9 a.m. Before the clinic opened, the assisting nurse cleaned the room and placed each patient's medical/psychiatric record on the doctor's desk in the order of their expected arrival. Then, s/he would call the patients from the lobby, one by one.

Generally, the psychiatrist would recommend hospitalization whenever a patient appeared acutely psychotic. In such cases the psychiatrist would ask the patient's parents about the patient's condition. S/he would also speak to the patient, providing comfort and support. "Let's get you hospitalized. You'll be fine." (If the patient was too excited and if the doctor found hospitalization imperative, the patient might be given an injection of a tranquilizer.) After persuading the patient to go into the hospital, the psychiatrist would call the closed-ward nurse and ask him/her to come take charge of the new inpatient. The psychiatrist would then explain to the parents (or other relatives) the prognosis and the possible length of hospitalization. The word *schizophrenia* was avoided by the psychiatrists when speaking to relatives.

The following interactions were recorded during and after my fieldwork. Recordings during the interactions were not permitted in the clinic. (Institutional and personal names appearing in this text are all pseudonyms.)

Interactions in the Outpatient Clinic: The Cases

The Interactional Context: the Clinic

In this section I discuss the interactions in the manner of interaction analysis. Because the data come from a single ethnographic setting, my interpretations may not apply to all other hospitals in Japan. My purpose here is to elucidate general patterns observed in psychiatrist-patient interaction in a particular Japanese hospital setting and to draw some tentative conclusions.

The outpatient clinic itself was a room, four by four meters in size. It was located adjacent to the hospital's pharmacy. The doctor's desk was in the center of the room, and there was a small, hard bed behind it. Except for a few small, round chairs, there were no other conspicuous pieces of furniture. Each patient entered the room and sat in the chair next to the doctor's desk, creating roughly a 90-degree angle between them. When relatives accompanied the patient, which was often, they would sit behind the patient.

The Cases

CASE A

On September 28, 1984, Mizutani *sensei* (physicians have this term, meaning "teacher" or "doctor" applied to their names) was serving in the clinic. *Kango-cho* was the assisting nurse. I sat on the other side of the desk to observe. The clinic opened at about 9:20 a.m. The first client was a middle-aged, slightly heavy-set man. The doctor started casually; he had seen the man before. "How are you doing?" (At this point, the man noticed my presence but didn't appear bothered in the least.) During the encounter, he talked mainly about his past and touched upon the topic of his welfare assistance, which was soon to expire.

After the patient departed, the doctor told me that the "patient might be on the brink of a breakdown." He explained that a "schizophrenic person often recollects his past when he is growing worse." The doctor picked up the phone and called the welfare office. The expiration of welfare meant that the patient would have to start working on his own. The possibility of a breakdown, coupled with the expiration of public assistance, seemed to have a symbolic meaning for the doctor. The expiration of his money seemed to also imply the expiration of the patient's health. The doctor reached the welfare office by phone and spoke to the appropriate agency staff seeking an extension of the patient's social assistance.

ANALYSIS

There may be a number of nonverbal cues from this setting that would influence the nature of interaction in this clinic. The furnishings of this clinic are simple and functional: the doctor's desk, a narrow hard bed, and a few small round stools. The stools for patients are not necessarily comfortable for sitting long, indicating the brief time normally allowed for each patient. Status differences are subtly conveyed through the difference between the doctor's arm chair and the patient's small stool. This stool, however, has a certain advantage for some patients in that they can adjust the distance from, and the angle with, the physician simply by moving the stool to a desirable position. Some patients pulled the stool slightly backward so that more of the doctor's back can be seen; some pushed the stool near the doctor's desk and rested their elbows on the desk while talking.

The seating angle can be another critical element in nonverbal inter-action. The 90-degree angle arrangements are reported to have six times more interaction than those where physician and patient are face-to-face and three times more than paralleled sitting (Tate 1983). In my own research, the 90-degree angle was found also to be prevalent in other domains of life in the Hiraoka Hospital. For example, one of the psychia-trists told me that he would often consciously create a 90-degree angle at *mensetsu* interviews with the patient.

When two nurses had talks about their work, they often maintained a 90-degree angle, sometimes around the desk and sometimes without one. In this cultural context, this positioning seems less confrontational and less intimate than facing each other. When the nurses talked to the patients, however, such a position was rare, and they tended to face the patient more directly. In the case of the nurses, the aim of conversation may be more or less cooperative, but with patients, the interaction is structured to convey its instructional premise.

In Hiraoka Hospital, the four psychiatrists took turns serving the clinic, and a nurse always assisted the doctor. The head nurse, Kango-cho, happened to be assisting on the first day of the interactions which are pre-sented here. The first patient, a slightly heavy middle-aged man, came into the clinic's room and was greeted by the doctor. The doctor initiated the conversation, "*Doh choshi wa?*" (How are you doing?)

Medical consultation forms an opportunity for doctor and patient to influence each other in identifying problems and choosing the appropriate actions for each problem presented (Kleinman 1980; Gaines 1979; Pendle-ton 1983). Because the consultations presented here took place not in the patient's home but in the hospital, the patient may be said to have had to enter into the doctor's "territory." The "possession" of this territory per-mits the doctor to enact certain interactional rules influencing the rights over turn-taking and over who can summon whom into talk and when one can be summoned (Goffman 1971).

The participants become aware of this territoriality and act within this framework to achieve their particular goal(s). In case A, the patient brought up two significant topics: (1) his past life and (2) his soon-to-expire welfare money. The doctor immediately responded to these comments, interpreting them as signs of a possible breakdown. To the doctor, they constituted a symbolic appeal indicating a link between the expiration of welfare money and that of the patient's health. It is the doctor's role to be empathic (*sasshi*) and to interpret the symbolic meaning of the patient's statement and act accordingly (i.e., making a phone call to the welfare office).

From a slightly different perspective, the patient's appeal can be seen as a "threat" to the doctor, as if he were saying: "If you don't permit me continued welfare benefits, I am going crazy again, which will be troublesome for you." The patient might learn of the best possible way of presenting his case during the brief moments of consultation. The doctor attempted, to the best of his ability, to read what he regarded as subtle cues of the patient indicative of a potential acute episode.

In this case, the doctor responds (overresponds?) to the patient's unstated desire (i.e., "Please help me!") and takes action according to the patient's wishes. The doctor's phone call, seeking an extension of the patient's benefits, seems to show that: (1) the doctor is expected to directly intervene to help create a desirable social, as well as medical, environment for his patient, and (2) the doctor nonverbally communicates that he takes the role of a guardian; that, as a guardian, he is a person upon whom the patient can depend. This response appears to be an example of what Caudill and Doi (1963) called the "passive dependency" of the patient and what Yamamoto (1972) called "benevolently paternalistic ties" with one's doctor which they found in Japanese psychiatric institutions.

CASE B

A middle-aged couple was called next by the nurse, Kango-cho. Before the couple entered, the doctor told me that the husband was an alcoholic and the wife had once been hospitalized for schizophrenia. As the couple entered the room, the doctor inquired, "How are things going since your last visit?" The man replied, "I have no work, so I'm playing *pachinko* all the time." (*Pachinko* is a kind of Japanese pin ball and is a minor form of gambling.) The talk turned to eating habits. The wife told the doctor that her husband often vomited at night. Upon hearing this, the doctor instructed the patient not to "eat at night."

Next, the three of them talked about an alcoholic man who had died recently. The husband opened the topic, "I heard E. *san* had passed away." [E. *san* had been hospitalized here for being an alcoholic. And, he and E. *san* were both "graduates."] Looking sad, the doctor said, "I didn't expect such a sudden death." They all knew the man.

The doctor then asked the wife about her husband, "Has he stayed away from alcohol?" She replied, "He occasionally buys a small whiskey bottle and drinks." The doctor then spoke directly to the husband and said, "It isn't good to drink secretly, you know." The husband had opened the topic and it went full circle back to him. The deceased man was alcoholic, so was the husband; the doctor included the wife in the discussion, asking about his condition. She revealed his secret drinking. Then the doctor made a suggestion to the husband. Finally, the doctor asked the wife about her own condition. She answered cheerfully, "The same as usual." The doctor said to the couple as they departed, "All right. I'll see you again. Take it easy." After they were gone, Kango-cho said, "They are doing well, aren't they?" "Yes," the doctor said, "I remember it was disastrous when they first came in to be hospitalized."

ANALYSIS

Doctor-patient communication at Japanese mental hospitals often shows a striking resemblance to teacher-pupil communicative patterns in Japanese elementary schools. I first noticed this interactional parallel in my observations of Hiraoka Hospital patients' outdoor activities. I found that the staff-patient interactions reminded me of my own school days in Japan. These striking parallels are noteworthy and considered at length elsewhere (Nomura 1987b).

In case B, we see that the alcoholic husband introduces the topic of another alcoholic who died recently. The deceased man was alcoholic, as is the husband; the doctor asks his wife about the husband's condition; his secret drinking is revealed; then the doctor gives an instruction to the husband. In this sequence, the husband is placed in a position of a misbehaving child. Instead of asking the patient directly, the doctor asks the wife about the husband's drinking, as if the wife were the patient's mother.

Then, corrective instructions are directed to the patient himself, expectedly serving to guide him with specifications of appropriate behavior. By not asking the patient directly, the doctor elevates the wife's position, from the position of a (possibly) co-equal wife to that of a parent. This action makes it easier for the doctor to address the patient with his role of "instructor" because the patient has been placed in the child's position in relation to his wife.

Several instances of this stance are repeated even in this short episode. Just before the topic of the deceased man is raised, we notice that the wife reports to the doctor that her husband "eats at night and often vomits." Receiving her report, the doctor then turns to the patient and tells him not to eat at night. This is the same pattern observed with reference to the topic of the deceased man. The interactional assumption, the regarding of the patient as one who needs guidance, is seen twice in this brief consultation. Ironically, the husband helps establish this interactional stance by voicing his own helplessness: "I have no work, so I'm playing *pachinko* all the time." He actively paints his own picture of passivity, of being dependent and socially immature.

CASE C

This case is a staff interaction occurring at the close of case B, above. The assisting nurse, Kango-cho, was wearing a white coat. In Hiraoka Hospital, there was no formal uniform for the staff. The nurses wore their everyday clothes or a type of sportswear. The female nurses put on an apron. Unlike other hospitals, the psychiatrists, including the director, did not wear white coats. Mizutani *sensei* was often in blue jeans. Interestingly enough, the clerks in the office wore white coats with name tags. After the couple had left, the doctor joked to her, "It's uncanny seeing you in a white coat!" Kango-cho said, "Why? Why? I think it's becoming." While this was a brief interaction, it tells us something of importance about the hospital and its staff.

ANALYSIS

The atmosphere of the Hiraoka Hospital was decidedly more informal than the hospital in which I had conducted my preliminary survey. One significant symbol was the staff's clothing. The doctors at Hiraoka wore neither neckties nor white coats. Dr. Mizutani was the most casual dresser, often wearing blue jeans. The informality of the doctors seems to have stimulated a comparable staff interactional stance indicated by frequent joking and a relaxed mood among the nurses. Some people reacted differently, however.

Kango-cho and the clerks in the office, for example, preferred formal white clothes as if to counterbalance the doctors' casual apparel. Today, however, the director of the hospital has changed, and the doctors appear more formal than when I did my fieldwork. It is interesting to note that the same clerks have stopped wearing white coats and now look more casual.

Generally speaking, people in Japanese organizations prefer formal apparel, including suits and ties; college professors and physicians are no exception. Unlike American academic conferences, Japanese academic meetings may resemble public official's or business meetings due to participants' formal attire. From the Japanese perspective, however, casual clothing is thought to give an impression of disrespect to the other and makes it difficult to assess his or her status, an all important aspect of proper interaction. In this sense, the situation at the Hiraoka Hospital at the time of my fieldwork was exceptional—perhaps due in large part to the personality of the director. Thus we see an influence on interaction of staff members from the directors.

CASE D

An elderly woman came in and the nurse took her blood pressure. "A hundred eighty-six," the nurse read. "It's high. It's really high today," said the doctor. There was talk about a recent incident in which the patient fainted. The woman was not a psychiatric patient. The doctor considered her case and wrote an order for medicine. The meeting was brief.

ANALYSIS

This old woman was the only nonpsychiatric patient on that day. The doctors' interactions with nonpsychiatric patients tend to be even briefer and more straightforward than those with psychiatric patients, evidencing little of the twists and entanglements found in psychiatric conversations.

The amount of eye contact (i.e., gaze) usually increased more with psychiatric patients than with nonpsychiatric ones. Interacting with psychiatric patients, the doctor may, consciously or unconsciously, attempt to pick up some unspoken cues to assess the mental patient's emotional state, as well as the validity of his/her statement.

The patients would also pay a great deal of attention to the doctor's nonverbal expressions. Partly due to their own anxiety and uncertainty over the illness, the patients even seek to pick up subtle clues from the doctor as to how and what they should or shouldn't be feeling (Friedman 1979). For winning the doctor's favor, the Japanese mental patients have to be particularly sensitive to this aspect—they are expected to act as if they were at the mercy of doctor's decisions.

CASE E

"Ikeda san! Ikeda Takeshi san!" the nurse called the patient. He looked defiant but greeted the doctor politely. "It's been a long time since you saw me last." His elderly parents came in after him. The patient was a tall, young man in his early twenties. The doctor introduced me, but my presence seemed irksome to the patient. The doctor read aloud from the record, confirming with the patient the details of what had been written. The patient agreed with the doctor at each point but in a defiant tone. His eyes showed discomfort at first and, gradually, hostility toward me. The father appealed to the doctor, saying that his son needed hospitalization because of "his abuse of the family." The patient didn't want to be hospitalized. They quarreled.

Mizutani *sensei* said, "I hear you've been drinking. How much do you drink?" "Beer, about three liters," replied the patient. The doctor asked the patient to lie down on the bed for examination. While the doctor was writing a comment, the father complained to the doctor, "He goofs off during the day and plays around at night." I sensed that there had been many earlier arguments. The hostility was clear. The patient said such things as "the world of the fourth dimension" or "seeing a priest in meditation." These puzzling remarks worked well to silence the "annoying" parents.

The doctor recommended hospitalization to the patient but he refused. Because other patients were waiting, the doctor suggested that the patient discuss it with his parents in the lobby. Later he came back with his parents and agreed to be hospitalized. He became cheerful and cordial and even gained weight, suggesting his overall improvement. During the hospitalization, however, this defiant young man was like a different person.

ANALYSIS

The defiant young man came into the clinic with his parents. Such a visit has a structural similarity with family therapy, where the therapist conjointly meets the family members. In this case, hostility between the father and the son was clear. They quarreled but the father frequently told the doctor how bad his son was and why hospitalization was necessary. The father's appeal to the doctor as authority and the son's polite greeting, regardless of his defiant look, both seem to suggest sensitivity to authority shared by the two. It might be possible to hypothesize that the father and the son played a tug of war at home regarding who had authority over whom. The patient's nonverbal expressions reflected such tension in himself and also in his relationship with his parents.

This young man's sharp staring eyes were impressive. Among all the nonverbal modes of communication, eye movement or gaze is one of the most expressive ones, particularly in psychiatric settings. People usually cannot fail to react when being stared at excessively. Japanese people usually avoid a long mutual gaze; instead they make very brief mutual eye contact and shift the direction of their eyes as soon as mutual eye contact has occurred. Brief mutual contact may occur again later in the interaction. Deviations from the normal range of gazing quickly introduces a certain tension among the Japanese which threatens the interaction.

The Japanese are, generally speaking, a very "eye-conscious" people in that they often assign negative meanings to eye contact between strangers. The Japanese always become conscious of other people's eyes at work in any public or private place. They cannot be too observant of other's behavior and appearances partly because of their overconsciousness about themselves. The Japanese more or less enjoy looking at others but do not enjoy being looked at and usually dislike mutual staring or eye contact, particularly with strangers.

Psychiatric patients at the Hiraoka Hospital, on the other hand, sometimes "stuporously" stared at the doctor for quite long stretches of time. Some patients stare at the doctor with sharp eyes, like this young man, often indicating dissatisfaction or anxiety. These psychiatric patients might have broken the normative pattern of the Japanese by showing a very objectionable behavior in the culture.

Another characteristic of Japanese psychiatrists that is noteworthy here is their interactional pattern toward the patient's relatives. When the patient's relatives or parents are present in the clinic, the psychiatrist more frequently interacts with them than with the patient. Carefully tuning into the relatives' reports and their facial expressions, the psychiatrist sensitively attends to the relatives' needs and complaints about the patient. This may be partly because the doctor can obtain more cohesive reports about the patient's condition from his/her relative, but it also serves to reaffirm the patient's social immaturity.

To the patient, however, it might appear that the doctor and his relative are forming a coalition to "gang up on him." In fact, the relatives usually actively seek the psychiatrist's approval and sympathy, explaining how unmanageable the patient is at home. When consultation ends and the patient goes out to the lobby, the relatives often remain in the clinic alone or come back to the doctor to ask questions or discuss problems that are not suitable to bring up in the patient's presence. These scenes may not be common in Western societies where the mutual trust between doctor and patient is the basis of their relationship. In the United States, for example, it is reported that a coalition is often formed between the patient and the hospital staff against the patient's family (Stanton and Schwartz 1954). The doctor-family coalition may be one of the most significant characteristics in Japanese psychiatric consultation.

CASE F

At 11:40 a.m., a middle-aged, thin male patient came in. The doctor asked, "How are you?" "The same as before," replied the patient. "Can you sleep?" asked the doctor. The patient answered, but after an awkwardly lengthy interval, "Oh, I can sleep." The doctor wrote something down on the patient's record, stopping for a few seconds to think. The patient looked at me once. While writing, the doctor asked, "Is your family fine?" "Yes, fine," said the patient, but his timing was off, again. As he finished writing the order slip, the doctor said, raising his voice, "All right." It indicated the end of the meeting. Then the patient began, "Well, Sensei. The medicine...I can sleep during the night..." The patient sounded as though he didn't want to take the night medicine; it appeared that he wanted to prolong the conversation.

Throughout the interaction, the patient showed psychomotor retardation. His replies were oddly delayed, but he began saying something serious when the doctor was about to finish the meeting. Bringing up an important issue at the end, the doctor explained, was characteristic of the manic-depressive. The patient's action might be in response to an exchange that had been too "instrumental" (note that the doctor's remarks had been brief).

ANALYSIS

One noticeable point in this episode seems to be the doctor's fatigue (as well as the observer's, perhaps). It was 11:40 a.m. and the previous case was quite time-consuming. The doctor's questions were brief and instrumental without obvious display of concern for the patient. The doctor might have had a time limit in mind as to when he wanted to finish up the outpatient clinic for the day. The patient, on the other hand, might have waited quite a long time in the lobby—it was close to noon when he was called in. The patient replied curtly with long, awkward intervals. The exchange went roughly as follows:

Doctor: How are you?

Patient: [Delayed] The same as before.

D.: Can you sleep?

P.: [Delayed] Oh, I can sleep. (The doctor writes on the record.)

D.: Is your family fine? (The doctor is still writing.)

P.: [Delayed] Yes, fine.

D.: All right! [indicating the end of consultation]

P.: Well, *Sensei*. The medicine...I can sleep during the night...

The doctor may perceive the patient's delayed responses as signs of the patient's unstable psychological state, or of some type of resistance against the doctor, or even of his, albeit socially constructed, immaturity. For the patient, these delayed remarks might simply be responses to the doctor's business-like questioning. Fatigue on the part of the doctor and the patient's irritation after a long wait in the lobby might have contributed to the patient's problematic interaction. To the doctor, bringing up important issues at the end was characteristic of the manic-depressive, whereas to the patient it was a response to the doctor's failure to inquire about medicine or to a perceived lack of empathy (*sasshi*).

It is also suspected that the doctor's use of the patient's medical record played a critical part in this episode. The doctor spent a large portion of time writing the medical record without observing the patient's non-verbal signs. Through careful video analyses of the medical consultations, Heath (1986) demonstrated how reading and writing the records can serve to undermine the patient's ability to disclose information and render the doctor insensitive to the moment-by-moment demands of the interaction. Pause can be used to elicit another's gaze; that is, a patient can withhold an utterance or pause within the course of a turn and thereby encourage a doctor to realign his visual orientation (Heath 1986). The patient's delayed responses are likely to be this type of pause to elicit the doctor's more considered attention.

The ideal tone of interaction between Japanese psychiatrists and the patients is that of an empathic and protective kin relationship. To minimize emotional distance thus seems one of the most important goals of interaction. The interaction may not turn out to be productive when participants fail to recognize or fulfill cultural ideals.

CASE G

A female nurse came in to deliver an envelope to the doctor while he was with the patient. The nurse said that the envelope was from the mother of the patient who was to be discharged that day. He looked inside and found cash. The nurse was gone but he shouted, "No! I can't receive this!" It seemed that the patient's mother had been with the nurse in the lobby earlier. But when the the doctor shouted, neither the mother nor the nurse responded.

ANALYSIS

This episode suggests the nature of role of the Japanese nurses. The nurse did not act as a mediator, she simply ran errands between the patient's mother and the doctor. Such passivity on the part of the nurses was observed often in the Hiraoka Hospital. The nurse relied upon the doctors for almost every decision about patients. Japanese psychiatrists would usually end up assuming the entire responsibility of treating and caring for their patients. Consequently, the doctor in charge often tries to have the last say in everything, even in matters that essentially concern nurses and caseworkers (Munakata 1986). The distribution of roles among the hospital staff may not be well-balanced in Japanese mental institutions (e.g., the doctor's phone call to the welfare office in earlier episode, which may very well belong in the domain of social workers).

CASES H AND I

The presentation of these two cases is combined as they are related.

CASE H

The next case was that of a woman who appeared with her small child. She seemed to be about thirty years of age. "How are you?" said the doctor to the patient. "Fine," replied the woman. She was a regular patient and was now quite improved. He continued without pause, "Is your husband feeling relieved, too?" (He was asking if her husband was relieved of his anxiety over her condition.) The woman replied, "Yes, he is...at the moment." The doctor followed humorously, "If so, I can also be relieved, at the moment, can't I?" "Yes, you can," she answered. "All right!" said the doctor.

CASE I

A few minutes after noon, the last patient came in. "How have you been feeling since your last visit?" asked the doctor. A slender, middle-aged woman replied, "I've improved a great deal." Neither this patient nor the woman before appeared bothered by my presence. He asked further, "Don't you feel dizzy anymore?" "Can you tell me what your improvements are?" The patient answered the questions, and the doctor told the nurse to take her blood pressure. As she extended her arm, her large wedding ring was noticeable. The doctor said, "Before, you fretted over many things, didn't you?" "Yes," she said while having her blood pressure taken, "I get easily absorbed. That is my character." The doctor meant to indicate her tendency to "indulge in worry," but the woman changed the angle and said that she was "easily absorbed in excitement."

While the nurse took her blood pressure and the woman spoke, the doctor wrote in the record. He glanced at the patient for a moment and continued writing. Then, he started reading what he had written. The nurse read the pressure, "110, 78." The doctor spoke to her, "It's a little bit low, but you'll be all right with this." He suggested that the patient come back in two weeks. The woman left with an expression of gratitude on her face. The nurse said, "Please take care" to the patient, who had already turned her back and had begun moving toward the door.

ANALYSIS

With returning patients, the doctors at the Hiraoka Hospital usually started with a greeting and question: *"Do desuka sonogo wa?"* The doctor would elicit information about the patient's condition since her last visit. Other typical questions by the doctors were: "Can you sleep at night?" and "What do you think is your present problem?" Eliciting information through short questions was the doctor's typical activity. Detailed explanations or discussions with the patient on medical decisions were infrequent, although such discussions were occasionally held with the patient's relatives. This is one of the ways in which interactions themselves communicate the Interacts' stance born of the paternalistic nature of doctor-patient relationships. The physician appears and is assumed to have superior knowledge; she or he seems to "understand" and "know" the patient, his or her problem and what the appropriate course(s) of action should be.

Conclusions

In this chapter I have identified a number of factors and showed their effect on doctor-patient interactions at Hiraoka Hospital. The factors delimited include: (a) the ecological factors, such as settings, clothing, and interactional angle; (b) the effect of gazing and eye contact in relation to the general ocular behavior in Japan; (c) the similarity observed in Japan between psychiatrist-patient and teacher-pupil interactions and the parallel in doctor and teacher status and role; (d) the cultural tendency of doctor-relative coalition against the patient; (e) interference of communication by the doctor's use of medical records; (f) the nature of hospital attire, and (g) the apparent imbalance of responsibility between Japanese psychiatrists and nursing staff.

I am unsure as to the extent of the generalizability of these observations beyond Hiraoka Hospital. Some of my observations might be unique to this institution. But, this paper has illustrated, through specific cases, some of the ways in which the cultural characteristics of Japan are reflected in psychiatrist-patient interactions and how the communicative elements can have a significant influence on the nature and outcome of the consultations in a single hospital outpatient clinic. This chapter suggests that Japanese cultural conceptions pattern medical interactions and shape the assumptions governing them.

References

Caudill, William

1958 The Psychiatric Hospital as a Small Society. Cambridge: Harvard University.

1961 Around the Clock Patient Care in Japanese Psychiatric Hospitals: The Role of the *Tsukisoi*. American Sociological Review 26:204–14.

Caudill, William and Takeo Doi

1963 Interrelations of Psychiatry, Culture and Emotion in Japan. In Man's Image in Medicine and Anthropology. Iago Galdston (ed.). New York: International University Press.

Doi, Takeo

1962 *Amae*: A Key Concept for Understanding Japanese Personality Structure. In Japanese Culture: Its Development and Characteristics. R.J. Smith and R.K. Beardsley (eds.). Chicago: University of Chicago Press.

Freidman, Howard

1979 Nonverbal Communication Between Patients and Medical Practitioners. Journal of Social Issues 35(1):82–89.

Gaines, Atwood D.

1979 Definitions and Diagnoses. Culture, Medicine and Psychiatry 3(4):381–418.

Goffman, Erving

1961 Asylums. New York: Anchor.

1971 Relations in Public. New York: Harper and Row.

Hahn, Robert and Atwood D. Gaines, eds.

1985 Physicians of Western Medicine. Dordrecht: D. Reidel.

Heath, Christian

1986 Body Movement and Speech in Medical Interaction. New York: Cambridge University.

Kleinman, Arthur

1980 Patients and Healers in the Context of Culture. Berkeley: University of California Press.

Lock, Margaret and Deborah Gordon, eds.

1988 Biomedicine Examined. Dordrecht: Kluwer Academic Publishers.

Munakata, Tsunetsugu

1986 Japanese Attitudes Toward Mental Illness and Mental Health Care. In Japanese Culture and Behavior. T. Lebra and W. Lebra (eds.). Honolulu: University Press of Hawaii.

Nomura, Naoki

1987a Ethnography of Interaction at a Japanese Mental Hospital. Unpublished Ph.D. Dissertation in Anthropology. Stanford University. Stanford, California.

1987b Japanese Mental Hospitals and Elementary Schools: The Parallel in Social Interaction. Paper presented to the American Anthropological Association Annual Meeting. November, Chicago, IL.

Pendleton, David and J. Hasler, eds.
1983 Doctor-Patient Communication. London: Academic.

Stanton, Alfred and M. Schwartz
1954 The Mental Hospital. New York: Basic Books.

Tate, Peter
1983 Doctor's Style. In Doctor-Patient Communication. David Pendleton and J. Hasler (eds.). London: Academic.

Yamamoto, Kazuo
1972 A Comparative Study of Patienthood in Japanese and American Mental Hospitals. In Transcultural Research in Mental Health. William Lebra (ed.). Honolulu: East West Center Press.

11

Attendants and Their World of Work[*]

Ellen Dwyer

Introduction

In America, attendants occupied an ambiguous position within the mental asylum work world. Nineteenth-century asylum superintendents liked to think of their institutions as homes, places of refuge which offered a healthy, happy domestic life to patients. Within this world of a family writ large, the superintendent was clearly the patriarch, a father with almost unlimited authority. His children were the patients; although adult in age, they lacked not only responsibility for their actions but also the right to self-direction. Attendants had a vital role within this family structure. Because doctors spent at most a few minutes a day with patients, attendants had the greatest opportunity to shape behavior. They cared for patients night and day, as one would for a sick spouse or child. They prevented patients from injuring themselves or others and retaught them the habits of adult self-control. Each ward or cottage was considered a distinct, if single-sex, family whose health as a unit depended upon attendants' unceasing vigilance.

Despite their awesome therapeutic responsibilities, attendants most resembled not members of the family but domestic servants, for whom the duty of child-raising had been added to their usual chores. Like nineteenth-century mothers, attendants were asked to provide a loving and moral environment for their patient-children, but they were deprived not only of the housewife's domestic autonomy but also of the many rewards of child-rearing. Many of the attendants' "children" never grew up; of those who left the asylum cured, few felt much gratitude toward the men and women who had overseen their darkest days. Finally, despite the limited legal position of nineteenth-century housewives, they had more social status, both inside

---

[*]This chapter is derived from a chapter in my book *Homes for the Mad* (1987). It was presented as a paper at the American Anthropological Association Meeting, Chicago, IL, 1987. It is reprinted here with the permission of Rutgers University Press which holds the copyright.

and outside the family, than did asylum attendants. Close to the bottom of the asylum work hierarchy, even the most devoted yet felt the burden of their public image, one of brutish abusers of helpless patients. In this paper, I will look specifically at the position of attendants during the nineteenth century at New York's first two public mental hospitals: the New York State Lunatic Asylum at Utica (an acute care facility) and the Willard Asylum for the Chronic Insane.

Conditions of Daily Work

Arduous and poorly paid, attendants' work seldom attracted the kind of skilled caretakers considered essential to the success of moral therapy programs. Asylum superintendents complained about incompetent attendants just as middle-class housewives complained about servants. They failed to perceive the contradictory nature of their expectations. While they required attendants to make beds, scrub floors, and bathe filthy patients, they also expected them to offer moral guidance and psychological counseling. The ideal attendant had, one New York State official proclaimed, "all the higher attributes of a refined nature, such as patience, benevolence, and sympathy...conjoined to a firmness that will not waver, a decision of character that will command respect in the midst of the wildest excitement, and a forbearance that cannot be thrown off its guard, even by personal assault."

Equally demanding was the Utica Board of Managers. Attendants, they proclaimed, must always be "tender and affectionate" to patients, calming the irritated and cheering the depressed. If abused or struck, they should never retaliate. In order to prevent suicides and escapes, attendants were never to leave their charges, even briefly, unless relieved by other attendants. Such individuals were not easy to find.

The board attempted to regulate attendants' lives as strictly as those of patients. Attendants had few personal freedoms and could not leave the institution without permission of the medical officers, to whom they owed total obedience. Forbidden to criticize the asylum or its officers, no matter what the occasion, they were enjoined never to forget that "the whole time of the attendant and assistants belongs to the asylum." In addition to such restriction on behavior, Utica's managers tried to control attendants' thoughts. "Let a smile habitually light up your countenance," they admonished; "Cultivate a humble self-denying spirit," they urged (a practical necessity given the conditions of work). The board's list of attendants' duties and responsibilities was endless. It was five times longer than the comparable list of duties prescribed for medical officers.

As a result of these rules, attendants had the heaviest work responsibilities in the asylum, but little formal power. Typical of the medical staff's attitude was the comment, "An attendant is good in proportion as he obeys the superintendent. The superintendent should be the brain, the attendants the hands." John Gray objected to hiring attendants older than forty, because, with maturity, men and women often lost the will to "spontaneous obedience and to the execution of fixed rules."

Gray was so obsessed with his own authority as to insist (to the horror of a legislative investigative committee) that attendants who visited wards other than their own without permission, even to investigate allegations of patient abuse, should be fired. Such unofficial activities, he contended, breed "insubordination and disturbance," for they usurped the prerogatives of the medical officers. In practice, because Gray and his fellow superintendents rarely appeared on the halls after 1860, attendants exercised many initiatives expressly forbidden them, such as ordering restraints and force-feeding for patients. Overworked assistant physicians acquiesced to, and even tacitly encouraged, these practices. Yet, attendants knew that such informal powers were theirs only by default and might be rescinded at any time.

While all attendants worked long hours for low pay, their experiences varied with their ward assignments. Work with convalescent patients could be pleasant and rewarding; that with severely disturbed patients in back wards often involved the threat of physical danger, in a chaotic and noisy setting. While the institutions' annual reports offered a wealth of detail about attendants' duties and work schedules, neither asylum doctors nor official visitors tried to capture the less formal aspects of attendants' lives: their friendships, amusements, and feelings about their work.

John Chapin's request to the legislature for funding of a new amusement hall at Willard was a rare exception. In it, he commented on the problems created by his many young unmarried attendants' social isolation, and suggested that an amusement hall might lessen the attraction of local taverns. Once built, the hall did indeed become the site of numerous events, organized and attended by staff members and the "better quality" of patients. In addition to frequent musical evenings, doctors, staff, and the townspeople of Willard also organized dramatic recitations, short plays, and presentations by the "Willard Minstrels."

Although such activities engaged many members of the staff, they did not eliminate the excessive drinking which created serious problems at both Utica and Willard. While Utica's administrators could not keep off-duty attendants away from city bars, Willard's fought a bitter political battle in the state legislature and with the governor to prohibit the sale of alcoholic beverages within several miles of the asylum. They also bought the only nearby hotel, primarily so that they could prevent its sale of alcoholic beverages to their employees.

The detailed "discharge list" for 1889 appended to the official Willard Employee Recordbook reveals that attendants drank not just during their free time but also while on ward duty. For example, three ward employees became so intoxicated and disorderly early one October morning that their antics drew the attention of a night watchman and one of the doctors. Initially all were dismissed for "intemperance," and the ward supervisor also was charged with patient neglect.

Insubordination, moral laxity, and patient neglect were considered by asylum superintendents equally serious threats to their institutions' authority structures. As a result, at Willard, employees were fired for attempting to organize a strike, conflicts with doctors, and insubordination, as well as for neglect of duties. Unfortunately, the steward in charge of employee records did not bother to note the issues which led to the threatened strike. When he dismissed a laundry attendant for "incompetency, insubordination, and improper language to the Superintendent," he also failed to record the circumstances under which this lowly drudge happened to encounter P. M. Wise.

Qualifications of Attendants

Asylum doctors frequently referred to such incidents as proof of their inability to find well-qualified attendants. Yet, beyond formulaic statements about attendants' importance, the superintendents at Utica and Willard paid little attention to the qualifications of those actually hired at their institutions. They delegated that responsibility to the asylum steward, whose hiring procedures were highly informal. According to Horatio Dryer, Utica's steward for over thirty years, during times of depression he was swamped with job applicants, but when the economy flourished he had none. Most often he judged candidates simply on the basis of their appearance. The matron used a similar process to hire female attendants. She looked first for evidence of "good health and a good nature." If applicants also could write their age and place of former employment and do simple sums, she employed them. While she preferred candidates with letters of recommendation, she often found herself forced to hire all those with a respectable and trustworthy appearance.

Although Willard's steward left no formal description of his hiring procedures, the information collected in his employees recordbook suggests the job qualifications he valued. Most of those he hired were relatively young: the median age for men was twenty-four and for women twenty-one. Like Utica's attendants, Willard's had little if any professional work experience. Most males had been farm laborers, and females, houseworkers. Only 9 percent of those hired between 1886 and 1890 reported previous asylum employment, thus suggesting that Willard was too isolated to attract the "asylum tramps" complained about by other superintendents. Such lack of expertise bothered neither the steward nor his superintendent. Even those with relevant job experience began at the bottom of the occupational ladder, as did 89 percent of all new employees. Those few applicants stayed only a short time, seemingly having turned to asylum work as a temporary expedient.

Between 1869 and 1886, Willard's steward noted little in his records about new staff members except their age. Beginning in the late 1880s, he also began to make occasional comments about their health. Also frequently noted in the post-1886 records of successful female applicants was their size. The steward divided them into two groups: those of "small stature," most often assigned to kitchen and laundry jobs, and those of "good size," more often made attendants. In the mid-1880s, the steward also began to note for the first time the nativity of those he hired. Increasingly, attendants' work, like domestic service, attracted newly arrived immigrants who lacked the social skills required for better-paying positions. Both the Utica and Willard asylums hired attendants who could not speak English, once again demonstrating their lack of concern (despite rhetoric to the contrary) for attendants' contributions to the therapeutic process. The resulting ethnic differences between patients and staff exacerbated ward tensions. Several Utica patients complained about being forced to associate with coarse, ill-bred Irish attendants. At Willard the situation was reversed; because most employees continued to be recruited from small towns near Willard, largely native-born Americans cared for the asylum's disproportionately foreign-born patient population.

A comparison of Utica and Willard attendants is not easy, for comparable records do not exist for the two groups. Yet, in general, Willard's attendants seem to have stayed longer and engaged in less patient abuse than did Utica's. Because both groups were poorly trained and overworked, such differences were probably due to the relative availability of other kinds of employment and the somewhat different supervisor-employee relationships at the two asylums. For example, the Utica Asylum after the Civil War experienced great difficulties in attracting and keeping high-quality attendants from the growing Oneida County area. Out of 583 attendants hired between 1869 and 1884, 493 left the asylum within a few years of having been hired.

Early in Willard's history, its managers bragged of the ease with which they attracted "first class attendants," but by 1882, its superintendent also complained that attendants seldom stayed even four years. Their restlessness, he claimed, was a peculiarly American trait, for English and Scottish asylums managed to keep excellent attendants for many years at much lower wages. Although Chapin's complaints echoed those of his fellow superintendents, they were not substantiated by his institution's employee records.

Of those nonprofessional workers hired at the Willard Asylum between 1869 and 1890, most worked at least four years. Twenty percent of the men and 10 percent of the women made a career of asylum work, leaving only upon death or retirement. Although most of those employees who worked for more than twenty years were males, women as a group worked longer at the asylum than did men, perhaps because they had few alternative job possibilities.

Whatever their persistence rates relative to workers at other asylums, Willard's attendants certainly stayed at their jobs much longer than did domestic servants, a group with whom they were often compared. Although nineteenth-century women complained about their servants' "restlessness" in almost the same terms as did asylum superintendents, household employers had more reason for dissatisfaction. Fifty to sixty percent of domestic servants stayed less than a year, and very few stayed as long as eight years.

Although asylum hours were even longer than those of domestic work, and the pay no better, perhaps working with chronically insane paupers was easier than with temperamental mistresses. Attendants had only limited formal power, but the overworked medical staffs were seldom able to supervise them as systematically as asylum rules mandated. In contrast, domestic servants had little privacy or independence. Domestic work also lacked the job security and occupational mobility characteristic of asylum employment. Almost all of Willard's employees started at the bottom of the asylum's occupational ladder, but more than half made at least modest moves up it.

Although far from typical, one long-term employee advanced her career in a fashion impossible in the most pleasant of households. When twenty-year-old Mary Ryan first came to the asylum in 1881, she began as a lowly dining room girl. After six years, she advanced to the position of attendant; four years later she became a supervisor, then a charge attendant. By the time she retired on a state pension in 1932, she held a high-ranking administrative position. Attendants at Willard also had ample chances for employment diversity. The frequency with which the steward offered exhausted ward attendants lateral moves when promotion was not possible may have helped the institution hold employees. Fewer than half of all nonprofessional employees held only one position, and most of that group left during their first two years of employment. At both Utica and Willard, promotions came from within the ranks, so that the longer individuals stayed, the greater their likelihood of job mobility.

Perhaps another reason rural New Yorkers sought Willard employment was the asylum's willingness to hire husbands and wives, and to rehire former employees with good work records (a boon for women who had left during their early childbearing years and for men who had experimented with but failed at farming).

For example, one woman who began working in the kitchen in 1879 left to be married in 1888. She was reemployed in 1889, left again in 1890, returned in 1893, and left again pregnant that same year "at the advice of her physician." The asylum was equally willing to hire widows with small children. Most of these mothers took jobs that did not require residency, like ironing and laundry work, but a few left their children with relatives and moved onto the wards. By the late 1880s, some of their children had joined the asylum work force as well. Such family ties among workers became increasingly common at the end of the nineteenth century.

As Willard's Irish community grew, young men and women began to migrate directly from Ireland to Willard, where relatives got them jobs at the asylum. The work force also included a small but cohesive group of Danes hired in the mid-1880s, most on the recommendation of a family patriarch, one Jens Jensen. In this manner, a tradition of asylum work emerged among certain families which persisted well into the twentieth century, and at the same time the size of Willard's work force stabilized. Although Utica, too, occasionally hired employees' siblings and children, it failed to develop the stable local work pool on which Willard depended. Not only were its superintendents markedly less interested in issues of employee morale, but the city of Utica and its environs offered a wider variety of alternative employment opportunities than did rural Ovid.

For the most part, attendants' wages were the same as those of day laborers and domestics and, in the best free-market tradition, Willard salaries clearly reflected fluctuations in the local demand for unskilled workers. When wages in Seneca county dropped in the early 1880s, Willard's cost-conscious board of trustees immediately reduced institutional wages as well. Although large numbers of attendants immediately left, the board attributed such defections to the "migratory disposition" of asylum employees. Nothing could have induced such unreliable employees to remain, they claimed, even higher wages.

Not surprisingly, Willard's salaries embodied the same sex biases as did the general labor market. Male attendants' salaries averaged 42 percent more than females and those of male supervisors were almost 100 percent more. Male cooks received double the stipend of their female counterparts. Those positions held only by women, such as dining room girl and chambermaid, were the lowest paying in the institution. Finally, men monopolized the highest paid, nonprofessional staff positions such as clerk, accountant, butcher, carpenter, and locomotive engineer (whose incumbent made $80 a month the same year kitchen girls made $9).

Equally striking as the gap between male and female salaries was that between poorly paid attendants (whatever the sex) and most other asylum employees, including such unskilled workers as teamsters and porters. Possibly attendants suffered financially from the frequent comparison of their work to domestic service. In any case, administrative rhetoric about the importance of their work was never translated into monetary rewards, even though state legislative committees several times recommended pay increases.

At Utica, the board of managers regularly raised the salaries of its professional staff but refused to do the same for attendants. On one rare occasion when they considered attendants' wages, discussion stalled when one manager insisted that no general wage increases be considered until female attendants were paid the same as males. When a number of Utica's most highly qualified attendants threatened to quit if they did not get either higher wages or additional privileges, John Gray angrily fired them. Such selfish and unreliable employees did not deserve a place within his asylum family, he asserted, for they were too self-centered to be entrusted with the care of others.

Late Nineteenth-Century Tensions and "Reforms"

Although attendants' wages remained low for the remainder of the nineteenth century, a number of other reforms helped to improve working conditions. In 1887, the Utica board for the first time gave two weeks vacation with pay to all attendants who had worked a full year, a much-needed reform. With the establishment of nighttime care at the end of the century, the state asylums also began to construct sleeping accommodations for attendants. These rooms were separate from patient wards. For the first time, attendants could retreat for short periods from the noise, confusion, and excitement. A reform somewhat less appealing to attendants were the uniforms adopted at Utica in 1887.

Even the managers divided over the issue of whether the wearing of uniforms was inherently un-American. However, Superintendent Blumer's arguments finally produced a four-to-three majority in favor of this innovation. Disagreeing that uniforms were a sign of servitude, he argued that they made easier maintenance of the "semi-military" discipline so essential in a large state institution. He also hoped that wearing uniforms would somehow improve attendants' estimation of their status and thereby encourage them to consider their work a lifetime profession.

After several legislative investigations of patient abuse at the Utica asylum in the 1870s and 1880s, a coalition group of social reformers, politicians, and neurologists campaigned for the improvement of asylum staffs. Yet reformers' proposals, even if implemented, would not have eliminated attendant-patient tensions. Reformers assumed that if "better sorts" of people became attendants, abuse would disappear. But patient abuse was rooted in social phenomena appreciated by few asylum outsiders.

Class and Ethnicity

Elitist critics often attributed attendants' brutality to their class and ethnic origins, but asylum records tell a different story. No matter what the class or ethnicity of attendants, they found working with violent, abusive patients difficult. Not infrequently, delusional patients saw attendants as demons and attacked them. Less threatening, but more exasperating, were those patients so demented that they could neither converse coherently nor control their bodily functions. Under such stresses, the metaphor of the asylum as a happy family broke down. Unlike parents, or even tutors and nannies, asylum attendants too seldom saw their "children" mature and grow up. Instead many found themselves trapped in situations similar to those which produced abusive mothers, seldom relieved from care of their difficult children. As a result, with a frequency impossible to estimate, overworked, harassed attendants responded impatiently, roughly, sometimes even brutally to difficult patients, even when their only offense was an unwillingness to eat or to sleep at night.

In short, while cries of outrage filled leading newspapers, those most agitated about the need for reform knew little about the social realities of patient care. They also made no serious effort to challenge asylum superintendents' almost total authority over their staff. At Utica, Gray's position on attendants changed little during the thirty-two years that he ruled the asylum. While he felt that their kind, loving care was vital to patients' recoveries, he fought bitterly all attempts to cut hours or raise pay. When reformers suggested that attendants might take better care of patients if freed from domestic duties, Gray again disagreed. Like many nineteenth-century asylum superintendents, he wanted attendants to be both loving companions to the insane and efficient domestic servants. Not infrequently, the second role (which best matched the attendants' social status within the institution) overwhelmed the first. Once attendants finished their housework, many considered their responsibilities met, and chatted with each other or read, instead of working with patients.

In contrast, Willard's superintendents personally attempted to strengthen staff morale. They also showed more interest in and concern for attendants' daily performances. Furthermore, Willard employee records suggest that, at least by the late 1880s, Willard's doctors monitored even relatively minor instances of patient mistreatment. When, in 1892, a twelve-year veteran handled an idiot roughly, he was warned that repetition of such behavior would lead to dismissal, despite his record of long and faithful service and the patient's lack of physical injury. Most often, Willard doctors presumed that an accused attendant was guilty, whereas Utica's took the opposite stance.

Until late in the century, neither Utica nor Willard offered their attendants formal training. The superintendents argued that training was a continuing, practical process. New attendants learned by watching their more experienced fellows, just as children emulated older brothers and sisters. Although asylum doctors frequently complained about parents' indifference to the socialization of their children, they failed to see their similar failures.

Yet, within the ward family as within the biological family, knowledge gained from slightly more experienced members was often inadequate. The first (and sometimes last) instruction of most attendants was in self-defense.

One Utica attendant best remembered lessons in how to kick recalcitrant patients in the stomach so as to leave no marks. Another candidly, if naïvely, described her limited "therapeutic" strategies: "If patients are refractory we try to hold them in a chair, and after awhile they will probably behave themselves, when we left them go again." She added that, while the doctors never officially informed attendants of their duties, they did so "whenever it is necessary." Not surprisingly, such haphazard education seldom produced attendants who could cope with mentally ill patients' diverse physical and psychological needs.

According to John Gray, journalists frequently aggravated the low status of attendants' work by their sensationalistic coverage of atypical patient abuse cases. (Certainly such articles reinforced public fear of asylums.) In the nineteenth century, as in the twentieth, those patients with the fewest resources were most vulnerable to attendant abuse. While Utica's doctors claimed its few widely publicized abuse cases were atypical, legislative investigations uncovered an institutional conspiracy of silence about abuse. According to one new Utica employee, when he saw his head attendant kick a patient, he did not report the incident out of fear that he himself would be discharged on a trumped-up charge. Once a patient was injured, floor attendants rehearsed together a manufactured explanation of the injuries. Most attendants felt that informing was as despicable as abuse.

When one horrified attendant saw a patient die from injuries inflicted by his fellow workers, he resigned rather than report the incident. As he told a senate investigating committee, "It is the general rule that if a person...makes it a practice to tell the doctors any thing, he is...well, he is called a sucker...and they all get down on him; so it is a general rule that one does not tell what happens."

Occasionally the prohibition within the attendant subculture against informing broke down, but those most willing to violate it tended to be marginal employees motivated by discontent about their work. For example, when a Buffalo State attendant reported an abuse case to his superintendent, he did so because, "Those Utica boys [his superiors] are down on me, and are going to get me out, and I am going to defend myself."

Many attendants considered the rough treatment of patients fully justified. Not uncommon (except in his frankness) was the Utica attendant assigned to the most violent ward (known colloquially as the "dead house") who claimed that everyone knew "a madman would kill you if he got the chance." Pointing out that fights disturbed his ward almost daily (one battle between attendants and male patients lasted three and one half hours), he argued that attendants should be allowed to "do a little fighting" when necessary. Such open acknowledgement of the need for physical force, he claimed, would eliminate the bleaching out process (whereby a patient was soaked in cold water so as to prevent the formation of bruises) which often produced more harm than a "thumping." This same attendant also gave the legislators a practical demonstration in how to choke patients with towels without leaving a mark.

Utica's administrators seemed to agree tacitly that three men could not care for twenty-five insane patients without some use of force, for they were reluctant to fire attendants accused of abuse or even to probe very deeply into patients' allegations of mistreatment. As even one ex-patient noted, if force were not sometimes used to control Utica's violent inmates, there would be no rest for the quiet men there. The excessive use of force was a particularly acute problem on the male wards, where general patient-staff tensions were exacerbated by male attendants' need to defend their masculinity. Most of Utica's male attendants seemed to share the attitude of a Philadelphia attendant who, when told by his superintendent that he should run and call for help when attacked rather than strike a patient, responded defiantly, "I'll never run."

While patient deaths at the hands of attendants were relatively rare, incidents of petty harassment, aimed at bolstering attendants' authority, were common. One victim of such treatment remembered vividly the feeling of being "unmanned" when forced to eat an extra bowl of soup, even though he was already full. Another, who had taught newly freed blacks in the South after the Civil War, complained that patients had no more rights than slaves and often were forced to submit to unreasonable tasks. Neither doctors nor attendants regarded them as individuals, she complained.

Tired and overworked attendants frequently lost their tempers. Ex-patients recalled feeling particularly vulnerable during baths, and several complained about the frequent forceful plunging of feeble patients into cold baths, where they were scrubbed with a cornstalk broom and soap so harsh that it blistered the skin. Patients also felt degraded when forced into bath water already used by four or five other patients. Once bathed, patients reported, they often received additional bruises while being dressed.

Whereas nineteenth-century newspapers attributed such incidents to inhumanity, Erving Goffman (1961) has suggested that mental patients are particularly vulnerable to abuse while being made presentable against their will. Forcible bathing and dressing, Goffman argues, violate the basic cultural rule that adults freely choose to present an appropriate physical appearance. When attendants take over that task, patients give up both dignity and deference. While nineteenth-century asylum superintendents lacked Goffman's insight, they, too, recognized the frequency with which patients were mishandled during bathing and, in a few instances, assigned doctors to oversee that activity.

Of course, not all patient-staff ward interactions were negative. Both John Chapin and George Blumer gave dedicated attendants credit for the successful implementation of a number of important reforms, including the abolition of mechanical restraints and the diversification of patient work opportunities. When a smallpox epidemic threatened the Utica Asylum, two Utica attendants voluntarily spent almost two months isolated with four smallpox victims in hospital tents pitched on a remote part of the asylum farm. Willard's attendants responded with similar bravery when an epidemic resembling typhoid fever swept the institution in 1871. Despite widespread apprehension, not a single attendant left the asylum service or refused to work around the clock. Other Willard attendants, including those assigned to chronic "dements," responded to their charges' helplessness and dependency with much pity and affection.

In addition to citing such individual achievements, both Willard and Utica doctors defended their attendants by noting the heavy physical and emotional demands of their work. The majority of attendants, doctors proclaimed, were hard-working, reliable, and compassionate. Their daily good deeds were too often overlooked when patient-staff tensions erupted into the popular press. Still, "good" and "bad" attendants resembled each other more closely than doctors cared to admit. Dedicated, energetic teachers of convalescent patients easily deteriorated into irritable, harsh autocrats after several weeks on a ward for the noisy, incoherent, and incontinent. The frequency with which the same individuals assumed the dual roles of loving parent and harsh patriarch reflected the conflicting demands of attendants' work. Like parents, attendants sometimes loved and other times struck out at their difficult children.

When asylums were small, superintendents managed to keep such erratic behavior within reasonable bounds. By the end of the century, the conceptualization of the asylum as a family in which attendants lovingly cared for the childlike patients was increasingly anachronistic. Amariah Brigham's cohesive Utica community, with its fifty employees, had mushroomed in size and complexity. To function efficiently, the institution required more than three hundred staff members. As they marched patients from activity to activity at the blaring of bugles, attendants more closely resembled prison guards than kindly companions. The Willard Asylum was even more overwhelming, a small world unto itself with a population of more than two thousand patients, doctors, and staff. Even the most preoccupied of Victorian patriarchs recognized his own children, but by 1890, Willard's superintendent knew few of his charges.

Such growth had been gradual, but asylum administrators never fully adjusted to it. In their annual reports of the 1880s, they experimented with a variety of new metaphors, e.g., medical, industrial, and military, to characterize their activities, but they had difficulty reconciling their therapeutic objectives, as well as their self-image, with notions of a military encampment or industrial plant. Therefore, they continued to rely most heavily on familial rhetoric. Both Utica and Willard administrators refused to abandon the vision of their institution as a home away from home, where patients and staff lived together in large and contented families. As a result, attendants remained trapped within the confines of what was at best an inadequate and partial vision of their work.

The medicalization of lunatic asylums at the end of the nineteenth century did little to improve attendants' status or to clarify the ambiguities of their position. When the 1890 legislature changed the names of New York's lunatic asylums to "state mental hospitals," asylum doctors hoped that the prestige of both their own work and their institutions would increase. Yet they never seriously considered redistributing internal asylum authority to accommodate their shifting mission. Instead, they emulated their colleagues at general hospitals. Despite the recent professionalization of nursing, large social and power differentials continued to separate doctors, nurses, and patients in general hospitals.

Within mental hospitals, this hierarchical structure was even more rigid. Hence, the continuing popularity of the family metaphor. It helped to blur power differentials exacerbated by the increasing emphasis given to a strictly medical approach to mental illness. The metaphor also facilitated institutional psychiatrists' justification of the continuing therapeutic differences between caring for the mentally and physically ill. For attendants, however, its effects were less benign. Although the most promising patients confined within the asylum family were encouraged by doctors to mature and break away, attendants were given few opportunities for change. The medical staff continued to show little interest in extending the benefits of professionalization to these lowly members of the hospital hierarchy, despite their vital role in patient care and therapy. Asylum doctors either could not or would not see the contradictions inherent in asking employees simultaneously to counsel and to clean, to befriend and to discipline, to follow and to lead. Even as mental hospitals moved into the twentieth century, attendants remained frozen in their old, conflicting roles: as children themselves in need of continual supervision by the medical staff, as the surrogate parents of patients, and as the domestic servants of all.

References

Primary Sources

MANUSCRIPTS

Chapin, John B. Scrapbook. Division of Manuscripts and University Archives, Cornell University, Ithaca.

Dix, Dorothea. Papers. Houghton Library, Harvard University, Cambridge.

Jarvis, Edward. Papers. Countway Library of Medicine, Harvard Medical School, Boston.

Kirkbride, Thomas S. Papers. Pennsylvania Hospital Medical Archives, Philadelphia.

New York State Board of Charities. Correspondence. New York State Library Archives, Albany.

New York State Lunatic Asylum. Records. Utica Psychiatric Center, Utica.

Willard Asylum. Records. Willard Psychiatric Center, Willard.

PUBLISHED ANNUAL REPORTS

New York State Board of Charities. *Annual Reports* 18–23, 1885–1890.

New York State Commissioner in Lunacy. *Annual Reports* 1–11, 1874–1885.

New York State Lunatic Asylum. *Annual Reports* 1–47, 1844–1890.

Willard Asylum for the Chronic Insane. *Annual Reports* 1–22, 1870–1891.

Secondary Sources

Adelson, Pearle Yaruss
1980 The Back Ward Dilemma. American Journal of Nursing 80:422–425.

Association of Medical Superintendents
1888 Proceedings of the Association of Medical Superintendents. American Journal of Insanity 45:146–47, 228–229.

Bucknill, John Charles, and Daniel Hake Tuke.
1858 A Manual of Psychological Medicine: Containing the History, Nosology, Description, Statistics, Diagnosis, Pathology, and Treatment of Insanity. Philadelphia: Blanchard and Lea.

Carpenter, Mick
1975 Asylum Nursing before 1914. In Rewriting Nursing History. Celia Davies (ed.). London: Croom Helm. Pp.123–146.

Chase, Hiram
1868 Two Years and Four Months in a Lunatic Asylum, from August 20, 1863 to December 20, 1865. Saratoga Springs, NY: n.p.

Church, Olga Maranjian
1982 That Noble Reform: the Emergence of Psychiatric Nursing in the United States, 1882–1963. Unpublished Ph.D. dissertation. University of Illinois at the Medical Center.

Clark, A. Campbell
1884 The Special Training of Asylum Attendants. American Journal of Insanity 40:326–343.

Davis, Phoebe B.
1855 Two Years and Three Months in the New York Lunatic Asylum at Utica: Together with the Outlines of Twenty Years' Peregrinations in Syracuse. Syracuse, NY: by the author.

Digby, Anne
1985 Madness, Morality, and Medicine: A Study of the York Retreat 1796–1914. Cambridge: Cambridge University Press.

Dwyer, Ellen
1987   Homes for the Mad. New Brunswick, NJ: Rutgers University Press.

Goffman, Erving
1961   Asylums. New York: Anchor Books.
1967   Interaction Ritual: Essays on Face-to-Face Behavior. Garden City, NY: Doubleday.

Katzman, David
1978   Seven Days a Week: Women and Domestic Service in Industrializing America. New York: Oxford University Press.

Kempe, Ruth S. and Henry C. Kempe
1978   Child Abuse. Cambridge: Harvard University Press.

Lathrop, Clarissa
1890   The Secret Institution. New York: Bryant.

Ray, Issac
1854   American Hospitals for the Insane. North American Review 79:67–90.
1851   Popular Feeling Towards Hospitals for the Insane. American Journal of Insanity 9:36–65.

Straus, Murray A., Richard J Gelles, and Suzanne K. Steinmetz
1980   Behind Closed Doors: Violence in the American Family. New York: Doubleday.

Walk, Alexander
1961   The History of Mental Nursing. Journal of Mental Science 1–17.

12

Psychiatric Institutions: Rules and the Accommodation of Structure and Autonomy in France and the United States

Helena Jia Hershel[1]

Introduction

In this paper I show how mental patient behavior is conditioned by both treatment ideology and social structure within the institutional setting. I discuss several treatment facilities and describe variations in both treatment practice and institutional expectations of the mental patient. Although many studies have examined psychiatric settings (e.g., Bloor & Fonkert 1982; Estroff 1981; Goffman 1961; Gurle 1974; Lebovicic 1978; Perucci 1974; Strauss et al. 1964), none deals specifically with the effects of variations within the institutional structure on patient behavior. Here, I argue that three specific factors: 1) treatment ideology; 2) the fit of the larger cultural setting to that of the treatment facility; and 3) patient-staff power relations all actually promote certain rules that limit or encourage patient expressivity.

Methods

The Sites

Four treatment settings are described: 1) a medicated hospital ward in France; 2) a medicated ward in the United States; 3) a nonmedicated hospital ward in the United States; and 4) a nonmedicated residential treatment facility in the United States. These settings vary greatly in terms of culture, use of medication, patient population, physical organization, treatment ideology and patient-staff power relations. The four treatment settings were selected to illustrate pronounced contrasts in present mental patient care. Though they are real facilities, the treatment settings are best seen as ideal types in the analysis of institutional contexts. For the sake of convenience, the medicated French hospital ward will be called Ward A; the medicated American hospital ward will be called Ward B; the nonmedicated American

Designation	Ward A	Ward B	Ward C	Ward D
Location	France	U.S.	U.S.	U.S.
Type of Facility	Hospital	Hospital	Hospital	Halfway House
Treatment Modality	Medication	Medication	Milieu Therapy	Milieu Therapy

Figure 1. The Four Treatment Settings

hospital ward will be called Ward C; and the nonmedicated American non-hospital treatment facility will be called Ward D (see Figure 1).

Fieldwork

I spent a total of two and a half years conducting fieldwork in these four psychiatric settings. The first year, I worked as an intern in Ward D. Several months later I spent my time observing American and French institutions. During a six-month follow-up period, I visited several public and private mental hospitals to verify the data I had collected.

The case material presented here is drawn predominantly from participant-observation on the wards during the second year of fieldwork. My various roles on the wards included leading group therapy in residential treatment centers as a volunteer; conducting family therapy with adolescents on inpatient psychiatric wards; and diagnosing French patients during psychiatric interviews. I made detailed observations of variation in the structure of different facilities both in conjunction with these duties and in periods when I acted solely as an unobtrusive observer.

My observations were taped recorded immediately after spending the day or night at the institution; I found this to be the most accurate and least intrusive form of recordkeeping. I then verified my observations by cross-checking them with hospital files, with staff, and by participating in supervisory meetings. Administrators and staff personnel were most helpful in allowing me entry into these facilities and providing information. This study could not have been completed without their full cooperation. The fieldwork led to a schema for understanding the nature of various treatment facilities. I first give an overview of this schema and define my terms; then I present the case studies from which the schema is derived.

Overview of Schema

The nature of any treatment facility is determined, in large part, by a model of mental illness. Practitioners in each of the four settings adhere to either a medical model or a milieu model of illness. The medical model is

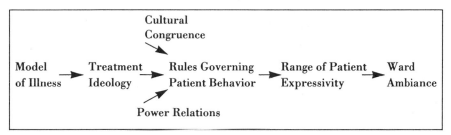

Figure 2. Factors Contributing to Varying Treatment Setting Ambiance

typified by the use of medication, the use of medical nosology, and the hierarchical patient-staff relations. The milieu model emphasizes nonmedication and attempts to provide therapy through patient support or patient-staff interactions that approximate "real life" interactions.

Each model of mental illness clearly implies a particular perspective on how mental illness should be treated. I will call this perspective the "treatment ideology" of the facility. The term "ideology" here is not used in a pejorative sense to imply falsehood or illusion, but to refer to a shared or collective set of psychiatric ideas (cf. Strauss et al. 1964). These sets of psychiatric ideas concern appropriate treatment and are established by the founders of any given facility. They are transmitted to staff members through training, meetings, policy directives, and instructions about staff duties and responsibilities. In this way, treatment ideology becomes a pervasive *a priori* assumption about appropriate patient care held by all levels of staff.

Besides treatment ideology, each facility has its own subculture that significantly has an impact on the nature of the facility. The degree to which the subculture either reflects or contrasts with the dominant culture is what I call the degree of "cultural convergence." The concept of "power relations" refers to who has the authority to sanction the patient. In combination, these three factors—treatment ideology, cultural convergence, and power relations—foster certain rule structures. The term "rule structure" refers to both 1) the content of the rules, i.e., what is allowable emotional expression and behavior, and 2) the form of rules.

The form of the rule structure has two components: the degree of rule rigidity and flexibility, and the degree to which rules are hidden or apparent. The first component, rigidity or flexibility, refers to the extent to which a patient can negotiate with a staff member about what is considered appropriate. Thus, the greater the degree of negotiation, the more flexible the rule structure. As to form, rules are considered hidden when they are so deeply assumed that there is no discourse about them; in contrast rules are apparent or visible when they are formally stated. Consequently, the emotional expressivity and behavior of patients is conditioned by both the content and the form of the rule structure (see Figure 2; also see Collett 1977; Hochschild 1979).

Designation	Ward A	Ward B	Ward C	Ward D
Location	France	U.S.	U.S.	U.S.
Type of Facility	Hospital	Hospital	Hospital	Halfway House
Treatment Modality	Medication	Medication	Milieu Therapy	Milieu Therapy
Degree of Rule Rigidification	++ Very rigid	+ Rigid	+/− Flexible	− Amorphous
Degree of Rule Visibility	Deeply Hidden	Mildly Hidden	Visible	Obscured

Figure 3. Rule Rigidification and Visibility

In the four case studies, I show that the rule structures resulting from various combinations of the ideological treatment model, cultural congruence and patient-staff power relations vary along two dimensions: rigidity and visibility. More specifically, I show that in France, the rule structure is extremely rigid and hidden; in the United States medicated ward the rule structure is less rigid but visible; in the United States nonmedicated ward it is flexible and visible; and in the American residential treatment facility, the rule structure is amorphous and obscure (see Figure 3).

Because each setting has a specific rule structure, each ward has a different ambiance, or general affective tone. Variations in tone result from the degree of rule structure limiting patient behavior to a given range. While there is variation within each setting due to differences in the individual patients, taken as a whole, each ward sets the conditions for specific behaviors and levels of expressivity, which define the setting's ambiance.

In summary, models of mental illness imply treatment ideologies. These treatment ideologies, along with variations in two other major factors, lead staff members to use specific, informal, and often a nonstated set of rules about what constitutes appropriate expression and behavior of the patients. The effect is that sanctioning limits patient behavior within a certain range of expression readily apparent as the distinct ambiance within each four settings.

Case Studies

The Medicated Settings

A critical determinant of the atmosphere within mental institutions is the degree of reliance on drugs for treatment and social control. The medical model, which relies primarily on the use of drug therapy, is the predominant form of psychiatric intervention in both American and French psychiatric institutions (Leifer 1970; Osmond and Seigler 1974; Wittman 1980). These medicated facilities tend to be more cost effective than nonmedicated units because demands on staff are lighter and patient stays within the hospital are limited. Despite the critical importance of treatment by drugs, medicated wards vary enormously in their overall ambiance and in the ways they manage the emotional lives of patients.

French Medicated Hospital: Ward A

The French hospital system has not fully integrated itself as a rational bureaucratic organization; rather, it conforms to a feudal model with centralized authority, protective rights, and a system of paternalism and patronage (FGDPA 1974) (as typically found in Mediterranean settings, see Blue, Katz, this volume—ed.). Still, extreme diversity among treatment styles, as might be found in the United States, is nonexistent.

Each wing of the large French hospital complex I describe is run by a psychiatrist who determines policies. Decisions regarding treatment procedure rest with the head psychiatrist and the personnel they themselves have brought to the institution, much like presidential cabinet appointees in the United States. In this way little fiefdoms are created by the head psychiatrists.

In general, the psychiatrists spend one hour in the ward in the morning, and patients see them privately once a week. Favorite patients may be seen more frequently to discuss philosophy, especially phenomenology, a specialty of French psychiatric schooling. Apart from dispensing medication, therapy does not occur on ward; therapy is not considered commensurate with hospitalization. The treatment of institutionalized patients is purely medical and pharmacological.

Unlike American psychiatric institutions, the social structure and organization of the French ward dictates a minimum of interaction between nurses and patients. The nurses, although central to the care of the patients and the running of the ward, relate little to the patients except for caring for their physical needs. It is not a matter of apathy; the psychiatrists monopolize communications with the patients. Communication regarding the patients' mental health is the sole domain of the psychiatrist.

Though the rules structuring communication between patient and staff are rigid and hierarchical, they are accepted by the patient as legitimate. Therefore, conflict on the ward is rare (see Ruesch and Bateson 1968). Patients maintain great deference for the all-powerful psychiatrists. In return the psychiatrist and staff treat the patient with kindness due a sick and deranged person.

The French, from early childhood on, are conditioned by strict patriarchal families, a rigid church, and a rigorous and inflexible educational system. The effect of these pervasive institutions is instrumental in conditioning the French acceptance of authority and hierarchy. Consequently, the patients in the psychiatric ward accept the authoritarian structure of the hospital setting, because its proscriptions and prescriptions parallel the expectations they have developed in the larger culture of France.

This hospital ward is in a metropolitan area and services a large region in the southwest of France. The facility is guarded and remote to visitors and anyone not directly involved in care of patients. The ward is locked, and the grounds are secured by a high fence and a guarded entry. Only the spaciousness of the quarters gives the appearance that one is not closed in. The induced docility of the patients by medication renders the population almost unaware of the sharp demarcation between themselves and the outer world:

> The main room of Ward A, the medicated ward, is large and sunny, lined with chairs of all sizes and description, not a one similar to the other and filled with patients equally diverse. Old and young, male and female, chronic and acute patients are spread thinly around the room chatting with one another. The patients have to stay in this day room with little activity but a T.V. mounted on a wall and a few board games. The bedrooms are locked during the day to force them out. Many patients are elderly and because of poor facilities for the aged they find themselves here. The more able and adjusted patients look after those who need care. Nurses participate with patients mainly for specific tasks such as serving meals and dispensing medication. The nursing staff enjoys a room away from the central room; they tend to congregate there except at meal time.
>
> Patients live together in a quasi-community and activities turn around the main event of the day, the noon meal. In this region of France, the noon meal is often the central and largest meal. Some more mobile and able patients set the table. All sit down together, showing noteworthy table etiquette, facing each other and sharing their common fate of being crazy but still acting civilized.

Because there is little interaction between staff and patients regarding their mental problems, close relations arise between patients. They offer each other support or sometimes scorn. They freely indulge in helping one another, giving advice on how to solve the mental or emotional problems that beset a particular patient.

The psychiatrist sees the patient only once a week; therefore, patients' anticipation of their interviews is frequently heightened. Though a patient's fate, i.e., length of stay and amount of medication, is determined in the initial interview, patients are typically compliant with respect to physician's directives.

The simple way in which the patient is led into the room and prepared to greet the head doctor creates an aura of sanctity. Thus, reinforcement of deference for the head psychiatrist initiates the communicative pattern. The following description of one interview illustrates some dynamics of the psychiatric interview and typical patient compliance with the psychiatrist recommendations (see also Heller 1968; Sullivan 1970).

> Two nurses hold the patient upright as she stumbles through the doors. The patient is heavily medicated and has been in the hospital and medicated for twenty days before this, her first psychiatric interview. The *medicin en chef* (chief physician) shakes her hand and with a calm, soothing voice tells her to disregard my five colleagues and me who sit in this small, cramped office. He draws the focus of her attention to him and only him. She knows this is an important occasion, her first chance to meet with the head doctor. There is a certain status attached to this event for which the nursing staff has carefully prepared her. This includes grooming and bathing, a change of clothes and the gentle goading by the nurses to behave.
>
> With impeccable skill, the head doctor secures her compliance with a persuasively gentle and resonant voice. The head doctor does not say much at first, but maintains constant eye contact. He waits to see what she will do with the silence around her. She begins to feel defensive and, as the patient gets agitated, her hands tremble. The doctor enters with a calming response. She is now already caught in a dilemma: the head doctor is placing himself in the position of creating a secure mooring for her, though it was he who intentionally created the stressful moment. (See Thibaut and Coules 1951)
>
> The initial conversation is somewhat unstructured. She knows she may be her own executioner and so is aware and careful in her conversation. She seeks the help of the doctor who is viewed with respect and assumed to possess knowledge about what she is experiencing. While it is the role of the doctor to offer insights, he is careful not to dispense too much information about her symptoms lest she learn more symptoms than cure those already present. The doctor must gain the confidence of the patient while maintaining distance. He must merge with her reality and then move away, confronting her to unmask her. He does this by creating the appearance of total understanding—empathy—all the while suggesting perspectives that are considered symptomatic of a particular diagnosis.

Rules about expressivity deny the expression of emotions in the psychiatric interview. Emotional expression is discouraged during the interview. The doctor is conducting a mental examination, but the patient is seeking an emotional relationship. It is perhaps the first direct social interaction she has had since arriving in the hospital. Emotional expression that is not significantly repressed by the patient is interpreted as symptomatic of greater mental and emotional disturbance, and medication is increased. So, expressivity by a patient on the ward is attended to not by staff, but by other patients in usually a supportive manner.

The treatment afforded patients as typified in the French ward stems from a strongly held attitude that these people are truly sick. This assumption is unquestioned, and when allied with the paternalistic system of care, a ward ambiance is created that is benevolent, yet static. There is no sense that people get better; the calm environment is aided by the ample use of medication and lack of intervention.

The American Medicated Ward: Ward B

In the United States, as in France, rule structure of the psychiatric hospital system reflects the values of the larger society. In France, the hospital system remains as part of an established feudal order. In feudalism, service to the state is given by the populace in exchange for protection of the powerful. In the French hospital, compliance of the patient is rewarded by paternalism of the psychiatrists.

Unlike the French, the American hospital system does not reflect the larger societal values. In the United States, the idealized values of the larger society include a pronounced sense of individualism and individual rights, autonomous action, and initiative. In contrast, the organization of mental institutions resembles a rational-bureaucratic society. Efficiency, recordkeeping and impersonality are some traits of the American mental hospital organization. Power remains with the office, not the person who occupies it, allowing for interchangeable personnel. In the United States, the authority of institutions is in direct contrast to the idealized values of the culture: the impersonal authority of the institution over the individual conflicts with a sense of individual rights. Therefore, in the United States, we see patient protest instead of patient compliance.

While the practitioners of the American medicated ward share the medical model of mental illness with their French counterparts (e.g., Hawkins 1969), the ambiance on the two wards dramatically differs. The American medicated ward I studied, Ward B, is one of two at a large hospital facility in a medium-sized California city. The patients come from all walks of life and accurately reflect both the middle-class composition of the city and the impoverished outlying rural areas. Both adolescent and adult patients are served by this hospital. Less than 10 percent of the beds are designated for the elderly.

Psychiatrists, psychologists, or social workers are rarely seen here. The hierarchy is a simple two-tiered system. Caretaking tasks are allotted primarily to members of a nursing staff, who are overworked and underpaid (see Dwyer, this volume). Hospital attendants are either on staff or on call to handle unruly patients. Staff is responsible for the maintenance of order and care simultaneously. These two functions often run counter to each other, and when they do, *order* takes precedence. For example:

> No one walks into Ward B without permission, not even staff. A nurse sits inside the door in a wooden chair, the kind with a writing arm like those in old school rooms. She holds a chart on which is recorded the comings and goings of all that pass by. Behind her are rows of tables and benches, mostly empty now, but that are used to serve meals and watch T.V. The room is bare. As you enter the room, the door locks behind you and the heavy metal screens on the windows diffuse the light from the outside. On one edge sits the nurses' station, sheltered by a high built-in desk that partitions this room from the rest of the ward, except for a narrow passageway. A nurse is stationed at the end of this corridor as a guard, similar to the nurse in the entry way. Just behind her are the sleeping quarters of the patients. Individuals share rooms of up to five beds.
>
> The patients are mostly to be found in their rooms dressed in hospital pajamas: blue for the men, pink for the women. They neither roam the ward nor chat in the halls. Instead they attach themselves to their particular bed either by lying in it or remaining close by. An occasional patient will shuffle up to the nurses' station to demand something.
>
> The atmosphere at first appears sedate except for the constant screaming at the end of the hall. There are six locked cells here. A third nurse is positioned in this location, where metal cells line a final tiny enclosure. Each cell is locked and dark. They afford little light except that from a small barred window on the door. The number of patients that inhabit these cells vary, but on a normal day three patients will be in locked cells. There are two kinds of sounds that come out of these cells: either the total silence of the sedated patient or an echoed pounding and screaming. The inside of the cell is completely bare metal. Each angry movement of a patient sends resounding tremors throughout the rest of the ward.
>
> As this ward is designed for containment, the three guard nurses speak neither to the patients, nor even with the rest of the staff. They tend to remain reserved and nonexpressive. Armed with clipboards, they take down notes on any behavior that comes to their attention. An undefined hostility pervades the atmosphere; the source appears not to be any particular individual, but an overriding fear and readiness to take action.

The physical structure and ambiance suggest a prison. The pervasive use of medication in the harsh atmosphere of the ward facilitates an atmosphere of authority and repression. From the vantage of the staff, medication is synonymous with the maintenance of order; patients often consider being medicated as a punishment. A typical patient-staff interaction illustrates how the staff's need to maintain order dominates the rule structure of Ward B, and, therefore, sets the conditions for behavior on the ward:

A young fellow, clutching a Bible in his left hand, pushes on the
door to the kitchen. He is denied entry and begins to scream at a nurse:
"God's word is more powerful than yours," pointing to his Bible he bel-
lows: "You must reckon with this force." Two nurses grab him. The
more they attempt to restrain him, the more his rage builds. He shouts
profanities and tries to break away from their grasp. It is a question of
wills and he will not succumb to their orders.

A big, burly hospital attendant approaches calmly. His mere presence arrests the conflict. Quickly, a male nurse arrives with a hypoder-
mic containing a tranquilizer. The hospital attendant orders the patient
to drop his pants so he can receive the shot in the buttock. The patient
pleads to receive the shot in his arm, but the male nurse insists. The
patient refuses and begs not to have his pants lowered, as if this is the
worst part of the treatment. He screams at me not to look, for being
seen is the greatest humiliation. Seconds after the injection there is
stillness, just a faint whimpering is heard from the young patient.

The nursing and attendant staff on Ward B have the power to interpret every word, step or gesture as a sign of sickness. All expressivity is primarily viewed as symptomatic of sickness. This is especially true for emotional displays or outbursts that gain attention. For instance, a complaining
patient who nags the staff to see the psychiatrist is likely to be interpreted
as more problematic than a patient whose inner depression inhibits social
interaction. The goal on this ward is custodial care through maximized
social distance and rigid spatial structure. Rule breaking, that is breaching
the social distance between staff and patient, is sanctioned by increased
medication and possible confinement in locked cells. There is little room for
compromise in conflict situations.

One major difference between French Ward A and American Ward B
is how authority is integrated into ward structure, and the ensuing relationship between staff and patient. Though both wards are medicated, the differing degrees of cultural convergence have a dramatic impact. The treatment ideology of the French hospital is not drastically demarcated from
French culture; therefore, the negotiation of special hospital rules is not
required. The patient is benevolently reduced to a nonentity, and the custodial care of the nurses insures a relative ease and acceptance of a sick role.
In contrast, in the American medicated ward, violence and disruption are
paramount. The degree of authoritarianism of the hospital ward is unparal-
leled in any other American setting except prisons. Authoritarianism is not
conferred benevolently but, rather, is used punitively. Rules about infrac-
tions are not readily defined nor carried out systematically. Variations in
medicated wards dispose the chronic patient to testing out the situation to
seek the boundaries of freedom. Yet the patient in this context is always
respected enough to be held accountable for his or her actions. For American patients there is some belief that things can be challenged; a sense of

hope exists with the greatest despair. In contrast, the French patients tend to internalize their misery, blaming themselves or others for their suffering but rarely blaming the institution.

In the United States, both patient and staff have, typically, been socialized in a society where emphasis is on individual rights. The staff members' basic orientation will be 1) to do their job, which is to protect the society at large from the potential irrational acts of the mental patient, and 2) to protect their interests in having an easier and more peaceful job situation. Similarly, American patients have a deeply inculcated view of their right to freedom of action. Thus, on the American ward, both staff members and patients are more likely than in the comparable French case to exert their sense of their rights. Clearly, the potential for conflict is greater when two equal and autonomous individuals are interacting than when two individuals of different status are interacting in an agreed-upon system of deference to the higher status person. Conflict is heightened on the American ward because those who interact with patients mostly are not privileged and protected, like the psychiatrists in France, but are low-paid members of the nursing and attendant staff. The workers who are responsible for interpreting the patients' behavior as mad and potentially disruptive, do so from moment to moment. Their interpretations often seem arbitrary and aimed at lessening their workload through the means of tranquilizing patients.

The Nonmedicated Settings

The two nonmedicated treatment centers resulted from "deinstitutionalization," a movement introduced in the United States as a labor-saving and cost-containment plan for the management of the mentally ill and concerns for patient freedom. In the 1960s, hospitals began emptying their beds with use of medication and limiting the duration of patients stays. Because many patients who were turned out of medicated facilities were disabled by the secondary effects of hospitalization, such as reduced networks, heavy medication and dysfunction, they often returned to their hospitals of origin. New types of facilities were then needed that would allow the patient to receive intense therapy but avoid lengthy and costly hospitalizations; experimental nonmedicated wards and halfway houses were the result.

A typical experimental nonmedicated hospital ward and a nonmedicated treatment facility will be described. These two nonmedicated facilities have a milieu model of therapy. So, the hospital ward provides family therapy and the residential treatment facility offers a loosely structured supportive environment. While both have a similar model of mental illness, the hospital ward, with its explicit rules and routines, is considerably more structured than the open-ended, amorphous orientation of the residential treatment center.

American Nonmedicated Hospital: Ward C

Though Ward C does not rely on drugs and is informed by a progressive therapeutic orientation, it shares certain aspects of organization and structure with the medicated wards analyzed in the previous section. Hospital wards are subject to certain administrative demands and exigencies. Caretakers in this setting are varied and many. Psychiatrists are on ward only to diagnose physical complications and prescribe drugs. Treatment coordinators work eight-hour daytime shifts; their job is to devise long-range treatment plans based on each individual patient's needs. The nursing staff has the main burden of care for the patients. When a new patient who is acutely psychotic arrives, the treatment coordinator may choose to put this individual "on special." "Specialling" demands that this individual be kept under eye contact twenty-four hours a day if necessary. All the staff members take turns specialling, rotating each hour. A patient may remain on special for up to seven weeks. No medication is given; the goal is for the patient to work out his or her problems under close supervision. Up to two people at a time may be on special. The nursing staff and hospital attendants get the brunt of this task, especially at night when treatment coordinators are not present:

> People mill about. The staff sits about very informally and discusses case histories or other matters. Although there are locks on the doors and windows that cannot be broken, a side door on the ward is left open to allow the free passage of patients and staff to the hospital grounds. While this is an experimental ward that espouses a humanistic approach to mental illness, still it has the formal organization of a hospital ward: one is either bedridden or confined to the halls. Activities are lacking. At the far end of the hall is a security room padded for the protection of the patient; the smell of urine is always present here. The room is lined with thick blue padding and patients who defy rules, act unruly, or become tiresome are placed here for a few hours, sometimes overnight.

The stated form of therapy here is family therapy. However, some patients do not have families who are either intact or available for therapy. "Milieu therapy" frequently replaces actual family therapy. The expressed goal of the therapy is for the patient to improve as a result of being in a supportive environment. Social interactions are intended to aid the patient in coping with his or her distress. Empathy is used as a therapeutic tool to indicate appropriate emotional expression and behavior. In this way the ward is family-like and naturalistic. "Reparenting" and regression are suggested as therapeutic devices when the patient's expression and interpretation of emotions are in contradiction with healthy behavior. In this setting expressivity is not only condoned, it is the focus of the therapeutic relationship. Senior members of the staff maintain that a certain amount of active expressivity, while it might be deemed "crazy" in the outside world, is necessary for effective therapy. Conformity to specific emotional rules is not required. Rules are flexible, and strange patient behavior is tolerated, if the action of the patient can be explained. For example:

> During an outing for the patients on a grassy field outside the main hospital building, Jeffery, a 15-year-old adolescent, begins to turn cartwheels, hoping to receive praise from an intern. Another staff member shouts at him to stop, as he might hurt himself and the liability costs would then fall on the ward. He stops, but utters an angry retort that includes swearing at the staff member, and he stomps off in a direction away from us. He is called in and upon questioning, responds that he is angry and is going to run away from the facility. He then changes his mind and heads off toward the ward.

This interchange is not considered disruptive by the staff; they explain that Jeffery's anger shows his desire to assume his responsibility for himself and is thus a natural, nonpathological response. If he had complied with the request to stop without anger, they would have interpreted this as proving overcompliance and a lack of ego development. In contrast on Ward B, a similar threat would have been interpreted as disruptive, and the boy would have been restrained. The staff member who reprimanded Jeffery works on both Ward B and Ward C. When asked about the differences between the two wards he answered:

> The patients in Ward B are not necessarily sicker. Many people in Ward C are actually sicker, with more elaborate delusions, but since they are not locked up, they don't have to act out. And if they feel as angry as Jeffery did they can express it as long as no one gets hurt.

American Residential Treatment Facility: Ward D

In the final setting, a residential treatment facility (RTF), the medical model is vehemently rejected. This facility developed out of a concern for the abuses of the medical model and institutionalization. Founders of the residential treatment facility tried, in as many ways as possible, to eradicate any semblance of a hospital setting. In contrast to the medical model, schizophrenia here is viewed as a positive, creative growth experience (cf. Laing 1967). Given this view, the resulting treatment ideology suggests free expression of illness and nonintervention by staff, as opposed to the more restrictive environment of the hospital.

The residential treatment facility as a workplace diverges greatly from the bureaucratic hierarchy of the American hospital settings. While there is a psychiatrist on staff, his sole duty is to fill weekly prescriptions. The staff supervisor is a "lay psychologist" with many years of experience in this type of setting. His main duties are to coordinate the activities of other staff

members and to conduct meetings where their grievances can be aired. The
remainder of the staff are paid and unpaid workers who spend time talking
with clients and supervising them in daily activities. Many of these staff
members have once been labeled mental patients or have close relatives who
have been in the mental health system as patients.

> Ward D is in a large house located in the poorer part of a suburban
> town, amid single-family dwellings and near small, rundown depart-
> ment stores. The inside of the center looks rundown and shabby, not at
> all clinical. The facility had not been run down by the residents but was
> purchased that way. Furniture and other goods came from donations.
> The building can accommodate approximately twenty-four residents; a
> staff supervisor and three or four regular staff members are present at
> any given time. Clients and staff seem to move about randomly. The
> residents are referred to as "clients" in an effort to reduce the stigma
> attached to the label of "patient."

At intake, clients are required to make a contract with a staff member
to fulfill certain obligations, including taking care of their personal hygiene,
cooking for themselves, and attending a certain number of structured activities per week. Those activities might be participation is men's or women's
groups, yoga, candle making, group therapy, dance or movement classes,
depending on the time and interests of the staff members. Still, many clients
prefer to lounge on the couches or wander aimlessly in the house.

Communication between staff and clients is mediated by some form of
work project or subject matter. Patient-staff relations, however, are disorganized, in part because neither the physical structure nor the appearance
of the staff aids in distinguishing them. For instance, in other settings staff
members have a specific place to work, an office or a desk. Here staff member intermingle freely in the household. Often the only way staff can be distinguished from clients is by the change in client behavior when a staff
member appears.

Staff members have the authority to reprimand clients if they do not
fulfill their contracts. Yet, besides specific duties spelled out in the contracts, rules for behavior and expressivity are unclear. This lack of clarity
regarding rules is justified by the treatment ideology. Rules regarding
appropriate emotional expression and behavior are not specified in everyday life in the real world; therefore, it is considered therapeutic to leave
many rules undefined.

Rules that are not set down in the contract are termed "boundaries."
A client only knows that boundaries exist when they are crossed. In fact,
neither staff nor patients are clear about what constitutes boundaries. A
senior staff member explained to me that he "is not going to define rules or
boundaries for the new staff." This is something that he wants them to

experience. Residents are also expected to sense what comprises the boundaries of appropriate emotional expression and behavior. Carol is a typical client trying to define boundaries: she has come from a medicated hospital ward, and she is sensitive to the change of context. She is always asking for or getting confirmations for her actions.

> Carol: Can I open a window? If people smoke under the fire detector the alarm will go off. Why don't they put signs on things? We need a sign over the stairs saying caution so that people don't bang their heads.
> Counselor: Well, this is not a hospital, we don't put signs on things.
> Carol: Well, I don't know what I am supposed to do and people say they don't like what I do.
> Counselor: Well, Carol, we don't like the way you are acting. You're playing games, your roles are inappropriate. Cut it out, you sound angry all the time.
> Carol: Well, you'd be angry too, if you didn't know.

Carol is frustrated by the general disorder in the facility and the lack of clearly stated rules. While she is seeking attention from staff, she finds that attention is only given when she gets angry. In this way neither her frustration at the rules nor her need for attention is sufficiently dealt with. If a client is able to deal with the ambiguity of boundaries, he or she is considered to be approximating conduct in the "real world." While the stated goal of the facility is to approximate the real world, this emphasis on vague boundaries makes interaction considerably more disorganized than it would be in real life. In this way, the subculture of the halfway house diverges from the larger culture. Because this setting is so amorphous, emotional expression and behavior are not limited to a specific range by the rule structure. The general ambiance on Ward D is chaotic. At times, the atmosphere is characterized by apathy and isolation. Clients are often enclosed in their emotional bubbles, focusing inward rather than interacting. A typical scene of isolation is as follows:

> Staff members and clients wander aimlessly in the house, going up and down the stairs. The clients are not supposed to remain in their rooms and therefore congregate in the downstair's den. Several clients are lying on couches; one is on the floor. Sally, a new arrival, is hiding in the corner in panic. As is often the case, clients aren't speaking to one another; most stare off into space, while others play nervously with a personal object such as a crucifix.

When emotions are expressed, patients often are neglected by staff. At other times, the house residents fuel each others' emotional outbursts, and the climate is disruptive. Understandably, such emotional outbursts tend to occur when the residents are compelled to interact:

Setting	Ward A	Ward B	Ward C	Ward D
Ambiance	Compliant	Rebellious	Familial	Chaotic
Staff-patient Relations	Deferential Interaction	Conflictual Interaction	Empathetic Interaction	Disorganized Interaction
Patient Behavior	No Questions About Protocol	Constant Protest About Rules	Mild Protest/ Negotiation About Rules	Protest Lack of Rules
Cultural Congruence	Congruent	Divergent	Congruent	Divergent
Degree of Rule Rigidification	+ + Very Rigid	+ Rigid	+/− Flexible	− Amorphous
Degree of Rule Visibility	Deeply Hidden	Mildly Hidden	Visible	Obscured

Figure 4. Summary of the Treatment Settings

The atmosphere of the house changes dramatically Wednesday nights. This time is set aside for the house meeting, where grievances are aired, clients' behavior is openly discussed, and boundaries are negotiated. Clients become animated as they are accused by and counter-accuse their fellow residents. "John took my radio, I saw him with it." "I was given that radio." "Why can't I have a cat in the house; you said we could have personal things," shouts another. "I hate cats." The pitch intensifies and even the most withdrawn client may join the confusion with a comment.

Discussion

The proposed schema (see Figure 4) allows us to understand how each ward described has a characteristic ambiance that results from the rule structure governing patient-staff interaction on the ward. The ambiance of the French medicated ward (A) is one of compliance. That of the American medicated ward (B) can best be characterized as rebellious. The American nonmedicated hospital (Ward C), on the other hand, is family-like; the non-medicated residential facility (Ward D), as we have just shown, is chaotic.

The ambiance of each ward, in turn, is the direct result of the emotional expressivity allowed by the rules. The rules in Ward A, for example, require deference to authority. In France, rules of deference on ward are overdetermined. First, the treatment ideology is to diagnose the patient in the initial interview and watch for the progression of the illness. Both psychiatrist and patient are well acquainted with this model of care, which parallels a patient's visit to a medical doctor for a physical illness. Second, the norms of deference and civility in the treatment setting converge with the norms of the larger culture. Finally, work roles are structured so that members of the nursing staff, who have frequent contact with the patient, are not allowed to intervene with patients. Rather their role is to uphold the order of deference paid the psychiatrists. Thus, compliant deferential behavior is generated by the general social order of the ward.

In terms of the dimensions of rigidity and visibility, the French rule structure can be classified as very rigid because the rules are a fixed, *a priori* assumption of the members of this society. Because the subcultural norms and those of the dominant culture converge, there is no need to make the rules explicit. Therefore, the French rule structure is classified as deeply hidden.

The rules of Ward B require constant negative sanctioning when staff functions are disrupted, when restricted areas are entered, and when there is any communication that involves swearing, confrontation, or resistance to staff demands. The rules of patient-staff interaction in Ward B, the American medicated ward, are also overdetermined. The treatment ideology requires containment of psychotic outbreaks or disruptive behavior by using medication and restraint; disruptive behavior and protest against sanctions are common, as the repressive norms of the treatment setting are in conflict with those of the larger culture. In addition, those charged with the burden of patient control are underpaid workers who find that medicating patients lightens their workload. The rules of this ward are classified as rigid, because they are nonnegotiable. Staff is given the power to repress patients, and that power is absolute. In contrast to the French setting, however, the rules in Ward B are classified as mildly hidden. This is because the rules become apparent once there is protest and resultant sanctioning.

The rules of Ward C require positive sanctioning of patient expression; such expression is seen as an indication that patients are working on their problems. In this ward, as in those described above, the treatment ideology, degree of cultural convergence, and the patient-staff power relations foster this structure. The treatment ideology is to allow patients to go through a psychotic break in a safe setting. It is believed that people get better by themselves; that expression, even if it would be considered crazy in the outside world, promotes healing. The subculture of the treatment facility is a family like atmosphere; patients readily adapt to this setting, as it is congruent with expectations of shared emotions in family life that are normative in the outside world. Patient-staff power relations also promote expressivity. Staff plays the role of parent and the patient plays that of the child. Thus, even regressive expression is condoned, if not encouraged, by the specific power relations on this ward. The rule structure of this setting is classified as flexible because rules are negotiable; also, because rules are discussed openly, they are classified as visible.

In Ward D, the residential treatment facility, rules are unclear because the treatment ideology maintains that unclear rules or boundaries approximate a real-life setting. The subculture of the ward is less structured than that of the outside world. The role of the staff members vis-à-vis the clients is also undefined; staff members often are untrained and tend to blend in with the patient population. They exert little authority over clients and are as unclear about rules and boundaries as the clients. The degree of rigidity here is classified as amorphous, for rules are so unclear that sanctioning sometimes seems arbitrary. The degree of visibility is classified as obscured because both patient and staff are unclear about the boundaries.

As Figure 4 shows, these rule structures are associated with characteristic patient behaviors. Patients on Ward A tend to be compliant, and their interactions with staff are deferential. Patients on Ward B tend to be rebellious, and their interactions with staff are conflictual. Patients on Ward C are expressive, and their interactions with staff are empathic. Patients on Ward D are apathetic, and their interactions with staff are disorganized.

A limitation of this study is that it is impossible to find populations that are exactly comparable in each of these different wards. Because of this limitation, some might argue that the variation in ward ambiance is due to the differences in the populations served rather than due to the variation in rule structures. The populations differ: the French ward contains a mixture of chronic psychotic, neurotic and senile cases, while the American medicated facility is largely populated by chronic schizophrenics in an acute state and readmissions. On the other hand, Ward C mostly serves patients who are experiencing a first or second psychotic break; Ward D offers its services to a mostly chronic population.

I maintain that it is the difference in rule structure, not the type of population, that accounts for the varying ward ambiance. For example, the French medicated hospital ward contains many patients who are just as sick as those in Ward B, yet the ambiance of the wards could not differ more. Moreover, the American nonmedicated ward usually filters in patients who are actively psychotic and often regressive, and yet their expressivity is fostered. In addition, at least in the American settings, patients are often transferred from one type of ward to another within a hospital or from a hospital to a halfway house. Thus, while people with given personalities and diagnoses are traveling from one setting to another, the ambiance of the wards does not tend to fluctuate with the appearance of new patients. Patients eventually adjust to their settings and begin to display the levels of expressivity and types of behavior—protest or lack of it—

engendered by the setting. The fact that patients have difficulty in making the transition from one setting to another testifies to the fact that the rules exert much force on the patient population.

Conclusions

By considering the schema presented in Figure 4, we begin to see the merits and drawbacks of each setting. Whereas the medicated hospital settings might be considered overstructured, with rules that are not subject to negotiation, the treatment facility is understructured and ambiguous with its notion of boundaries.

Finally, the schema makes it apparent that the norms of the institutional subculture and those of the larger culture need to be matched, to some extent, to minimize outbursts, protest, and disruptive behavior. In wards A and C, where there was a degree of cultural convergence, violence and confused behavior generally was not seen, though it was on wards B and D. After considering over- and understructured contexts, we might ask: What is a useful rule structure within an institutional setting? The answer may be a rule structure like that of Ward C. While the regulations of a hospital ward are clearly apparent, the rule structure emanates from human concerns, not institutional ones. The treatment ideology requires that patients be rewarded for their ability to enunciate their wishes. A pro mium is placed on expression. The use of empathic understanding here adds a personal dimension and flexibility to rules. This setting prepares patients to adapt and conform to life outside the hospital better than does the others.

Notes

1. A version of this paper was presented at the symposium on "The Ethnography of Psychiatric Institutions," at the American Anthropological Meetings, Chicago, IL, November 22, 1987.

References

Bloor, M. and J. Fonkert
1982 Reality Construction, Reality Exploration and Treatment in Two therapeutic Communities. Sociology of Health and Illness: A Journal of Medical Sociology 4(2).

Collett, P., ed.
1977 The Rules of Conduct: Social Rules and Social Behavior. Oxford: Basil Blackwell.

Estroff, Sue
1981 Making It Crazy: An Ethnography of Psychiatric Clients in An American Community. Berkeley: University of California Press.

French Government Department of Public Assistance.
1974 Étude Sur la Psychiatrie en Région Ile de France. INSERM. French Government Department of Public Assistance.

Goffman, E.
1961 Asylums: Essays on the Social Situation of Mental Patients and Other Inmates. New York: Doubleday.

Gurle, L.
1974 Dimensions of the Therapeutic Milieu: A Study of Mental Hospital Atmosphere. The American Journal of Psychiatry 131:409–414.

Hawkins, D.
1969 Treatment of Schizophrenia Based on the Medical Model. Journal of Schizophrenia 2:3–10.

Heller, K.
1968 Ambiguity in the Interview Interaction. In Research in Psychotherapy, Vol. 3. J. Schlien (ed.). Washington, D.C.: American Psychological Association, Inc.

Hochschild, A.
1979 Emotion Work, Feeling Rules and Social Structure. American Journal of Sociology 85(3):551–575.

Laing, R.
1967 The Politics of Experience. Middlesex: Penguin Books.

Lebovicic, S.
1978 L'Organisation des Soins Psychiatriques en France. La Révue du Praticien 28 (May 21):229–235.

Leifer, R.
1970 The Medical Model as Ideology. International Journal of Psychiatry 9:13–21.

Osmond, H., and M. Seigler
1974 Models of Madness, Models of Medicine. New York: Harper and Row.

Perruci, R.
1974 The Circle of Madness. New Jersey: Prentice-Hall.

Ruesch, J., and G. Bateson
1968 Communication: The Social Matrix of Psychiatry. New York: Norton and Co.

Strauss, A., M. Sabshin, R. Bucher and D. Ehlich
1964 Psychiatric Ideologies and Institutions. New York: Free Press of Glencoe.

Sullivan, H. S.
1970 The Psychiatric Interview. New York: Norton and Co.

Thibaut, J., and J. Coules
1951 The Role of Communication in the Reduction of Inter-personal Hostility. Journal of Abnormal and Social Psychology XLVII:770–777.

Wittman, F.
1980 Task Force Report: Sociophysical Settings and Mental Health: Opportunities of Mental Health Service Planning. Community Mental Health Journal 16:46.

13

The Rise of Greek Professional Ethnopsychiatry

Amy V. Blue

Introduction

For the initiated and uninitiated tourist (and anthropologist), Greece conjures up images of ancient ruins, villages colored in whites and blue, sunlit seas and beaches, and ebullient Greeks whiling away hours at *tavernas* and *kafenions* (cafés). However, hidden behind this festive, "no problem" atmosphere is a harsh reality of mental asylums inhabited by abandoned individuals. Just as the modern Greek nation, a unique blend of East and West, has struggled for an identity during her turbulent history, so has her professional psychiatry.

My informants were often eager to emphasize that there is no "Greek psychiatry," but rather a "soup" composed of German, French, British, and American traditions. This is certainly true, as one psychiatric faction draws its philosophy and practice heavily from one of these others, i.e., one center is American in its orientation; another sees itself as the "French (psychoanalytic) school"; one institution is primarily Anglo-Saxon (British) in its organization and activities, etc. In this chapter, I shall demonstrate the links of Greek professional psychiatry (a biomedicine) to its cultural, socioeconomic, and political contexts[1] through a brief historical examination.[2] Some key facets of modern Greece's history[3] such as the importation of foreign institutions, foreign interventions, and periodic repression, are elements which have directly and indirectly influenced the development of the country's professional psychiatry. Tsoucalas has written, "Domestic social and political forces have never been able to develop or function autonomously" (1969:15). In my presentation, I will emphasize legislative and institutional developments.

History and Politics

Greece's Declaration of Independence from the Ottoman Empire in 1821[4] eventually resulted in a political stalemate. Her plight began to draw international attention and Russia, France, and Great Britain intervened, destroying the Turkish-Egyptian fleet at Navarino in 1827. Though now an independent nation, due to foreign intervention, Greece was at the mercy of these protecting powers to determine the size and sovereignty of her statehood.[5] The powers chose for her to be a kingdom, placing the young Otto of Bavaria on the throne in 1832.[6]

Small in territory (it excluded Epirus, Thessaly, and all islands except those immediately adjacent to Greece), the country was devastated after the nearly ten years of war for independence. Of the three million Greeks, only about seven hundred thousand were residing within the state. Athens, named the capital in 1836, was a small village with about five thousand inhabitants at the time. In fact, no city of significance existed within Greece's boundaries; religious, cultural and economic centers were all abroad. Constantinople was the center of the Greek world, housing Greek schools, publishing houses, a university of high prestige and a Greek population of over 200,000. Greek society was based upon an archaic, semi-feudal structure, with 95 percent of the inhabitants peasants (Tsoucalas 1969). Industrial development was extremely limited, handicapped by the primitive communication system (Sherrard and Campbell 1969).[7]

The merchant navy rapidly expanded (tripling after 1838), and commerce began to grow, thereby creating a small bourgeoisie. The reign of King Otto came to be characterized by a total disregard of the real needs and aspirations of the Greek people. The revolution of 1844 resulted in the first Greek constitution, based on the French model (Mouzelis 1978) and which slightly alleviated the difficult local situation (Tsoucalas 1969). Near the end of her first thirty years of independence, Greece had been subjected to foreign intervention and had initiated a course of borrowing ideas and institutions from European nations' Western institutions (e.g., her education system was based on French and German models [Clogg 1986]).

Within the Greek nation itself, no specialized institutions accepted mentally disturbed individuals for residential or outpatient treatment at this time. All such institutions were in Constantinople, which had the main mental asylum of the Ottoman Empire and three Greek hospitals.[8] Mentally ill persons were accepted by these hospitals. Interest for a disturbed person occurred only when he or she had committed some form of disturbance. Families commonly resorted to binding the agitated person in the basement for short or extended periods of time. When wandering around villages, the disturbed person was met with a range of behavior, from respect[9] to being the object of jokes or stone throwing (Ploubidis 1981).

Informal ecclesiastical interventions, such as prayers and exorcisms, occurred sporadically, and some monasteries gained renown for the treatment of mentally disturbed individuals.[10] The monasteries of Meteora and Athos certainly accepted mentally disturbed individuals, but information regarding their practices is not available (Ploubidis 1981). The patron saint of Cephalonia, St. Gerasimos, is known as the protector of the possessed and mentally disturbed. Thus, pilgrimages to the island were (and continue to be) a treatment avenue (Hartocollis 1958).

Common elements of the religiously based therapeutic regimen were: strict fasting and prayer by the disturbed person and his or her family; binding the person inside or outside of the church to control the agitation (in old churches, the rings for this purpose can be seen); beating the devil believed to reside within the person but which simultaneously acted as a tranquilizer; and the internment of the sufferer at the monastery (Ploubidis 1981). Customary care of the mentally ill person who was bothersome or wandering around in the city was to place him or her in police station basements (Ploubidis 1981).

Not until about 1860–1861 did the issue of care for the mentally disturbed in the nation appear in the government.[11] The lack of specialized institutions obliged the government to pay a total of 320 drachmas a month to different monasteries for the maintenance of twenty-one mentally ill individuals at this time: these monasteries played an elementary and relatively insignificant asylum role. Extensive plans for the construction of a mental institution for Greece were devised by A. Georganta and announced in a small medical journal of the period, *Asklipious*. The design was based upon European hospital models, primarily Italian and French examples, that he had visited. The requested expense surpassed the amount the government was willing to provide, however, and the dream of the institution was never realized (Ploubidis 1981).

Another solution for a mental institution was the utilization of an abandoned orphanage of Aiginas, proposed by royal order in 1860. From the nation's total of 422 mentally disturbed men and women, it was considered that 153 were "uneasy," that is, "violent, rowdy and dangerous." Of these, the institution was to accept, in its first phase, sixty persons, thus the basic admission criteria for a mentally disturbed person was some form of socially bothersome or dangerous behavior. Legislation, intended to oversee the functioning of this proposed hospital in Aigina, was subsequently presented to Parliament in October 1861. Shortly thereafter, in 1862, the unpopular King Otto was dethroned. Subsequent governments rejected the plans for the establishment of the institution. Whether or not it was purely for economic reasons that the effort was abandoned remains a question (Ploubidis 1981).

The proposed legislation did survive, passed by the government in 1862. Reconcilable with existing Greek legislation and constitution, the French Law 1838 regarding the mentally ill was adopted. This act was Greek psychiatry's first importation of a foreign institution. The law placed the mental institution (the proposed facility of Aiginas) under state supervision: 1) to insure families the security, personal freedom and care (treat-ment) of their unfortunate members, and 2) because the institution would be maintained through public expenditures[12] (Ploubidis 1981).

The state undertook the obligation to cover the deficit from a person's care, and hospitalization of the poor was paid through public funds. The minister of the time recognized the inability of a large number of citizens to pay for care, but hoped private individuals and the public would prosper again. In reality, after 1864, the government paid the greatest portion of expenses for poor mentally disturbed individuals.

The title of "patient" for the mentally ill person, and hospitalization and treatment as the purpose of the confining institution, was legally safe-guarded by the legislation. Emphasis was placed upon the legal substantia-tion of the admission and freedom of the patients from the moment the doc-tor certified their cure or improvement or their family demanded them. Despite this, the legislation appeared similar to that of developed European countries. A discrepancy existed in that the legislation appeared before its actual object, that is, the institution for the mentally ill: legislation usually regulates established practices.

Corfu

Upon Otto's departure, the three protecting powers once again searched for an appropriate head of state for the Greek nation, finally selecting as the new King, Prince George Glucksberg of Denmark. This change in monarchy marked a definite shift of Greek policy from the Russ-ian to the British orbit, and as a gesture of friendship, the British-occupied Ionian islands, possessing a mental institution, were handed to Greece in 1864 (Tsoucalas 1969). This hospital, Greece's first mental hospital, was inherited from a foreign power. It was not organized by the Greek state itself.

The hospital of Corfu was founded in 1838 by the British Governor, Sir Edward Douglas. Established in abandoned army barracks, it had eight patients at its inauguration and thirty-eight by the end of the year. Accord-ing to its charter, the institution was intended exclusively for mental patients and had a therapeutic purpose, based upon physical, pharmaceuti-cal, and moral therapies. The mentally disturbed person was recognized as being ill. The text of 1838 stated that "idiots" would not be accepted unless they provoked bothersome or dangerous behavior, an indication that the institution was intended originally to accept the most difficult cases of men-tal illness (Ploubidis 1981). Other basic concepts of nineteenth-century psy-chiatry were introduced: work as therapeutic; the concomitant belief that the hospital's location should provide patients with a rural setting, and; the institution should be shielded from the outside world (Bairaktaris 1984).

When it was inherited by the Greek state, the hospital was officially declared to be in extremely poor condition and was insufficiently staffed to care for patients. Renovations were initiated by the government. The internal charter of the institution was published in the Government Paper in 1866, in which the text of the charter voted in 1860 by the Senate of the Ionian States remained intact. This charter had been greatly influenced by European legislation and therefore was reconcilable with the existing Greek legislation of 1862 (Ploubidis 1981).

Patients and Staff at Corfu

No public authority, apart from the Senate of the Ionian Islands, was permitted to decide the admission of a person, unless that person was declared an emergency case. In such instances, the police requested the admission, which subsequently required confirmation by the Senate. Otherwise, a written application by the family regarding the case of mental illness, the financial situation and a medical certificate was sent to the Senate. The head-director of the philanthropic facilities of Corfu, or the doctor-director of the institution, accepted the patient and decided if admission was necessary. For the other islands, the decision was taken by the leader of each island (Ploubidis 1981).

The supervisor (a basic person of European psychiatric hospitals of the nineteenth century) had great power over the other personnel. He was responsible for the benevolent treatment toward those admitted and the execution of the doctor's decisions. Violent behavior against patients was strictly forbidden, and punishment by dismissal was possible. Each guard was to be in charge of less than ten to twelve patients, as well as to maintain order and peace during meals and to separate the sexes. Some of these guards were to possess knowledge of another profession in order to instruct the patients. A position of an underdirector was foreseen, who would have the same duties as the guards and would teach the female patients to be suitable in their gender and social position. One guard was obligated to do night duty and each guard, in turn, had the right to spend a night out of the institution (Ploubidis 1981).

Personnel consisted of the following: 1) the leader of philanthropic facilities of Corfu (a high office established in 1850); 2) the doctor (doctor-surgeon) who directed the institution; 3) the supervisor (head nurse), under orders of the preceding two; 4) a priest; 5) a guard-farmer to direct the agricultural works; 6) a cook.

The institution's doctor not only had responsibility for the treatment regimen of patients but also for the administration of the institution. In addition to monthly accounts and annual statistics, the following books were to be maintained by him: 1) monthly bills; 2) correspondence; 3) observations of the patients and the employees; 4) histories of the patients and their illness; 5) expenses; 6) admissions and releases of patients.

The therapeutic regimen of patients was described as "pharmaceutical and moral." The pharmaceutical regimen was established by the doctor during daily visits. The patient's time working in fields, in workshops, and in water therapy assisted the moral therapy (its dictates not clarified in the charter's text). The patients were to be kept reasonable without chains and whips, an earlier practice, but with kind manners. The good behavior of the personnel was to contribute to the calmness of the patients. However, if these methods were not sufficient, sudden showers or, in emergencies, hand binding, was used (Ploubidis 1981).

Morning wake-up and nightly rest differed according to the category in which the patient opened. The patients were placed into six categories and their clothing and food was described in detail. For example, the needy and poor had to wear the same clothing and were accepted free of charge, with a certificate of welfare by the police. The well-to-do had separate rooms and the right to have a servant, with the approval of the institution's director. The discharge of a patient was decided by the director of the philanthropic facilities of Corfu or by the institution's discharge of one of its members.

The first director of the hospital of Corfu was an English military doctor, followed by a Maltese and, from 1842 on, only Greek doctors.[13] From 1874 until 1887, X. Tsirigotis was director of the institution. Considered the father of Greek psychiatry, Tsirigotis published four booklets on his experiences and on scientific thoughts. From Corfu, he was educated at the University of Pisa in Italy (Simatis and Moros, n.d.). Upon arrival at the institution, he recognized its reality was not as that described in its charter. He believed it served primarily the criminally insane and did not employ any scientific principles (Bairaktaris 1984). The absence of showers and hydrotherapy for patients, the mixing of patients "higgledy-piggledy," and the hospital's inability to organize occupational activities for patients because of the arrangement and condition of the building were his chief complaints.

He therefore initiated a campaign to improve the institution's conditions according to other European countries, traveling to Italy to visit asylums there. His consideration of the appropriate physical arrangement of the hospital as a therapeutic measure reflects one of the basic ideas of European psychiatry of the nineteenth century. For example, the building should have an entrance and a first floor with bars on the windows; for the manics and dangerous, cells were envisioned with walls covered with cotton quilts of dark colors. Another of his convictions was that the hospital should be closed and have extensive lands at its disposal for patients to work (Ploubidis 1981).

Tsirigotis considered the institution's cure rate of 12–13 percent low and attributed it to the faulty building, the poor habits of care, and the family's delay to admit a mentally disturbed member. A rise in admissions was noted by 1878, and he believed an improvement in the institution was responsible, as well as a lessening of superstitions and the custom of maintaining mentally ill persons in monasteries. Those generally hospitalized were workers and artisans or well-to-do dangerous. Persons exhibiting simple *monomania* or *monomania accompanied with homicidal or suicidal tendencies*, and those presenting sensible paranoia of Briere de Boismont, were to be isolated at the hospital. General paralysis did not necessitate immediate admission. The small number of old people, mentally retarded and alcoholics is associated with the characteristics of the Greek society of the period. For the classification of patients, Tsirigotis relied upon the system of the Italian professor A. Varga, presented in 1876 (in Ploubidis 1981).

In the statistics of 1878, Tsirigotis notes that pharmaceutical measures were utilized sparingly because he had not observed their action in treatment of the mentally ill. Preferred therapy was moral treatment based on the fatherly relation to be created between the doctor and the patient. Within this relationship, the mental and emotional abilities of the patient were to be manipulated. The doctor was to serve as the complete master of the institution, establishing family visits, patient strolls, care of patients' bodies, use of hydrotherapy, medications, and restraint. The personality and philosophy of the doctor and, to a degree, of the other personnel, played a fundamental role in the application of this moral treatment. At its worst, it could become a system of military discipline (Ploubidis 1981) (see Hershel, this volume on local authority of physicians in France—ed.).

From 1869 until 1877, 1,292 patients were hospitalized at the institution of Corfu, an average of 143 per year; the number of chronic cases did not surpass one hundred in 1878. In 1877 and 1878, admissions from the Ionian Islands and Corfu were 32 percent and 36 percent, respectively, of the total. The local character of the only psychiatric hospital in all of the country is clear: for the same years Athens and Pireaus gave only 17 percent and 5 percent, respectively, of admissions.

The hospital of Corfu, despite its insufficiencies, was representative of European psychiatry of the nineteenth century. It was not an asylum but a hospital: an institution with therapeutic purposes. Basic concepts of the period were introduced: the recognition of mental illness as a disease and the capability of the disturbed person to form an interpersonal relationship; the use of moral treatment and work, particularly field labor, as a positive therapeutic influence; the importance of the institution to be properly physically arranged and organized for effective treatment; and preference for a rural or secluded location. The inclination for importing ideas from Western Europe, occurring from independence, appears in this early era of Greek psychiatry: the Law of 1862, based upon the French Law of 1838, hospital plans modeled upon those of other European countries, nosological classification systems, and of course the establishment of a mental hospital.

The period after 1864, when the first democratic constitution was promulgated, until the end of the nineteenth century, was characterized by the first major effort to modernize economic and administrative structures. Far from being an industrialized country, a small bourgeoisie gradually appeared and the greatest change in the social structure was the expansion of the urban population during this time (Tsoukalas 1969).[14]

An oppressive problem of the mentally ill had not been manifest, due primarily to the still relatively small, homogeneous urban population and the traditional customs and understandings of mental illness. The hospital of Corfu was to offer the nation's psychiatric care for nearly twenty years until the initiative of a donor created another mental institution[15] (Ploubidis 1981).

Dromokaition

Tz. Dromokaiti, followed by later donors, provided a gift responsible for the construction of *Dromokaition*, a mental hospital located outside of Athens. For at least twenty years, Dromokaition was to act as a role model for the country's psychiatric care. Thirty-two thousand square meters of land were granted by the government, and building began in 1883, based on the plan of the French psychiatrist Lunier. With Tsirigotis appointed director, the hospital had eighty-five patients the day of its grand opening in 1887 (Ploubidis 1981).

A new series of laws regarding mental hospitals, referring specifically to Dromokaition, appeared in 1887. These permitted its functioning under the control of the Ministry of the Interior, with the Law of 1862 as a basis. The internal statutes of the institution were published in the government newspaper later in 1887 in the form of ministerial acts. In general, the administrative committee and its president had extensive powers (Ploubidis 1981).[16]

The doctor-director was to live within the institution. To acquire the position, a doctorate degree and proof of experience with mental disease or as a doctor of a mental hospital for two years was necessary. All nurses were allowed to leave the institution for twenty-four hours once a week. The head nurse was to follow the doctor during visits and note in a small book the treatment he dictated (for example, immersion, cupping by glass, baths). She was responsible for the equipment, the maintenance of cleanliness and order, and the execution of night services, and she was to supervise all the nurses in the performance of their duties. The abuse of patients was strictly forbidden and punishable by dismissal.[17] The nurses did not have the right to smoke or accept gifts, and those who had knowledge were obligated to shave the patients and lower personnel twice a week. The residency of the nurses inside the institution and the lack of any kind of preliminary training (in other cases they were simply called guards) is common with other European mental hospitals of the nineteenth century and the hospital on Corfu (Ploubidis 1981).

Patients were differentiated into three classes: I, paying 700 drachmas bimonthly; II, 400 drachmas; and III, 120 drachmas. The charter foresaw free care, in class III, for five indigent patients. One article gave authorities the right to send a certain number of mentally disturbed for a fifteen-day observation period. In reality, the authorities were obligated to maintain in the institution a significant number of poor mentally disturbed, and the right of admission for observation was rarely used. Work therapy was established quickly, with the organization of workshops, vegetable cultivation, and elementary stock breeding in the yard.

The statistics of Dromokaition from 1887 to 1901 present the diagnosis of *frenopathia of degeneration* as the most frequent, 49.3 percent of the total (in contrast to those of Corfu during the years 1877 and 1878). Concentrated under the same diagnosis were pathological conditions which, at the present time, have nothing in common. From a total of 587 "degenerates," there existed only ten "idiots" or "fools." The others belonged to the category of mental (*pnevmatika*) patients or of superior (*anoteroron*) degeneration, that is, persons with multiple delusions or systematic degenerative delusions, rarely with forms of idealism, delusional ambitions, mysticism, persecution, or childhood anomalies.[18] The small number of idiots or fools constitutes evidence for the maintenance of mentally retarded persons of the period by their families. Also, from the statistics of Dromokaition disappeared the diagnosis of monomania and lipomania (of Esquirol), which had received intense debate in Europe (Ploubidis 1981).

The diagnosis of *"simple (primitive, protogonou) dementia"* was second in frequency, with 19.9 percent of the total. This diagnostic category of simple (primitive) dementia was introduced in Greece in 1905 by G. Zillanakis, subdirector of Dromokaition until 1907, and Dr. Oikonomaki.

From a total of 185 admissions in 1903, two-thirds were well-to-do persons, while one-third were poor, maintained by public authorities. All social classes and all provinces, including those of the Ottoman Empire, were represented among those hospitalized. Of the 1,060 admitted between 1887 and 1902, 229 were left treated, 125 improved, and 476 remained stable. The low number of cures was attributed by M. Gianniris, director at the time, to the large amount of general paralysis among the admissions and the family's reluctance to send a patient for treatment (Ploubidis 1981).

Other Institutions

Small institutions, of an asylum character, were founded in the provinces about this time. In Keffalonia, an asylum established by the British authorities about 1840 in old barracks was renovated in 1918, through a donor, Vegio. The institution's name changed to reflect the benefactor and it continued to maintain a local character. In national statistics of 1938, its recognized capacity was one hundred beds. The earthquake of 1953 destroyed it and the few remaining patients housed in tents were transferred in 1958 to Leros (Ploubidis 1981).

On the island of Xios, which had possessed a hospital until an earthquake in 1881 finally destroyed its remains, the family of Skilitsi donated funds for the construction of a new facility, which opened in 1886. The various departments of the hospital were housed in separate buildings, one being a mental asylum. In 1899, seven male and eight female mentally disturbed patients were admitted, while the hospital had sixty-six men and seven women. In 1938, the asylum had a capacity of sixty beds and was classified as a community institution. Its functioning discontinued with the foundation of Leros in 1958.

The Asylum of Mental Sufferers of the Cyclades was founded in 1908 with the initiative of Philanthropic Committee of Ermopolis. In national statistics of 1938, it was considered a philanthropic institution with sixty beds. In 1948, fifteen patients were overseen by an elderly man who played the role of director, nurse and steward. A doctor visited occasionally. With the foundation of Leros, the asylum was abolished.

An asylum for the mentally ill of the Jewish community in Thessaloniki was founded, as a ward of the Hospital Hirs, in 1907. Statistics of 1938 refer to it as a community institution with seventy-five beds. After the disappearance of the Jewish community after World War II, the hospital of Hirs lost its original character and after 1945 functioned as a public hospital. Reference has also been made to an asylum on Mytlini that up until 1940 had a capacity of twenty beds (Ploubidis 1981).

By the beginning of the twentieth century, estimates of mentally ill persons in the nation were two thousand to three thousand, but how these figures were obtained by authors of the period is unclear. The mental hospitals of Corfu and Dromokaition had a total capacity of about four hundred, the majority of patients presenting severe mental illnesses of an incurable and chronic nature. These institutions were representative of nineteenth-century European psychiatry, and reports from visitors of the period indicate they stood fittingly well (particularly Dromokaition) next to their European counterparts. Traditional patterns of care persisted, i.e., community and family indifference unless precipitated by an outburst, religious interventions, and the internment of the mentally ill poor in police station basements.

In 1903, the journal *The Psychiatric and Neurological Review* published a questionnaire regarding mental illness in Greece. There were only four responses. A picture of the mentally ill person in the community at this time is given by Z. Lellou, from Gavalou in Mesolonghi. In the last twenty years, he had not observed more than eight mentally ill persons in a population of eight thousand. The inhabitants' behavior towards these individuals was benevolent, he thought, except for the children, who bothered them with the idea they were possessed by demons. A philanthropic basis for care had not yet developed. No monasteries existed in the region to accept them, and only two churches provided food and shelter.

Local factors believed to contribute to the development of mental illness were the abuse of alcohol and tobacco, and malaria. He considered malaria to be one of the basic causes of the great frequency of degeneration, unbalancing, and mental retardation in the area. Young women who abused alcohol and suffered from malaria presented simultaneously severe forms of hysteria. He thought that in one hundred women there were not more than ten to twenty with good health, the others suffering mainly from nervous conditions. In neighboring poor mountain villages, where the consumption of alcohol and malaria were infrequent, he believed hysteria to be less frequent and other nervous conditions to be lesser in severity.

At the time, mental patients were sent with difficulty to a mental hospital. He did not regard the hysterias and mental retardation as main mental illness, an understanding seen in hospital statistics. Of the eight individuals, only two had been hospitalized for a time in Corfu, none of them members of an upper class. One left the hospital under normal circumstances, while the other had escaped. Despite that he was thought dangerous for his family and originally police intervention had been necessary to send him to Corfu, no one thought to send him back. The primary criterion of families and authorities for admission was the dangerousness of the mentally ill person and whether the environment had been terrorized for a period of time. All the ill of the peasant class remained with their family, and medical presence was episodical. The majority, particularly peasants, spent most of their time wandering around mountains and villages, usually in an acute phase of their illness. A common folk treatment for acute periods was binding to beds and withholding of food for days (Ploubidis 1981).

Within Athens during this time, a small upper and middle class began to emerge. Numerically and economically able to obtain the services of private institutions, they were ideologically prepared to accept medical treatment of their mentally ill in specialized institutions. Hence, the private psychiatric clinics were born. The psychiatrist who opened such a facility would have not only an Athenian clientele, but, if the clinic developed a good reputation, it also could attract the well-to-do Greek families of other Greek cities and colonies (Ploubidis 1981).

Private Clinics

The first private clinic opened in 1904, in Athens, owned by S. G. Vlavianou. He had studied in Paris and his clinic followed a French model. Therapies relied upon at this clinic were various, including the medication of the period (Bernali, Kina, and Bromirini, etc.), suggestion and hypnosis, tepid showers, and music therapy. Psychotherapy is also mentioned, with no clarification of its principles. The name of Freud was not mentioned in any correspondences (Baslamatzi 1983; Tzavaras and Kirtata 1983).[19] The functioning of private clinics was not regulated explicitly by the Law of 1862, and legislation addressing them was not in existence before 1923. G. Papdimitriou considers that the number of private clinics did not surpass ten until World War II (Ploubidis 1983).

Other psychiatric events were occurring during this period, notably the establishment of the university clinic. M. Venizelos, from 1851 to 1861, and A. Vitsaris, after 1862, had taught university lectures on nervous and mental diseases. The organizer of university-based neurology and psychiatry was professor M. Katsaras. With his initiative, the legacy of A. Eiginiti was used for the construction and organization of a university clinic (Royal Order of 19.7.1904). At the inauguration in 1905, the facility had twenty-four beds, and in 1938, according to the national statistics, had 112 beds. It functioned as a center of diagnosis and therapy for neurological and psychiatric patients at the acute phase of their condition. When the French psychiatrist Libert visited in 1911, a great advantage was seen in the size of its staff, which numbered twenty-five nurses for forty-four patients. The patients were separated into three classes, and they paid for care.[20]

Few and scattered were psychiatrists at this time. In the first and second decades of the twentieth century, the total in Greece, Constantinople, Smyrna, and Alexandria could not have surpassed twenty or thirty. Each had studied at European universities but had great difficulties in establishing their professional and scientific reputation for the public. Hence, it is not by chance that the Neurological and Psychiatric Association was not founded until 1936. Here I will point out that psychiatry as a separate medical entity did not exist at this time. Doctors were trained only as neurologist-psychiatrists and were known only by this title, a practice that existed until the 1980s. By the turn of the century, the reliance upon European psychiatric institutional concepts, particularly hospital construction, was commonplace. This continuous borrowing from European psychiatries began to infiltrate in a problematic manner, i.e., in the translation of foreign words and the creation of Greek psychiatric terms and the utilization of different nosological classifications. An initial indication of the emerging "soup" character of Greek psychiatry appears in G. Zillankis's reference to statistics from the hospital of Corfu. Comparisons were impossible because the medical director there, Dr. Skarpas, "followed the German nosography" (Ploubidis 1981).

Greece's participation in the Balkan Wars, 1912–1913, resulted in an increase in territory (notably Epirus, Macedonia, including Thessaloniki, and Crete) and its population. The population exchange between her and Turkey after defeat by the Turks in 1922 proved to have a greater effect on the fabric of the Greek population. Barely able to maintain her own population, 1.5 million Greeks were transferred into the country as refugees. The urban population was greatly augmented, Athens nearly doubled in size between 1920 and 1928, with a number of shanty towns springing up around her (Clogg 1986, Tsoucalas 1969).[21]

With the formal addition of Thessaloniki and Crete in 1913 to the Greek nation, two other institutions were admitted to the psychiatric-care network. Historical information regarding the mental hospitals of Thessaloniki and Soudas, near Chania, Crete, is sketchy. The hospital of Thessaloniki was founded about the time of World War I (Bairaktaris cites 1917) and that of Soudas, 1910.

The statistics of Dromokaition indicate a small increase of admissions in 1915 in relation to the years 1906–1910 and for the first time, the number of indigent patients surpassed the number of well-off. This could be attributed to a sudden rise in the number of mentally ill from the lower classes (parallel to the population increase after the Balkan wars?), a transfer of wealthier clientele to the private clinics, or both.

Nevertheless, an increase in the mentally ill, particularly the poor, became visible. In Athens, those held in the basement of the police stations were transferred to a house in Moschato in 1914–1915 by the Ministry of the Interior. Then, in 1918–1919, about fifty to sixty patients were transferred to a villa, *Agia Eleousa*, in Kallithea, and, by 1923, three hundred persons (mentally ill, vagabonds, addicts) resided in bestial living conditions, without medical supervision (Ploubidis 1981).

Recent History

The mental hospitals passed into jurisdiction of the director of hygiene of the newly established Ministry of Welfare in 1924. At this time, the systematic organization of the hospitals of Thessaloniki and Soudas occurred. The hospital of Thessaloniki was transferred to its present site in Stavropoulis in 1925, formerly horse barracks of the French Army (Bairaktaris 1984). An administrative committee was created for the situation at Agia Eleousas. Numbering four hundred in 1926, the residents had placed tents and wooden huts in the garden, and a psychiatrist, along with four doctors of other specialties, had been appointed. By 1928, the situation was more congested and miserable, with five hundred patients inhabiting the villa. This situation prompted the arrangement and equipping of some larger wooden huts by fifty to sixty of the calmer patients and two to three nurses under the supervision of a leader-nurse. These "buildings" consisted of the first core of the Public Mental Hospital of Athens (Daphni). In 1923, the "better" patients were transferred, and in 1936, the chronic and incurables were moved (Ploubidis 1981).

The next legislation concerning the mentally ill, Law 6077, was published in 1934. One of its basic innovations was the conversion of the public mental hospitals into agricultural colonies. (This reflected two basic concepts from nineteenth-century psychiatry: the therapeutic value of working and the institution's subsequent ability to be relatively self-supporting.) At Daphni, the appointment of an agriculturalist was the fruit of this legislation (Ploubidis 1983). A second innovation of the law refers to the administrative organization of public hospitals and personnel. Administrative committees were to be composed of representatives of the ministry and judicial authorities. Doctors lost the administration of the mental hospitals when the doctor-director (a basic idea of the nineteenth-century psychiatry) was abolished. A differentiation between guards and nurses occurred. The title of nurse was based upon previous experience in service in a hospital or clinic. The need for previous experience comes from the fact that nursing degrees could not be earned in the country (Ploubidis 1981).

The law also set the maximum capacity per institution:

The Public Mental Hospital of Athens	1,500 beds
The Public Mental Hospital of Corfu	650 beds
The Public Mental Hospital of Thessaloniki	600 beds
The Public Mental Hospital of Chania	300 beds
Total	3,050 beds

National statistics of 1939, which did not account for beds in private clinics, gave the following figures:

Public Mental Hospitals:	
Athens	1,809
Corfu	325
Thessaloniki	250
Chania	309
Community Mental Hospitals:	
Dromokaition	645
"Hirs" Thessaloniki	75
"Skilitseio" Chios	63
Eginition (University Clinic)	112
Philanthropic Institutions:	
"Vegio" Kephalonia	100
Asylum of Syros	60
Total	3,740

A small asylum on the island of Mytilini also functioned, but was not mentioned in the national statistics. These statistics indicate that the hospitals of Athens and Chania reached or surpassed their maximum capacities, while the others grew at a slower pace. The capacity of an institution was measured by the number of beds, but many patients slept on mattresses placed on the floor or shared a bed with two or three others (Yfantopoulos 1988).[22] Nursing personnel also lived in the institution and slept in its beds (Ploubidis 1981, 1983).

By the time of these national statistics, a military regime under General Metaxas had been in power since 1936, and the country was thrown into an "unprecedented obscurantism" (Tsoucalas 1969:53).[23] Further tragedy was to unfold in the country with the Axis power's occupation, 1941–44. During the notoriously cold winter of 1941–42, thousands died in the streets of Athens from lack of food. Mountain villages, frequently burned, also suffered famine, and the country eventually relied upon foreign sources for food (McNeill 1978).[24] Resistance groups sprang up, along Communist and non-Communist lines. Immediately after the occupation, a civil war resulted in a bitter struggle to gain control of the nation. Cease-fire was declared in October 1949, with official figures stating that 40,000 lives had been lost and unofficial estimates ranging up to 158,000. Hundreds of thousands of people were homeless and material damage was as extensive as it had been in 1944 (Tsoucalas 1969).[25]

Information regarding the mental institutions and mentally ill during the war period is scarce, though certainly those in the hospitals suffered more than the general population. The number of patients at Daphni was reduced to half within a few months after the occupation. The institution became chaotic (especially during the winter of 1941–42), and with the doctors all at the front, no medical treatment was available. Some of the personnel hid resistance fighters as the insane in the institution, to shield them from the Germans, who then threatened to blow up the buildings with patients in them. Daphni was again drawn into the civil war, the Left assuming control of the hospital to use it for their wounded (Bairaktaris 1984).

Although Tito's closure of the Yugoslavian border played a significant role in the Communists' eventual defeat, the American Truman Doctrine provided the country with an unprecedented amount of military and economic aid.[26] Again, Greece was rescued by foreign intervention, this time by a power which was not pleased with any suspicion of Communist infiltration. The popularly elected rightist regime following the civil war subjected the nation once again to a repressive atmosphere. Thousands of the nation's progressive elite were killed, imprisoned, or exiled during this period (Tsoucalas 1969). Opponents of the regime also found themselves in Daphni, as is evidenced by a rise in admission:

1939:	2,000 patients
1943:	1,000 patients
1953:	3,000 patients.

Some political prisoners were labeled mentally ill to defame and destroy their reputation, while others declared themselves so to escape imprisonment (Bairaktaris 1984). During the 1950s and early 1960s, the expression of innovative ideas was greatly discouraged. Tsoucalas (1969) writes that this accounts greatly for the inward-looking and nonpolitical character of non-Communist culture in the years after the civil war:

> It is no coincidence that, while Greeks forged ahead in the visual arts, in music and in poetry, there were no major achievements in the social sciences, literary criticism or prose writing. Not merely political opposition, but any kind of dissident progressive outlook, was at once identified by the dominant bourgeoisie with Communist-inspired subversiveness. (Tsoucalas 1969:116)[27]

A more liberal social and political atmosphere arrived with the election of the Centre Union in 1964. Coercion by police virtually disappeared, educational reforms were proposed, and new ideas in general fomented.[28] This climate of freedom was short-lived: the military coup of 1967 plunged the country once again into a repressive period, this one lasting seven years.

While up to World War II Greece's psychiatric care and services probably differed little from the European neighbors from whom she borrowed, a retardation or stagnation is the overall characteristic of Greek psychiatric and mental health care after World War II and continuing until the 1980s. This is attributable in part to the formal link of neurology and psychiatry, which focused treatment on biological (pharmacological) therapies and inhibited the exploration of socially and psychologically based treatments. Also implicated are economic obstacles and social and political periods of repression (which probably assisted the continued link of neurology and psychiatry). It cannot be mere coincidence that while other Western nations forged ahead[29] in developing new therapies (biological and psychosocial) for the mentally ill, revising and creating new services apart from institutional care, Greek psychiatry's answer to her pressing problem of institutional overcrowding was to simply transfer "incurable" and "abandoned" patients to army barracks or sanitariums renamed as mental hospitals.

Nearly every decade after World War II, the Ministry of Health formed committees for the revision of the 1862 legislation. The committee of 1948 introduced the concepts of regional sectorization of mental hospitals and voluntary admission of patients. In 1957, the Ministry of Health requested legislative ideas from a committee of the Panhellenic Union for Mental Hygiene (created in 1956). The committee developed a complete package replacing the anachronistic Law of 1862. It included sectorization, psychiatric services in general hospitals, mental health centers, day hospitals, alternative patient rehabilitation solutions based in the community, legislative reforms for the professional preparation and employment of patients, and training schools for nurses and psychosocial workers. An inherent flaw in this legislative effort was the compulsory entrustment of its application, which required money, to ministerial decisions. The plan was subject to one reduction and modification after another through the bureaucratic path and was never realized in the original form (Lyketsos 1988).[30]

Nongovernmental efforts for the improvement of mental health care appeared with the creation of the Mental Health Center in Athens in 1957 (Lyketsos 1981, 1988). (The Center of Mental Hygiene in Thessaloniki was established in the late 1960s.) Attempts to improve institutional conditions were initiated in pockets. At the 'A' clinic of Dromokaition, cooperation between psychiatrists and the nursing staff and the development of biological therapies created a confidence with patients so that the deeply entrenched iron bars could be removed from the windows and the doors could be opened in 1953. All physical restraints (iron cages, chains, straitjackets) were abolished. Later, the gate of the hospital was opened to permit the free interaction of patients in the large garden and the surrounding area of Dromokaition (Lyketsos 1981, 1988). Conditions were certainly better here since the institution, not a state facility, was able to regulate admissions according to its facilities. The majority of the patients did not pay for care and were referred by the Department of Social Welfare (Hartocollis 1966).

A description of Daphni at this time is provided by Rasidaki (1983), who arrived in December 1953 as director of the 'D' Psychiatric Clinic (with 250 patients). A total of two thousand patients were hospitalized at the institution, two or three persons frequently sharing the same bed. The buildings were not yet heated and suffered from poor drainage systems. A fence or other marker of the hospital's boundaries was nonexistent, as was a front gate or formal entrance. Thus, all the patient pavilions were permanently double-locked and first-floor windows were fenced with iron bars. None of the patient pavilions had telephones, and the hospital communicated with the rest of the world through only two phone lines.

The few doctors employed at the hospital were brought from a central point in Athens by a truck each morning. They worked a total of two or three hours, arriving about 10:00 and departing; as today, about 12:00 or 12:30 (Blue 1991).[31] The medical pyramid of assistants, registrars, and directors had been reversed: many directors, fewer registrars, and few assistants. There was no social worker (the term had not yet appeared in Greece) and, of course, no psychologist. Nursing staff was composed of "practicals" (persons without a nursing degree).

Always in agreement with the Law of 1862, patients were admitted to the hospital following an opinion by the Services of the Ministry of Social Services, or a decision by the police or the public attorney. The patient was to be discharged after the doctor's opinion of cure had been sent to the prefect or the person who had requested his admission sought his release.

Three occupational therapists attempted in a small room to occupy fifteen to twenty patients. Of course, many more patients were occupied with cleaning the pavilions (cleaning people did not yet exist or were very few) and knitting for the nurses.

Eventually, with the continued institutionalization of persons and no programs for their rehabilitation and release into the community, an impasse was reached. The traditional answer to overcrowding by simply constructing more buildings with more beds was not working.

"Every voyage with a ship is possibly the last"
(Foucault 1981, quoted in Bairaktaris 1984:81)

A solution to the increasingly congested conditions was the creation of a colony for the mentally ill on the island of Leros. One of the Doecannese Islands given to Greece by Italy after World War II, Leros is about twelve hours by ship from Pireaus. Small, semi-arid, with typical inlet beaches and sparkling Mediterranean bays, the island suffered heavy damage during World War II. The Minister of Commerce wanted some form of income for his constituency, as the withdrawal of the Italians and English had left many islanders without employment and prompted them to leave for Athens or abroad (Bairaktaris 1984). Because the island already possessed empty Italian army barracks, a colony for the mentally ill would be an easy solution to a variety of problems: employment and income islanders would derive from an institution, its distant location conveniently placed unwanted mentally ill patients away from their families, society, and the press, and the relief of the congested conditions at the public mental hospitals. Through convincing the party in power and the vice minister of health, the decision to found a colony for the mentally ill on Leros was made in 1957. Though introduced by the ministry, the psychiatric community raised no strong objections to the plan as it considered creating an institution more pertinent than examining the consequences of its location (Bairaktaris 1984).

Shortly thereafter, the most severely ill and incurable patients from Daphni and Thessaloniki, who had no contact with their families, were shipped to the island, for "hospitalization." An informant stated that those who arrived were "not exactly like humans, animals or plants." Clothing and identification of the patients had been mixed up during the boat journey, thus regaining their identity was an initial task. Personnel at this time was lacking. There were two doctors and one assistant. When the responsible doctor complained to authorities in Athens, he was told not to ask so much for the mentally ill person; it was a waste of money and the country had more pressing needs (Bairaktaris 1984). Patients would help each other, they suggested, the schizophrenics would help the epileptics, thus additional personnel was not required.

A new charter, granted in 1964, renamed the institution and infused it with a medical character. It was named the Psychiatric Hospital of Leros. The bed capacity was officially raised to 2,683. The level of care was described as miserable and unbearable, with a completely untrained, unprepared nursing staff. As more and more incurable patients arrived (a large group was transferred from the institution of Soudas in 1966), the answer to the staff's cry for assistance from the ministry was bunk beds for the patients. Baglesos, a psychiatrist at Leros for more than twenty years (from Bairaktaris 1984), cites the following reasons that Leros achieved its miserable status and long-range plans for improvement were not initiated:

> The island is an exile. The region is very small and cultural activities for an educated person are extremely limited. The salary is low. There is no possibility to maintain a private practice or moonlight in a private clinic as another income source.

According to Baglesos, despite the institution's misery, its achievements included the other state hospital's release from chronic patients, permitting them to concentrate care on acute cases. The aim of Daphni, a bed for every patient, was fulfilled. Thousands of families were freed from the load of caring for their ill and thus could preserve their own environment. The institution provided Greek society three services: assistance for the ill person and his or her family, the employment of the people working in the institution, and support and the furthering of commercial interests of this border island (i.e., defense purposes as it is off the Turkish coast).

The situation on Leros was to remain obscure until the beginning of the 1980s when young psychiatrists went to the island for their community service intern and were horrified by the conditions they encountered: women chained to trees, patients naked during all seasons and showered en masse with hoses, rotten meat served, patients chained to metal beds in basement, total isolation, routine giving of medication, and minimal treatment. In 1982 there was an initiative by doctors to halt further admissions to the island and a movement to shut the institution completely. This move has been supported by the European Economic Community.

By 1970, the hospital in Thessaloniki continued to be overcrowded, and an answer was found in an old sanitarium, a former monastery, isolated some twenty-six kilometers from the small town of Katerini. Regardless of their region of origin (whether close to Katerini or not), the most severe cases from Thessaloniki and those abandoned by their families were sent to this institution, *Petras Olympou*.[32] Down in the Peloponnese, another public hospital had opened in 1968 in Tripolis (Kriaras 1982). Also about this time, the asylum of Soudas was relocated in new buildings a little outside of the town of Chania.

The Junta fell in 1974, and Greece again tasted democracy. One of the goals of Karamanlis, the elected Prime Minister, was the updating of Greek society and her infrastructure. Another aim, the entry of Greece into the European Economic Community under full membership, was realized some four and a half years after negotiations began in 1976. A desire for change (*allaqi*) was voted into power in 1981 with Papandreou, the leader of Greece's first socialist government. Further efforts toward secularizing the nation (such as introducing civil marriage) occurred (Woodhouse 1984), as well as the creation of a National Health System in 1983.[33] A new Mental Health Law, Law 104, which contains a provision for voluntary admissions and the sectorization of mental hospitals, was passed in 1973.

During the 1970s, psychiatric care remained highly centralized, paralleling the centralization of Greek health care (Mavreas 1987) and the centralization of Greek services in general.[34] Most inpatient facilities (63.5 percent of beds) were located either in Athens or in Thessaloniki, although only 40 percent of the population resided in these areas (Stefanis and Madianos 1981).[35] Mental health care catchment areas were nonexistent. Inpatient services were available through the large mental hospitals or through small private hospitals. Private clinics had developed in great numbers after World War II. A result of the poor care offered by the public sector, they also reflected a changing social structure: the breakdown of extended families, the relative isolation of rural areas and increase in urban populations, group emigration, etc. Naturally, these clinics were located primarily in Athens and Thessaloniki.

Outpatient facilities, in general, were scarce. In Athens and Thessaloniki a few mental health centers operated, not based upon a catchment area. Primary care was also offered through the Social Insurance Organization (IKA), which had an agreement with the existing private hospitals for inpatient care. Private outpatient care, primarily in Athens and Thessaloniki, was provided by neurologist-psychiatrists. Services other than primary care, such as psychotherapy, family therapy, rehabilitation, day care, drug and alcohol treatment, were virtually nonexistent.

By the end of the 1970s, some psychiatric care innovations for Greece began to appear. Through Eginition Hospital in Athens, a mental health center with a catchment area in the Byrona-Kaisariani districts, has been functioning since 1979. The first psychiatric department in a general hospital opened in Alexandroupoulis in 1979 with the first day hospital (connected with Eginition Hospital in Athens) started. A basic problem developing day or part-time care was linked to the legislation of 1862, which permitted adult psychiatric patients hospitalization only on a 24-hour basis (Mantonakis 1981).

A significant change for Greek psychiatry was the official separation from neurology in 1982 and subsequent alterations in training requirements. After six years of medical school, specialization in neurology-psychiatry consisted of three years, one year of general medicine, one year of neurology, and one year of psychiatry. University residency programs existed, though the majority of practitioners have been trained in nonuniversity affiliated general hospitals for neurology and in the state hospitals for psychiatry. Training requirements are now six months of internal medicine, six months of neurology, and three years of psychiatry. The years of psychiatry are to be spent in a rotation between psychiatric departments of general hospitals, the large state hospitals, and mental health centers, but because these services are not uniformly developed around the nation, once again a directive exists prior to its object.

The development of ancillary mental health care services has greatly and rapidly expanded since about 1985. There are now psychiatric departments in general hospitals; residential hostels, primarily for chronically ill patients; more mental health centers, some concentrating services on psychotherapy; mobile units visiting patients in their villages; and efforts to deinstitutionalize patients who have spent lifetimes in institutions.

Although the return of many senior university psychiatrists from abroad certainly fueled new ideas, the separation from neurology and the longer training period in psychiatry has permitted new residents the opportunity to develop treatment skills other than medication and to explore efforts for patient rehabilitation. A general philosophy exists throughout the country to avoid hospitalization whenever possible and to treat the individual on an outpatient basis. This renaissance of psychiatric care is attributable to the break from neurology and the freer social and political climate to actively pursue patient rehabilitation and mental illness prevention. Greece is once again in a position to emulate her European neighbors, as she did in the last century and the beginning of this one. Her participation in the European Economic Community has resulted in the allocations of vast sums of financial support for mental health care programs. Thus, the economic obstacles and lack of focus on psychiatric care, present since the beginning of the nation and the birth of her psychiatry, have temporarily been relieved—through the traditional avenue, intervention of a foreign power. And, as new ideas and services are disseminated through her contact with Europe, the soup of Greek professional ethnopsychiatry will continue to be stirred (Blue 1991).

Notes

1. The full link with the wider cultural context has been set aside here as it is a focus of a larger work, see Blue (1991).

2. Historical sources regarding Greek psychiatry have been drawn primarily from Ploubidis (1981, 1983) for the period up to the foundation of Daphni, the appropriate citations and informant interviews. Historical material in English is nonexistent at this time.

3. I have relied upon Tsoucalas (1969), believing this to be the best analysis of Greek history up until the period of the junta. Other histories of Greece include Woodhouse (1984), Clogg (1986), and McNeill (1978). Mouzelis (1978) provides an excellent analysis of capitalist development in the country.

4. The revolution was fueled more by Greeks of the diaspora, primarily a Western trained intelligentsia, than the peasants and artisans within the Ottoman lands. Mouzelis (1978) writes that the diaspora bourgeoisie assisted the effort by providing leadership and material resources. They also introduced French revolutionary ideas and Western science and culture to a society underpinned by Greek Orthodoxy and its anti-Enlightenment, anti-Western orientation. Shortly after war broke out, internal conflicts developed. A "traditionalist" policy was favored by the landowning-cum merchant class who wanted to assume the power that the Turkish had, maintaining a political status quo. The Westerners, the intelligentsia and diaspora bourgeoisie with wealth abroad (and not much to risk through a progressive policy) wanted to "modernize" Greece through a strong centralized state, inhibiting regional fragmentation and the politico-autonomy of local notables.

5. The policies these powers pursued were as follows: Russia wanted a large Balkan Greco-Slav state established under her protection to ensure her a position in the Mediterranean after the collapse of Ottoman power. These aims were supported by the fact that the majority of the Balkan population was Slav, all ascribing to the Orthodox faith. Great Britain desired the existence of the Ottoman Empire, as a counterbalancing power against Russian expansionism. However, with the Ottoman's impending demise, Britain favored an independent Greek nation which would be politically and economically dependent on her, and thus serve as an antagonistic force toward other ethnic groups in the Balkans (Tsoucalas 1969:17–18).

6. The protecting powers had agreed to prohibit the placement of any member of their own royal families on the throne (Clogg 1986:66; Woodhouse 1984:169).

7. Few roads existed for wheeled traffic; goods were carried by pack animals, and many of the Turkish bridges destroyed in the War of Independence were not repaired (Sherrard and Campbell 1969).

8. In 1780 there were three Greek hospitals in Constantinople: the Hospital of Galata, the main hospital for the Greeks; the Hospital of Stavrodromiou; and the Hospital of Eptapirgiou. In 1839, a new hospital was built, housing inhabitants of the older Hospital of Galata. Around the building and its church a high wall was erected because of certain categories of inmates and the fear of invasion by vagabonds. The hospital accepted the following categories of individuals:

a.   ill men and women;
b.   needy elderly;
c.   mentally ill men and women;
d.   suspects and "the depraved" men and women enclosed by patriarchal orders;
e.   malefactors sent by the police;
f.   depraved children wandering the streets who had displayed tendencies to refuse the traditional religion;
g.   certain women sent for punishment as a reprimand of the patriarch and local church leaders.

In 1850, a new building was added in which the elderly and the mentally disturbed were housed together on the entrance and the children of the institution, orphans and naughty, were placed on the above floor. The plan for this separation, initiated by the Patriarch Gemanos, was the removal of the weaker and mainly children from the "intercourse of cunning men and depraved women" (Ploubidis 1981:47–49).

9. In the Byzantine tradition, as well as Islamic, certain displays of insanity were considered godly messages (Ploubidis 1981).

10. In the Balkan region, three Rumanian monasteries acquired fame as asylums and were to be cores for future hospitals (Ploubidis 1983).

11. Greece had been induced to support the Russians during the Crimean War (1853) in Thessaloniki and Macedonia. The British and French responded to this action with an occupation of the port of Pireaus for three years (1854–57). After the troops departed, it was declared for the nation to be under economic control by the powers. This economic control ended in 1860 (Tsoucalas 1969:20–21). A link between the end of this economic control and the fact that the government began to discuss state care of the mentally ill is a possibility.

12. Further details of this law state: This state supervision will be assured through the selection, by the Ministry of the Interior, of the doctor-director of the institution and inspections conducted by administrative and judicial authorities. In addition, the mayor has the right to visit an interned person and request information regarding his or her condition.

Specifically, application for admission is to be written and accompanied by a medical certificate underwritten by a doctor who is not a relative of the person seeking admission or of the director or another employee of the institution. The written directive, accompanying the medical certificate, must then be sent to the prefecture within twenty-four hours. The prefect is then obliged to give notice of the admission to the court attorneys and person's town mayor. Since the standing diagnosis requires a patient observation period, the institution's doctor is required to submit a second certificate within fifteen days. The cure of the patient must be declared in written form, and the director, if other than the doctor, must permit an immediate discharge. If treatment has not been successful, the family may request release of the patient from the hospital. If the patient is considered dangerous, the institution's director may request the person's continued stay in the hospital from the prefect. If there is no response from the prefect within fifteen days, the director is then obliged to release the patient to whomever legally asks for the discharge. Public officials, such as the prefect and the police chief, have the right to send disturbed individuals disrupting the community and its residents to the mental hospital. According to the ministry, articles 13, 15, 16, and 17 of the law make abuses of this right relatively impossible. For example, a mayor does not possess this right. In addition to the twenty-four-hour certificate and that of the first fifteen days, the institution's director is to make a presentation every three months to the prefect. The judicial authority has the freedom to control what occurs in the institution. The law included the temporary removal of the patient's property by judicial authorities if necessary (Ploubidis 1981).

13. These doctors and dates of their service at the hospital are as follows: A. Kogevinas (1842–46); X. Lavranos (1846–54); S. Neratzis (1854–66); A. Agiovlasitis (1866–69); K. Kefalas (1869–74); Tsirigotis (1874–1887). (Simatis and Moros n.d.)

14. Between 1863 and 1909 road mileage multiplied tenfold, foundations for a modern railway were laid, ports for large steamships were built, and the Corinth Canal opened. A thorough reorganization of the civil service, and the Army and Navy, occurred. Several large banks opened, creating a basis for a modern credit system and industrial production advanced. However, the number of industrial workers at the end of the century was only 200,000. The urban population increased from 8 percent in 1853 to 28 percent in 1879 (Tsoucalas 1969:23).

15. The mental hospitals, unlike the general hospitals and educational institutions, took little advantage of the tight relationship during all of the nineteenth century between Greeks within the national boundaries and those residing in the diaspora which resulted in large endowments and legacies bestowed on the foundation or renovation of public institutions in Greece. However, the foundation and completion of Dromokaition, the hospital of Skilitseiou of Chios, the renovation of the asylum of Kephalonia, Vegio and other small institutions were due to endowments (Ploubidis 1981:80).

16. The second article stated that the institution would be directed through an administrative committee of four members (president, vice president, treasurer, and secretary). It would not be able to make a decision without the presence of at least three members, and in the case of a vote, the vote of the president would overrule. The decisions must be undersigned by the president and the secretary. A member of the administrative committee must visit the institution at least once a week. The administrative committee had the handling of property of the institution and is obligated to submit annual accounts to the Ministry of the Interior. The accounts must be published by the press. The doctor-director was responsible through the Law of 1862. The admission had to be approved by the president of the administrative committee, because payment for the first two months of care had to be previously put down. If a patient had not placed payment ten days before the expiration of two months, the doctor-director was obliged to release him. If the patient was dangerous and he who had sought admission was not present or refused to accept him, then the doctor communicated to the prefect (in agreement with Law 1862). If the prefect did not answer within ten days, then the doctor directed the person to the police (Ploubidis 1981:86).

17. Professional misdeeds were punished by the administrative committee with reprimand, holding from one to five days' worth of salary, and dismissal. The amount held for punishment was distributed as a reward to the other employees (Ploubidis 1981:132).

18. The discussions of degeneration, its indications and contents, preoccupied European medicine, forensic medicine and psychiatry during the last quarter of the nineteenth century and the beginning of the twentieth century. Greek doctors and lawyers, to a significant degree, used the meaning of degeneration (Ploubidis 1981:133).

19. Psychoanalysis has never entrenched itself within Greek psychiatry. The first presentation of its principles in a medical context was in 1928 with the publication of an article, "Psychoanalysis," by D. Kouretas in *Hellenic Medicine* (Tzavaras and Kirtata 1983:39; see them also for more information regarding the psychoanalytic bibliography in Greece).

20. The classes and charges are: A' class, 360 drachmas per month; B' class, 210 drachmas per month; C' class, 120 drachmas per month.

21. Greater Athens grew from 452,919 inhabitants in 1920 to 801,622 in 1928. Hundreds of thousands of refugees crowded around the main cities, unemployed, penniless, and homeless (Tsoucalas 1969:36).

22. The first appearance of outpatient care in Greece was in 1938 when the insurance association IKA established a basic organization and operation for the development of outpatient services. Therefore, outpatient care began in Greece covering only the bourgeoisie, who made up 32.8 percent of the total population. The rest of the population remained "uncovered" without basic hygienic services (Yfantopoulos 1988:64).

23. The new state participated in imprisonments, book burnings (titles by Freud, Zweig, France, Gorki and others), abolished labor unions and imprisoned dissidents (Tsoucalas 1969:52–53).

24. The war had impoverished Greece so much that the country could not possibly support the urban-based administration and professional armed forces necessary for internal security. This inhibited economic recovery, so that the Greek urban population remained dependent on food delivered from abroad or charity (McNeill 1978:65).

25. In the last year of their occupation, the Germans burned hundreds of villages and executed 70,000 people (Tsoucalas 1969:69).

26. Tsoucalas (1969) provides an excellent analysis of the politics involved in the creation of the civil war and its termination. See also McNeill (1978:81–137) for the role of the United States in post-war assistance.

27. While the political and ideological neutralization of the organized Left continued, repression assumed new forms. After 1955 open terrorism had decreased, the machinery of pressure remained constant. A "certificate of national probity" was required as a condition for a variety of things, such as being employed by the state or any private or semi-public firm controlled by the state, acquiring a driver's license or passport, getting into the university, hunting or fishing, and numerous other everyday activities requiring for one reason or another an administrative authorization. In a country where unemployment was the most urgent problem for the majority of people, the threat of not being able to find a job was probably the most effective method of political control. Elaborate lists of "nonnationalists" were kept by the police, based upon those who had been refused a certificate. It has been estimated that around one million persons were on this black list (Tsoucalas 1969:146).

28. The elections of February 1964 brought the Centre Union into power and a more liberal atmosphere and climate of freedom. Coercion by police and gendarmerie virtually disappeared, a number of extremist right-wing bands were dissolved, the majority (but not all) of the political prisoners were released and the "certificate of national probity," though officially maintained, fell into disuse. An unprecedented ferment of ideas, debates, political and cultural activities created a totally new climate. A completely reformed educational program was proposed. The creation of a third University in Patras and the establishment of two others in Crete and Epirus, gave a great impetus to the antiquated cultural and educational scene.

Compulsory schooling was extended from six to nine years, and free school meals in all primary schools in the countryside (partly supplemented with limited scholarships for secondary schools) made the law's provisions realistic in a country where poor parents would rather use their children's labor. This was a popular reform by Papandreou as it was a chance viewed by peasants for their children to become "civilized human beings" (Tsoucalas 1969:183–184).

29.   Despite its secular essence, modern Greek culture remained imbued with religion and no major anticlerical trend appeared from the prevailing conformity (religions marriage was the only legal form until the 1980s). Though oriented to the West, Greece refused to partake of the flourishing of critical and demystifying thought following World War II in Western Europe (Tsoucalas 1969:116).

30.   In 1953, legislation was passed regarding the creation of health districts differentiated into thirteen hygienic districts and termed the organization and administrative unions of services between central, peripheral and prefectural levels. The function of Social Hygiene Stations was the covering of necessary outpatients from the rural population of the country. The criteria used at the time were one hygiene station for 5,000 to 8,000 inhabitants. Hygienic services and medical care for the population were to be offered through a doctor, a visiting nurse, a midwife, and two assisting employees. Following this, in 1955 the population bases were altered and for populations over 3,000 inhabitants, an "Agricultural Surgery" would be created. The "Community Surgery" would be staffed by a doctor of general medicine (having just completed basic medical school), a midwife, and a visiting nurse. The "Rural Surgery" would have a general doctor. In 1964, a rural doctor would serve populations of 2,000 or more. The outpatient care of the rural population was completed in 1961 by establishing the Organization of Farmer's Insurance to handle the funding of outpatient care for farmers. At the same time, the extension of social insurance for more groups of the bourgeoisie population covered a greater portion of outpatient care which was offered by the consulting doctor with the insuring agent or the policy of the insurance organization. The outpatient care was also offered by the outpatient surgery of the hospital (Yfantopoulos 1988:65).

31.   Some things (i.e., the working hours) have not changed.

32.   Bairaktaris (1984:80) writes that since the opening of Petras Olympou, the hospital of Thessaloniki has not exceeded its bed capacity and has been able to maintain statistics.

33.   The National Health System places an emphasis upon decentralizing Greek health care services (see below) and promoting primary health care. Many health centers have sprung up around the country. For physicians there is now the employment choice of either working for the ESY (the National Health System) on a full-time basis, or maintaining a private practice on a full-time basis. It is illegal for a physician of ESY to accept remuneration separately from patients, consulted either in the ESY setting or privately.

34.   This centralization of Greek life in Athens is a result of the rapid urbanization of the country experienced in the post-war period. Between 1952 and 1963 an unprecedented growth in the urban population occurred, making it, for the first time in Greek history, slightly larger than the rural population. In the 1951 census the urban population was 37.3 percent and by 1961 it had risen to 43 percent; the

rural population had fallen to 44 percent; and the semi-urban had remained constant at 13 percent. Athens rapidly grew, which absorbed 62.7 percent of the total population. By 1961 the region of the capital provided over one-half of industrial employment, received 80 percent of imports, paid 75 percent of direct and 65 percent of indirect taxation, had an income more than 40 percent higher than the national average, absorbed more than half of total newspaper circulation, accounted for a majority of hospital beds and 85 percent of specialist doctors, and housed the bulk of the fairly excessive civil service personnel (Tsoucalas 1969).

   35. Mavreas (1987) demonstrates how even this statistic is misleading because two of the psychiatric colonies are included in the provincial area, thus the figure becomes even greater (78 percent of beds).

References

Bairaktaris, Konstantinos
1984 Anstaltspsychiatrie in Griechenland (in German). Munster: Lit Verlag.

Baslamatzi, Grigori
1983 Psychiatry and Prevailing Ideology (in Greek). Contemporary Issues 9:107–112.

Blue, Amy
1991 Culture, *Nevra* and Institution: The Making of Professional Greek Ethnopsychiatry. Unpublished Ph.D. dissertation in Anthropology. Case Western Resserve University. Cleveland, Ohio.

Clogg, Richard
1986 A Short History of Modern Greece. New York: Cambridge University Press.

Hartocollis, Peter
1958 Cure by Exorcism in the Island of Cephalonia. Journal of the History of Medicine. July, pp. 367–372.
1966 Psychiatry in Contemporary Greece. American Journal of Psychiatry 123:457–462.

Kriaras, K. D.
1982 Observations of Admissions Under Compulsory Order at the Mental Hospital of Tripolis (in Greek). Encephalos 19:225–226.

Lyketsos, George
1981 Prevention of Chronic Mental Disorders in Greece (in Greek). Bibliotheca Psychiatrica 160:105–109.
1988 Lessons from the Past. Encephalos 25:2–5.

Mantonakis, John
1981 Problems Related to the Organization and Opening of the First Day Hospital in Athens. International Journal of Social Psychiatry 27:151–153.

Mavreas, V. G.
1987 Greece: The Transition to Community Care. International Journal of Social Psychiatry 33:154–164.

McNeill, William H.
1978 The Metamorphosis of Greece Since World War II. Chicago: University of Chicago Press.

Mouzelis, Nicos
1978 Modern Greece: Facets of Underdevelopment. New York: Holmes and Meier
      Publishers.
Ploubidis, Dimitris
1981 Contribution to the Study of the History of Psychiatry in Greece: the Tradi-
      tional Behavior Toward the Mentally Ill and Mental Institutions of the 19th
      Century (in Greek). Athens: Unpublished Dissertation in the Psychiatric
      Clinic. University of Athens.
1983 (An) Introduction About the Establishment of Psychiatry in Greece (in
      Greek). Contemporary Issues 19:21–30.
Rasidaki, N.
1983 As I Remember: Memories of the House of Shame (in Greek). Athens: E.M.
      Moraitou-Sideridi.
Simatis, P. and N. Moros
n.d.   Mental Hospital of Corfu 150 Years Since its Foundation (in Greek). n.p.
Stefanis, C. N. and M. G. Madianos
1981 Mental Health Care Delivery System in Greece: A Critical Overview. Biblio-
      theca Psychiatrica 160:78–83.
Tsoucalas, Constantine
1969 The Greek Tragedy. Baltimore: Penguin Books.
Tzavaras, Thanasi and Dimiri Kirtata
1983 The Psychoanalytic Bibliography in Greece (in Greek). Contemporary Issues
      9:39–44.
Woodhouse, C. M.
1984 Modern Greece: A Short History. London: Faber and Faber, Ltd.
Yfantopoulos, John
1988 Health Planning in Greece: Some Economic and Social Aspects (in Greek).
      Athens: National Center of Social Research.

14

Conflicts of Cultures in
a State Mental Hospital System

Pearl Katz

Introduction

In the past decade, the State of Maryland has received national recognition for a "revolution" in its mental health system (see McGuire 1982; Miller 1983; Psychiatric News 1984; Russell 1983; Sergeant 1983). A key aspect of this revolution has been the more than two hundred, young, university trained psychiatrists who have chosen to work in the state mental health system since 1976. More than half of them have remained in the system for more than five years. The majority of these psychiatrists have assumed positions in one of the twelve state inpatient facilities.

Most are now ward chiefs, but some have taken up posts as superintendents and clinical directors at various hospitals. Several of the psychiatrists have assumed high administrative positions in the State of Maryland Mental Hygiene Administration, as directors of the state's Mental Hygiene Administration, regional directors, assistant directors, and one Assistant Secretary for Health. A few are working in the community mental health centers.

The addition of the university-trained psychiatrists has resulted in significant improvements in all mental hospitals, emergency psychiatric care, and community mental health centers in Maryland. It has improved the caliber of the nurses, psychologists, and social workers who work for the state hospitals. It also has led to the remedicalization of the mental health system. Links among many state and private institutions which serve the mentally ill have expanded in number and density (cf. Harbin et al. 1982; Russell 1982).

The improvements in the quality of care in the mental health organizations in Maryland have been unique. These changes were possible largely because of bureaucratic linkages that were formed between different "cultural" traditions. The two major "cultures" were the state mental hospital system and the University of Maryland Medical School's Department of

Psychiatry. Both of these cultures (university and state) had historically different and separate political, institutional, and psychiatric traditions. The contact between these two cultures initially provoked great resistence in the state hospitals and, subsequently, improvements in the delivery and quality of mental health care for patients in the state hospitals. Throughout the United States, previous attempts to merge university and state cultures were short-lived, highly resisted, and ultimately unsuccessful (Faulkner and Eaton 1979; Katz 1984a).

The historical underpinnings of these cultures is necessary to an understanding of the conflicts that these changes generated. State mental hospitals had state-trained psychiatrists who were older, mostly foreign medical graduates practicing custodial institutional care; on the other hand, university psychiatric practice consisted of university-trained psychiatrists, young, mostly American medical school graduates practicing therapeutic institutional care (Katz 1984a).

Methodology

Anthropologists and other social scientists who have studied mental hospitals in the past have traditionally examined them as homogeneous, local-level phenomena that were virtually isolated from outside influences (cf. Caudill 1958; Caudill et al. 1952; Stanton and Schwartz 1954). Most identified with the patients. Some, like Caudill, pretended they were patients. The combination of both perceiving the hospital as isolated as well as identifying with the patients restricted researchers' perspectives; they assumed that the society beyond the hospital was homogeneous and oriented to exploitation of the disenfranchised. One consequence of this perspective has been that anthropologists have neglected to examine the dynamics of interrelationships between the "micro" and the "macro" structures.

The study reported here explicitly focuses upon those dynamic processes. It is a part of a larger study which examined the effects of the state structure (e.g., the governor, the legislature, the federal and state legislative and reimbursement picture, the power structure in the universities, and the educational and manpower background of psychiatrists) upon the micro-structure (staff and patient behavior and morale on the wards). It also examined the effects of the local social structure and organization (such as the interaction among staff and its effects on patients, increased chronicity of the patients, or increased violence on a ward) on the state structure and organization (such as the support for a new clinical director).

The larger study examined the ways in which the changes in the state central mental health office affected the administration of the hospitals, the implementation of changes in the hospital, ward staff morale, and the therapeutic character of the wards. It examined how low patient morale and increased patient violence on a particular ward both affected, and were consequences of, turmoil at the hospital administration level, which, in turn, both affected and was a consequence of turmoil at the state political level. This perspective led to interpreting local processes, such as resistances to implementing change and the cultural conflicts in a hospital as part of the dynamics of a changing state mental health structure (Katz 1984a, b).

The methodologies employed were ethnographic participant-observation and the techniques of in-depth, open-ended interviews. The participant-observation consisted of the following: a) intensive work in six wards in three large hospitals (two wards in each hospital), for three weeks in each ward, plus three weeks in two of the wards after a three-year interval; b) periodic participant-observation in six wards, for a total of one week each; c) observation of a clinical director in Ken Oak Hospital, every day for seven consecutive months; d) observation of three superintendents, three clinical directors, two regional directors, and the director of psychiatric training, for two to four nonconsecutive days each; e) attendance at committee meetings; discussions with state mental health directors and legislators and other politicians, state executive mental health committees, clinical directors' committees, university psychiatric education and training committees; and f) attendance at psychiatric education classes, including Tavistock groups, and clinical case conferences.

Open-ended, recorded interviews, ranging in length from three to nineteen hours, were conducted with 131 mental health professionals. The majority of interviews were with psychiatrists and psychiatric residents. A minority consisted of talks with active and retired state and hospital administrators, psychologists, social workers, and psychiatric nurses. Some psychiatric patients were interviewed about their perceptions of events on the wards. The two fieldwork methodologies took place over thirty-nine months.

State Mental Health Culture and History

Before the mid-nineteenth century, local communities, such as counties and municipalities, cared for their dependent and impoverished citizens, including the mentally ill (Deutsch 1949; Sarbin and Juhasz 1982). By the late nineteenth century, states increasingly assumed a wider role for care (Grob 1983:72–107). Although a large number of state mental hospitals were built during the latter half of the nineteenth century, problems of overcrowding, inadequate buildings, and low morale of staff members persisted (Dwyer, this volume; Grob 1983:8). The population in mental hospitals continued to increase during the first half of the twentieth century. In 1903 there were 150,000 patients in the United States; by 1940 there were 445,000 patients (Grob 1983:180). The population in state mental hospitals peaked in the mid-1950s at 559,000 (Grob 1983:317).

By the end of the nineteenth century, and into the first four decades of the twentieth century, state hospitals housed aged, senile, retarded, and impoverished people, in addition to the mentally ill. Legal, rather than medical, criteria for hospitalization predominated and custodial goals predominated over therapeutic goals. Patients received most of their care from low-paid attendants and nurses (see Dwyer, this volume). At the same time, psychiatrists and laymen believed in a "cult of curability" through medical and human intervention (Romano 1975:29). These two contrasting cultural influences resulted in an "ambiguous organizational character" of state mental hospitals (Morrissey, Goldman and Klerman 1980:48). In Maryland, under the influence of social reformers such as Dorothea Dix, the first hospital to care exclusively for the mentally ill was established in the late eighteenth century (Hurd 1911).

Custodialism in the State Hospital Culture

The state mental health culture in the United States has always been dominated by the large state mental hospitals. Since their inception, state hospitals have been notoriously resistant to change (Dunham and Weinberg 1960; Greenblatt et al. 1955). The reasons for their rigidity include their embeddedness in the state bureaucracies, their dependency upon state legislatures for their funding, their geographic remoteness relative to urban centers, their "total institutional" culture for the patients and employees, their isolation from the rest of medicine and from academic psychiatry, and the social undesirability of the people they traditionally served (e.g., the insane, impoverished, aged, and retarded).

Since the late nineteenth century, these hospitals had been overcrowded, inadequately staffed and underfunded. They were, "dirty, dingy, and poorly staffed by barely prepared, demoralized, and overwhelmed staff members" (Talbott 1980:69).

Greenblatt described his first psychiatric rounds at Boston Psychopathic Hospital in 1941:

> At the back of the ward were seven seclusion rooms from which emanated most of the noise, confusion, and odor. One peered into these cells through narrow windows at revolting pictures of deteriorated life...naked persons living in their own excretement (sic), terribly hostile, repressed, or crushed.
>
> (Patients) were physically overpowered, dragged screaming and kicking through the wards, protesting in panic. (Greenblatt et al. 1955:55)

The overcrowded state hospitals were always short of personnel, particularly psychiatrists. In the 1960s, thirty-two states had an average of two psychiatrists, or less than one per one hundred state hospital inpatients

(Thompson et al. 1983). There were so few physicians that each of them generally carried responsibility for several hundred patients. And there were proportionately still fewer qualified psychiatrists. Care was largely in the hands of attendants (Greenblatt et al. 1955:1–2).

Until the 1970s, the role of the state hospital staff was one of providing custodial care. The ideology of custodialism was

> saturated with pessimism, impersonalness (sic) and watchful mistrust. The custodial conception of the hospital is autocratic, involving as it does a rigid status hierarchy, unilateral downward flow of power, and a minimizing of communication within and across status lines. (Gilbert and Levinson 1957:22)

Custodialism provided,

> a highly controlled setting concerned mainly with the detention and safekeeping of its inmates. Patients are conceived of in stereotyped terms as categorically different from "normal" people.... In consequence, the staff can-not expect to understand the patients, to engage in meaningful relationship with them, nor in most cases to do them much good. (Gilbert and Levinson 1957:22)

Dunham and Weinberg described custodialism in a typical hospital of the 1950s:

> On the wards...the picture is often one of degrading poverty. The number of attendants on duty is minimal, and most of them have been taught to view their role as that of watching patients, taking care of the latter's basic physical needs, and either supervising or doing the daily ward housekeeping. (1960:10)

The culture of the state hospital was sustained by its geographical, social and intellectual isolation (see Blue, this volume). Isolation affected the staff by sustaining the rigid social structure and reinforcing role behavior. Maintaining staff routines took priority over the therapeutic needs of the patient. The culture was one which turned inward with an atmosphere consisting of suspicions, gossip and mistrust. As Dunham and Weinberg noted:

> The hospital employee culture...is analogous to the paranoia of a mentally ill person (which is)...reflected in the suspicions, the ideas of reference, and the backbiting. (1960:247)

Dunham and Weinberg also noted (1960) that state hospitals fiercely resisted changes:

> (T)he most significant feature of this paranoid social structure is its resistance to change.... New ideas, new practices, new forms of therapy, new research viewpoints, are difficult to introduce if they interfere with existing hospital routines.... (p.64)

The hospital culture has become so encrusted with traditions of the past that it provides little opportunity for originality and spontaneity. The weight of tradition is too strong (pp.30–31). They make every attempt to preserve, to foster, and to enhance this hospital culture even though their actions prove to be inimical to the therapy of the patients (p. 248).

Since the early 1940s, there has been a preponderance in state mental hospitals of foreign-born psychiatrists who were graduates of foreign medical schools (see Varma 1984). Many of these physicians chose psychiatry as a profession because psychiatry was the only field in which they could receive residency training. Although state hospital psychiatrists were paid much lower than those in private practice and had considerably less prestige, many remained for years in the state hospitals after their training. Those who were able to begin private practices left state service. From the late 1930s until the late 1940s, the majority of foreign psychiatrists were German-speaking. Most of them left the state mental hospitals after a few years to go into administration, private practice, or academic psychiatry. They were followed in the 1950s and 1960s by physicians from the Third World, particularly from Asia, and later, from South America.

The opportunities afforded foreign physicians in state hospital psychiatry contrasted with university psychiatry residency programs' preference for Americans. This resulted in invidious disparities between American medical graduates and foreign medical graduates. The custodial culture of the state can be understood not only as a result of its embeddedness in the state political structure, but also of the adaptation of the state psychiatrists to a low status within medicine and psychiatry, and to the demands for caretaking of thousands of patients with minimal staff.

Until 1976, Maryland's treatment of the mentally ill has been representative of all states. The few changes that were instituted in the state hospitals in Maryland were the result of widely publicized scandals. Each of these scandals was initiated by state mental health leaders who were desperately frustrated in their attempts to get legislative support to improve the system. In each case, a leader invited outsiders, often newspaper reporters, to examine and expose shocking inadequacies in the hospitals. In each of these situations, the investigation and the publicity resulted in improvements in the state mental health system, and led to the resignation of the leader who initiated the investigation (Katz 1985).

For example, in 1946, the Commissioner of Mental Health, in an attempt to get appropriations from the Maryland Legislature for expansion and for salary increases to compete for qualified personnel, invited reporters into the hospitals. His action resulted in a series of newspaper articles entitled, "Maryland's Shame," and in the commissioner's losing his job. It also resulted in an increase in the mental health budget by the legislature, improvements in mental health care, and a complete reorganization of the state mental health system. The scandals were exceptional and traumatic events which initiated short-term changes in a culture characterized by opposition to change.

The significant changes in the state mental hospitals since the 1960s have included major psychopharmacological advances which paved the way for both a more controllable, more hopeful, and less numerous inpatient population, and, therefore, the initiation of community-based programs, following deinstitutionalization, for the chronically mentally ill. However, in spite of important innovations in the treatment of the mentally ill, there nevertheless has remained a state mental hospital culture whose ethos and social structure rendered it virtually impervious to change.

Psychiatric Residency Programs and Two Psychiatric Cultures

The psychiatric profession in the United States, although sharing the same background as that of physicians, developed along two different and separate paths. These paths are called here "state psychiatry" and "university psychiatry." With few short-lived exceptions, these two psychiatric traditions remained separate in their respective cultures, institutional homes, and relationships to the rest of medicine until the 1970s. They refer, first, to the residency training programs for practitioners, and, second, to the organization and organizational cultures in which the respective graduates practice psychiatry.

Virtually the entire training and all subsequent practice of state psychiatry took place in state mental hospitals. State psychiatric residency training was often indistinguishable from service. In contrast, university psychiatric residency training was one in which residents learned psychodynamics and long-term therapy of neurotic patients, and for which standardization of education in a university medical school leading to Board certification was sought. University-trained psychiatrists rarely received any training in the state mental hospitals because of the custodial philosophy, the chronicity of the patients, and the reputation for inferior psychiatric care there.

Before 1900, virtually no effort was made to provide systematic instruction in psychiatry in medical schools. Before World War I, teaching programs in psychiatry existed in several state hospitals, in university-based psychopathic hospitals with limited outpatient services, and in a few distinguished private mental hospitals. Lack of training in psychiatry was not a serious impediment to becoming a psychiatrist. Physicians interested in psychiatry had to serve long apprenticeships in a mental hospital:

> After completing a course of study either as an apprentice or at a medical school (the physician was appointed) as an assistant physician in a mental hospital.... Typically an assistant physician in a mental

hospital had never seen an insane person, nor visited a mental hospital. If the physician did not wish to go into another medical specialty, he could become a superintendent.... To a considerable extent, psychiatry consisted of managerial and administrative chores. (Grob 1983:31–32)

State Psychiatric Culture

To a great extent, state psychiatric culture reflected that of the state hospitals because residency programs were carried out in state hospitals. The American psychiatric profession originated in state mental institutions. The overwhelming majority of psychiatrists were originally public employees. Unlike other medical professionals, psychiatrists were institution-based (Starr 1982). They were dependent upon the local and state political system, which frequently changed leadership and policies. They were dependent on legislators, who had little knowledge of, nor serious commitment to, the mentally ill for their budget and policy priorities. Their prestige in the eyes of other physicians and the public was low.

State-trained psychiatrists interpreted their mandate as running hospitals smoothly and quietly, with little interference from the public. State-trained psychiatrists had staying power and tenacity, retaining their jobs through seniority. Many of the participants' commitment to mental health was so encumbered by its entrenchment in the state's bureaucratic tradition that they tenaciously protected the status quo. One university-trained psychiatrist described the situation: "In the state you have to wait until people die, retire, or kill themselves."

Those psychiatrists who sought change in state hospitals "find themselves powerless to put their newer ideas into action" (Dunham and Weinberg 1960:30–31). Attempts by individual state psychiatrists to initiate changes and improvements encountered stubborn resistance, and the results were short-lived (see Katz 1984b). Dunham and Weinberg note:

> To the extent that (the doctors) are immersed in (the state hospital culture), their therapeutic usefulness is proportionally diminished.... Their work, thus, sooner or later takes on a routine character...their authority and knowledge will hardly be utilized if these threaten in any way the customs and traditions of the employee group. (1960:248)

Maryland had two separate residency programs until 1976. A few carefully selected physicians, mostly born and educated in the United States, were in university schools of medicine psychiatry residency programs, particularly the University of Maryland and The Johns Hopkins University. Most psychiatry residents, however, were in the state psychiatry residency program, serving in overcrowded state hospitals. Few of these state psychiatrists were born or educated in U.S. medical schools. Given the heavy service demands of the state system, education in all its forms for state residents received low priority. A Maryland psychiatrist who was a resident in one of the state hospitals in the 1950s reported that there were ten physicians for 2,400 patients. He spoke only of working conditions: "There was no opportunity to know the 240 patients under your care. Only the nurses knew them. With that many patients, you had to choose what is important to do."

The service demands were so great that they precluded structured learning or accessible psychiatric supervision. Learning was defined as "what is important to do."

University Psychiatric Culture and Residency

The university culture in the departments of psychiatry in medical schools encouraged change and promoted learning and free enquiry into the nature, causes, therapeutic modalities, and psychopharmacological interventions of mental illness. University psychiatry residents were exposed to a broad range of educational experiences which, in addition to didactic courses, included supervision and participation in the diagnosis and care of patients suffering from mental illness. The university culture stressed teaching, learning, and inquiry over service obligations to patients.

The university culture was also an elitist culture. University psychiatric admissions programs had the luxury of limiting and choosing their patients according to criteria compatible with its culture. Until recent years patients were primarily selected on the basis of their potential contribution to psychiatric education, in contrast to the state system, which was required to treat all patients. The elitism of the university culture resulted in a higher socioeconomic class of patients, shorter term patients, and fewer chronic patients. Most importantly, university residents' learning requirements took precedence over their service requirements. The culture of elitism in the university was also reflected in the selectivity of psychiatric residents; the universities were the most selective of the pool of applicants, and rarely chose foreign-trained physicians. Consequently, foreign medical graduates, regardless of their ability and their previous training in the countries of origin, were almost inevitably relegated to state residencies.

In the university culture, research was closely linked with diagnosis and treatment of patients, and with teaching. The system of promotions in university psychiatric culture was based upon academic-therapeutic skills, while in the state hospitals promotion was based on seniority, friendships, or political considerations.

University psychiatry culture received its impetus in 1921 when the newly founded American Psychiatric Association (APA) attempted to upgrade training and education in psychiatry through professional certification. This led to the creation of the American Board of Psychiatry and

Neurology in 1934 (Starr 1982:345). In 1929, the APA attempted both to integrate psychiatry into the general medical curriculum as well as to establish separate departments of psychiatry within medical schools. This led to formalization of the educational requirements in psychiatry and to the creation of a specialty board.

After World War II, there was an exponential increase in the number of university psychiatry residency programs. In 1945, there were fewer than 200 full-time psychiatric faculty appointments. By 1972, there were 2,500 full-time psychiatric faculty appointments (Romano 1975:31). In 1935, virtually all psychiatrists served on the staffs of mental hospitals. After 1945, the role of state hospital psychiatrists in the APA was sharply reduced. By 1956, only about 17 percent of the 10,000 members of the APA were employed in state mental hospitals or Veterans' Administration facilities (Grob 1983:287).

Maryland's Psychiatric Cultures

Before 1976, Maryland was similar to other states in that it had two separate residency programs with a few carefully selected United States-born and -educated psychiatrists in the university schools of medicine psychiatry residency programs. The smaller residency programs in the state hospitals had a preponderance of foreign-born and -educated psychiatrists. The state psychiatric culture evidenced a cumbersome, bureaucratic machinery. By 1975, leadership was lacking at every hierarchical level, from the commissioner of mental health and others in the Central Mental Health Office, to the leadership within the state mental hospitals, to the regional and county mental health programs. The culture's ethos was characterized by a lethargy borne of frustration and hopelessness at being able to improve or change the system.

Even as late as 1975, when the APA evaluated the residency programs in Maryland, it referred to serious limitations in the training in the state hospitals. It wrote:

> (T)he three State Hospital Psychiatric Residency Training Programs encompass about twenty-five foreign-trained residents who go to Baltimore one-half to one day a week to participate in an "acculturation program," and attend seminars and didactic lectures. (APA 1976:30)

In 1976 a young, brash, ideologically motivated "child of the sixties," university-trained psychiatrist became the director of the Mental Hygiene Administration in Maryland. He appointed other university-trained psychiatrists in the State Central Office and began to link some state institutions, large mental hospitals, an inner-city community mental health centers, and a research center, with the university. Thus began the joint university-state residency training program, in which university-trained psychiatrists and residents began to work and train in the state hospitals. By 1981, three university-trained psychiatrists assumed positions of superintendent and clinical directors of two of the three large state mental hospitals. An active collaboration with the university developed where university residency training took place in state hospitals, and university psychiatrists were placed in important leadership positions, such as clinical directors and superintendents. These changes served as catalysts for changes in a system which had traditionally been committed to resist most changes.

Ken Oak State Hospital

Ken Oak State Hospital was one of the four large inpatient facilities in Maryland. It was also the most neglected hospital in the state. Like the other large state hospitals, Ken Oak's early history reflected periods of immense neglect both of the human and the physical conditions within it. Whereas substandard conditions were the norm for all of the state hospitals for much of their existence, the particular history and geographical location of Ken Oak contributed to its greater neglect.

An evaluation study authorized by the governor in 1976 found that the conditions for patients at Ken Oak were uniformly more restrictive than the other three large Maryland hospitals. The evaluation study found that 40 percent of the overall treatment was poor to marginal, patient records generally lacked medical history, and staff and patient morale was low. The evaluation study stated: 1) violations of state and hospital policies regarding working hours, physician presence and treatment documentation had been going on since 1968, and continued to occur (p.150); and 2) "a number of employees schedule work hours and work days purely for the convenience of the employee" (p.146).

Only one of twenty-two psychiatrists at Ken Oak in 1982 was board-certified. The majority of the psychiatrists were male, state-trained, over forty years old, and had come to the United States during the 1950s and the 1960s from countries in the Third World, particularly the Middle East, to take residency training in psychiatry. The state hospitals were the only option for them to practice medicine.

Culture Conflicts in Ken Oak Hospital

In 1982, a university-trained female psychiatrist in her thirties, Dr. Burke, was appointed Clinical Director at Ken Oak. The arrival of a university-trained psychiatrist in a position of authority was not greeted with enthusiasm by most of the staff. Because Ken Oak had been more isolated and neglected, it was also more resistant to change than the other state hospitals in Maryland. Ken Oak was noted for its close-knit networks among nonpsy-chiatrist staff members, some of whom were third generation employees.

Three days after Dr. Burke became Clinical Director at Ken Oak, she became dramatically aware that the state psychiatrists were not taking responsibility for their patients. A nurse on an acute admission ward called to inform her that no physician was available for that ward. Dr. Burke then discovered that the psychiatrist in charge of that ward was on vacation for three months. The psychiatrist who was covering for him was on vacation for two months. And the psychiatrist who was covering for the second psy-chiatrist (and therefore for two wards) was also on vacation, for two weeks. Thus, three wards, with a total of over 100 patients, had no doctor.

Many staff members informed Dr. Burke of the unavailability and irresponsibility of the physicians at Ken Oak. Some examples highlight these points.

- The hardest thing in this hospital is to try to call a doctor. (Nurse)
- The doctors only look in the book about the patients. They don't look at the patients. They should talk to the patients to find out what's happening. (Nurse)
- Doctors do not read their notes. You have to find the doctor and tell him in person because you cannot rely upon him to read it. So you have to find him, and he is rarely there to find. (Dietician)
- A lot of staff members are afraid of patients, especially the doctors. The doctors lock themselves in the room and leave the violent patients on the ward for others to deal with. (Social worker)

A state auditor's report referred to the unavailability of psychiatrists to telephone operators' calls. Many only spent four or five of the required eight hours a day in Ken Oak. They engaged in paid private practice during hours they were required to work at Ken Oak. They did not arrange for coverage for their patients when they were not in the hospital.

The unavailability of physicians was highlighted on an occasion in which a sheriff came to Ken Oak to deliver a summons to a psychiatrist. The sheriff said, "I've been coming here for thirty years. You never find doctors around. I'd come and no one knew where they were. I'd come back two or three more times. Sometimes I tried at their homes. But so often I'd return the summons as 'undeliverable'."

When Dr. Burke first arrived as Clinical Director of Ken Oak, she discovered that the 1976 Evaluation Study had understated the problems of Ken Oak. The Evaluation Study did not report on the psychiatrists because the evaluators could not obtain access to them. During her first three days at Ken Oak, Dr. Burke came to understand the reasons for the psychia-trists' secretiveness.

The psychiatrists did not comply with state policies, and no one systematically enforced them. Dr. Burke found no written records of physicians' meetings, correspondence, or ward activities. Patient records revealed that many psychiatrists rarely saw their patients, they neglected to read or act on staff notes, and their secretaries wrote progress notes because the psychiatrists themselves did not see the patients. Many psychiatrists neglected to fill out discharge summaries and write transfer notes. They signed certificates, discharge summaries, and incidence reports without seeing the patients. Many progress notes only contained a half a line, such as, "medication prescribed." The majority of the patients were diagnosed as having chronic undifferentiated schizophrenia, which had a poor prognosis. Few were diagnosed as having manic-depression, as many patients in modern psychiatric hospitals were found to have, and which has a promising prognosis. The psychiatrists tended to keep patients in the hospital for long periods of time.

There was virtually no therapeutic monitoring of drug levels. The physicians rarely monitored drug levels or changed the drugs they prescribed during patients' long stays; nor did they review or change patients' privilege levels during patients' stays. In the pharmacy, no new drugs had been requested or ordered from the formulary for the past five years. Fifteen-year-old drugs still sat on the pharmacy shelves. Many of the physicians practiced polypharmacy, often prescribing subtherapeutic doses of multiple drugs.

Ken Oak had a bad reputation in the legal community because promises had been broken, letters had not been sent, responses to court orders had either not answered questions, or had provided incompetent responses. When the Joint Commission for the Accreditation of Hospitals (JCAH) came to Ken Oak in 1982, they did not grant accreditation. They commented critically about treatment plans, among other things. The commission said:

- Conceptually (the psychiatrists) do not understand about treatment plans, how they fit together and how you use them. They have no idea how the whole process flows.

- Treatment plan addresses same issues month after month, in spite of the fact that goals and methods are ineffective, without change or progress notes to support continuation of plan.

- Treatment plans are present but goals are not related to treatment. Some individual treatment plans included the following:

1.
Target Problem: Probably depression.
Goal for Patient: Reduce depression.
Corrective Approach: Supervision by nursing staff.

2.

Target Problem:	Patient is aggressive.
Goal for Patient:	Patient will be more cooperative.
Corrective Approach:	Nurse will supervise patient for aggressive outbursts.

One patient's record read, "He has no acute medical or psychiatric problem." Yet the patient had been hospitalized for years and was medicated on high doses of neuroleptics.

As a young, female, American university-trained, and board-certified psychiatrist, Dr. Burke contrasted significantly with most of the psychiatrists at Ken Oak. Their education and cultural backgrounds, particularly their beliefs about rates of change and modern Western bureaucracies, as well as about women, age and authority, were at great variance with the cultures, symbols, and values which Dr. Burke represented.

The psychiatrists feared and resisted her largely because she represented an unwanted and threatening incursion into their culture. They also resisted her because they feared that although they were state employees, they might lose their jobs. They had noted that in the other state hospitals in which the university gained a foothold, there were many changes in the roles of the state psychiatrists. Some of those psychiatrists had left the hospitals and university psychiatrists were hired or promoted to replace them.

The state psychiatrists perceived that the university psychiatrists condescended to them and/or denigrated them, thus ignoring all that they had "achieved" for the hospital in the past, under "very difficult" circumstances. Indeed, the university psychiatrists did look condescendingly and in a denigrating manner upon the state psychiatrists; they believed that "nothing happened in the state system before 1976." Some of the state psychiatrists explicitly told Dr. Burke of their reluctance to have her and her culture in Ken Oak: "I don't want the university to bring their world to ours. They are different."

For the first year, the state hospital staff unrelentingly resisted Dr. Burke's attempts to initiate changes. They continued to call in sick on Fridays and Mondays. They continued to sign in and out at times other than when they actually came in and out. They continued to leave before the physician on night duty arrived. Most of the resistance to Dr. Burke was in the form of opposition, both overt and covert, to innovations she attempted to implement. They continued to remind her of her newness to the state system, her lack of experience in the state hospital. They repeated that their long experience in the state gave them knowledge of what could be done. A typical response to an innovative suggestion was, "That's not going to work. We've been here longer." When she tried to implement a schedule for night duty, they opposed each alternative she suggested. When she tried to promote the more able of the state psychiatrists, they resisted. For example, one replied, "I feel too tired to go to a pressured area and with fast turnover. I am trying to ease down." When she mandated that the "somatic doctors" talk with the patients (they did not feel it necessary to talk to patients), the Director of the Somatic Service resigned.

When Dr. Burke talked about some plans for introducing new therapeutic modalities in Ken Oak and tried to encourage the physicians to learn them, there was considerable resistance. For example, a state psychiatrist said, "We've been doing this for a long period of time, and we've been doing quality patient care. You are new here."

Dr. Burke sent a memo to the physicians to write a diagnosis when they requested laboratory tests, and the doctors protested. One said, "You may not have a diagnosis. It may be a routine admission." She responded, "Put down the admission diagnosis." Another psychiatrist replied, "We'll put in 'admission' for diagnosis." One psychiatrist asked, "What if they are normal?" She responded, "You mean to say that people come to this hospital and they are perfectly normal?" One psychiatrist said, "The nurses know more about the diagnoses. We don't know." Dr. Burke answered, "Do you talk to the patient?" The psychiatrist, in all earnestness, said "No." Dr. Burke replied, "If you don't talk to the patient, you do not know the patient." A psychiatrist responded, "If a patient is here for a long time—a chronic—with no change, there is no need to see the patient often." One psychiatrist told her, "The doctors are united in their anger against you."

The state people were fully aware of the events that had occurred in the two other large hospitals where university psychiatrists assumed leadership positions. Many state psychiatrists left, and university psychiatrists were hired or promoted to replace them. The state psychiatrists were acutely aware of the low esteem with which the university psychiatrists regarded them.

A state psychiatrist described his perceptions of the university psychiatrists:

> Everyone who comes from the university, they feel so grandiose, as if they took a course in grandiosity. They know everything. No one else knows anything. I find it difficult to have university psychiatrists. Whatever they say is beyond everyone's head. They assume that we have a very primitive hospital where no one knows what he is doing. He tries to impress. The best person to teach us is someone who has worked in the state system. All American doctors are not brilliant. Over the years it has always been us at the bottom.

Many of the state psychiatrists believed that they had been deprived and exploited in the past. Their preoccupation with personal and occupational deprivation led them to de-emphasize their professional obligations to their patients. They had a strong feeling of entitlement, believing that the state system 'owed' them. One psychiatrist said,

Nonrational Bureaucracies (State Culture)	Rational Bureaucracies (University Culture)
Professional activities revolve around personal relationships.	Professional activities revolve around written rules.
Tradition and the status quo are valued. The past is revered.	Newness is valued. Past is to be changed.
Age obtains authority, prestige, and status.	Ability obtains authority, prestige, and status. Youth is more current.
Males hold all authority, prestige, and status.	The sexes are (ideally) absolutely equal.
Past experience is important.	Newness is better and takes precedence over past.
Time flows, passes, exists, and is to be experienced.	Time flies. Time is money. Time is to be used.
Rules, time, and numbers are not definite, but negotiable.	Rules, time, and numbers are definite.

Figure 1. Bureaucratic Characteristics

> We've been working here for a long time with poor salaries and poor working conditions. We've been through a lot in this hospital. Whoever comes in from the outside, they try to punish us. We took care of this hospital up until now and no one appreciated it.

Their statements are reminiscent of the "rhetoric of complaint" found in social interactions in Mediterranean countries (Gaines 1982; Gaines and Farmer 1986). This involves the use of self-portraits of suffering that demonstrate one's worthiness as a social person (also see Lee 1959) and which simultaneously suggests one's psychological depth (Good, Good and Moradi 1985). Table 1 illustrates some of the ways in which the values of the state-trained psychiatrists in Ken Oak hospital contrasted with the values of the university-trained psychiatrists. The cultural values of the state-trained psychiatrists were based upon a state mental health culture of the past. Its cumbersome, static, inefficient bureaucracy had much in common with the values and operations of the bureaucracies of the countries from which these psychiatrists came. As noted, most of them were older (over forty) male psychiatrists from Third World countries. The majority were from Middle Eastern countries, and a small minority were from Southeast and East Asian countries. When they came to the United States, the only residencies open to them were those in psychiatry at state hospitals.

In nonrational bureaucracies, as well as traditional Middle Eastern cultures, a person's reputation was based more upon ascribed status, such as age, sex, and kinship, than upon his achieved status, such as education or social mobility (Patai 1983; Weber 1968). A person's reputation determined not only his own behavior but also the ways in which he expected others to behave. Often little distinction was made between behavior and expectations of behavior of near-equal males enacted in personal domains from those enacted in professional domains. Kinship, friendship, and business or professional relationships (the latter of which were often also kinship) between near-equal males were considered to be personal relationships based upon trust.

In Ken Oak State Hospital, the values about the authority of age and sex conflicted sharply with those of the university-trained psychiatrists. The latter valued authority based on education, training, motivation, achieved leadership, and, frequently, youth. The presence of a young woman in the authority position of clinical director represented a serious threat to the values and status hierarchy of the state-trained psychiatrists.

The psychiatrists responded to Dr. Burke in a highly personalized manner because of her sex, age, and limited experience. They often told her that she was so attractive that they could not concentrate in her presence. They frequently complained that she, personally, was punishing them, not, for example, that the policies she implemented (which were usually existent policies which had never been enforce) were restricting or controlling. They often accompanied their use of the word "punish" with a quick, chopping gesture, suggesting a particular form of female retaliation.

Their responses indicated that they regarded her behavior as personalized through her femaleness and not as universalized through her professional role. A typical personalized response by a state psychiatrist toward Dr. Burke occurred at an introductory meeting, her first week at Ken Oak: "It's not going to work with you. You are a woman. You are much younger. You are an outsider, not from the state service."

In Ken Oak State Hospital, the state-trained psychiatrists revered tradition and regarded age, experience, and the passing of time as bestowing wisdom and status. They perceived Dr. Burke's youth and short tenure in the state hospital system as invalidating her authority. They often referred to these values in their objections and resistance to her. One psychiatrist told her, for example, "When you get older, you will do better." When Dr. Burke referred to the timeliness of a medical intervention with a patient, a state psychiatrist said, "Time never made any difference to me. We are accustomed to do things without thinking about time."

In the nonrational bureaucracies, professional activities frequently revolved around personal, friendly, face-to-face relationships based upon trust (cf. Weber 1968). The specific nature of each relationship was negotiated between the parties. In contrast, in rational bureaucracies, professional activities revolve around written rules, not personal negotiation. The state-trained psychiatrists at Ken Oak frequently complained about the "impersonal" style of communications between Dr. Burke and themselves. For example, when she began to write memos enforcing existing policies, the psychiatrists took great personal offense. They perceived that she was attacking their person, not that their behavior violated regulation.

For example, Dr. Burke wrote a memo to one of the psychiatrists who had been absent from the hospital during working hours because he was engaging in private practice outside the hospital. That psychiatrist approached her with the "impersonalness" of the memo and how he was singled out "personally." He first complained that he was the only physician who supported her. Then he complained that the memo was "very impersonal."

The psychiatrists complained that Dr. Burke was not being "friendly" when she attempted to enforce the rules. For example, one said, "things should change, we agree. But the way to handle things, you need to be friendly." Another addressed her in the third person in his threat to resist her: "We are sorry that Dr. Burke has no friends." One psychiatrist told Dr. Burke, "We want to comply with rules and regulations. But we'd like a little bit more 'affection'." Dr. Burke responded, "If I didn't care or have affection for this work, I wouldn't be here." A psychiatrist said, "I object that the medical director is taking the responsibility of the personnel department. How do you expect us to cooperate with you when you check my time."

The psychiatrists frequently rephrased substantive issues as personal issues. In response to the enforcement of their prescribed working hours, one said, "You can't do that, Doctor. This regimentation is stifling and unnecessary. We are more than willing to assist you to do this job." When Dr. Burke reminded the physicians that they had to spell out treatment plans, they responded, "Do you want all of this included?" and "Do you want me to spend an hour or two writing up treatment plans?" One psychiatrist who came in two hours late in the morning and left two hours early in the evening responded to the time regulations by saying, "I personally don't mind coming late. It doesn't really matter, whether it is 8:30, 9:30 or 10:00. However, if you want me to come at 8:30..." Dr. Burke responded, "It's not what I want." The psychiatrist responded in an exaggerated compliant tone, "Whatever you want."

The psychiatrists suggested that all regulations were personally negotiable and that time was never precise, but approximate. Modern rational bureaucracies place value upon precision and specificity, such as represented by time or numbers (Weber 1968). In personalized bureaucracies, such as the traditional state hospital system or as Middle Eastern bureaucracies, everything is negotiable and dependent upon the personal attributes of the leader (see Blue, this volume; Patai 1983; Weber 1968). One psychiatrist said, "It seems to me that rules and regulations are guidelines. Instead of just messing around with the time, if I come late, it'll be time that I owe you."

A conflict between precision and negotiation was illustrated when several somatic physicians requested that their work load be reduced because they had too much work. Dr. Burke asked them to document their time and activities. They refused to document their activities, accused her of not believing them, and implored her to trust them. In the discussions it emerged that these physicians never made rounds. Dr. Burke suggested that they should, indeed, examine patients. They responded angrily:

> You didn't spell out that we have to go on the wards to examine patients. One person has an idea, another person has an idea, and you decide in between.

Dr. Burke told the physicians:

> There should be a definite time and place to meet with the psychiatric consultant. Twice a week with each set of physicians, and on a regular basis the four of you should meet to address yourselves about patients.
> Physician A: Each time we see each other we'll discuss the patient. Why the four of us? Why not two of us?
> Dr. Burke: The more you know about each other's patients, the better their care.
> Physician B: We always talked whenever we see each other. But to meet at a specific time, and to go especially to meet...
> Physician C: It's not good to get together in a group.
> Physician D: We discuss it automatically.

Rational bureaucracies depend upon the dissemination of and adherence to written rules; nonrational bureaucracies value oral communication and personal interpretation (cf. Weber 1968). One psychiatrist told Dr. Burke, "Most of the information on the patients is not on the charts. It is passed on orally." When Dr. Burke asked a psychiatrist about a particular policy, he answered,

> There is no written policy. It is customary. What we've been doing is what we routinely do. It becomes an unwritten policy. It has been going on for over fifteen years.

Dunham and Weinberg described the rationale for the state psychiatrists' resistance to innovations:

Getting something done quickly, accurately, and efficiently is perhaps the most basic sin anyone can commit within the hospital society.
This is particularly true because the desire of any person to introduce
something new is likely to be disturbing to someone else who has a vested interest in some aspect of hospital life. (1960:64–65)

Conclusions

Despite the strong resistance, Dr. Burke was able to institute significant changes at Ken Oak Hospital. A university culture crept more and
more into the state culture, as the combined state-university psychiatric
residency program became institutionalized. Teaching seminars and rounds
were integrated into the routines for all staff. The university psychiatric
residency program, encompassing four wards, became firmly established at
the hospital. It was staffed by university-trained psychiatrists and third-
year psychiatry residents from the combined state-university residency
program. Ken Oak was also able to attract more highly educated psychologists and nurses.

Within two years of Dr. Burke's arrival, resistance against her and
the university culture weakened considerably. Many of the state psychiatrists improved in their knowledge base and in their patient care (see Katz
1985; Katz and Kirkland 1990). In 1985, three years after Dr. Burke's
arrival, two acute-admissions' wards (one with a state-trained psychiatrist
and one with a university-trained psychiatrist) were restudied. Although
some aspects of psychiatric leadership and patient care differed, the state-
trained psychiatrists had improved considerably. In 1987, Ken Oak State
Hospital was given JCAH accreditation, a demonstration of local influence.
(For which, see also Maretzki, this volume.)

However, many aspects of the state hospitals have not changed drastically. The conflicts lie dormant and are expressed largely by long-term state
psychiatrists who continue to perform the minimum legally mandated
actions. The state system of seniority still protects long-term employees
from losing their jobs.

The complex network of state-university linkages has resulted in a
much wider interpretation and implementation of the state's ability to care
for the mentally ill. Patients receive better care in some parts of all twelve
state hospitals (Katz 1984a, 1985). Increased commitment to the mentally ill
in public hospitals by recently trained psychiatrists is represented by their
increased exposure to and recruitment into public-service psychiatry. The
cultures of both the state and the university are changing, although many
parts of the state mental health system have acculturated to that of the university.

References

American Psychiatric Association
1976 Maryland Department of Health and Mental Hygiene. A Study by the Consultation and Evaluation Services Board. Washington, D.C.

Caudill, William
1958 The Psychiatric Hospital as a Small Society. Cambridge, MA: The University Press.

Caudill, William et al.
1952 Social Structure and Interaction on a Psychiatric Ward. American Journal of Orthopsychiatry 22:314–334.

Deutsch, Albert
1949 The Mentally Ill in America: A History of Their Care and Treatment From Colonial Times. New York: Columbia University Press.

Dunham, H. Warren and S. Kirson Weinberg
1960 The Culture of the State Mental Hospital. Detroit: Wayne State University Press.

Faulkner, L. R. and J. S. Eaton
1979 Administrative Relationships between Community Mental Health Centers and Academic Psychiatry Departments. American Journal of Psychiatry 136:1040 1044.

Gaines, Atwood D.
1982 Cultural Definitions, Behavior and the Person in American Psychiatry. In Cultural Conceptions of Mental Health and Therapy. A. Marsella and G. White (eds.). Dordrecht, Holland and Boston: D. Reidel Publishing Company.

Gaines, Atwood D. and Paul E. Farmer
1986 Visible Saints: Social Cynosures and Dysphoria in the Mediterranean Tradition. Culture, Medicine and Psychiatry 10(3):295–330.

Gilbert, A. and Daniel J. Levinson
1957 The Patient and the Mental Hospital: Contributions of Research in the Science of Social Behavior. Milton Greenblatt et al. (eds.). Glencoe, IL: Free Press.

Good, B., M. -J. DelVecchio Good and R. Moradi
1985 The Interpretation of Iranian Depressive Illness and Dysphoric Affect. In Culture and Depression. A. Kleinman and B. Good (eds.). Berkeley: University of California Press.

Greenblatt, Milton, et. al.
1955 From Custodial to Therapeutic Patient Care in Mental Hospitals: Explorations in Social Treatment. New York: Russell Sage Foundation.

Grob, Gerald, N.
1983 Mental Illness and American Society, 1875–1940. Princeton, New Jersey: Princeton University Press.

Harbin, Henry T., et. al.
1982 Psychiatric Manpower and Public Mental Health: Maryland's Experience. Hospital Community Psychiatry 33:277–281.

Hurd, Henry M.
1911 The Site of Johns Hopkins Hospital. The Johns Hopkins Nurses' Alumnae Magazine 19:5–20.

Katz, Pearl
1984a A Comparison of University Trained and Non-University Trained Psychiatrists on State Hospital Wards. Unpublished manuscript.
1984b History of the Public Mental Health System in Maryland: 1773–1976, Unpublished manuscript.
1985 Effects of Changes on Patients in State Hospitals. Paper presented at the American Psychiatric Association Annual Meeting, Washington, D.C.

Katz, Pearl and Faris R. Kirkland
1990 Violence and Social Structure in Mental Hospital Wards. Psychiatry.

Lee, Dorothy
1959 Views of the Self in Greek Culture. In Freedom and Culture. Dorothy Lee. Inglewood Cliffs, NJ: Prentice Hall.

McGuire, Patrick
1982 Young Idealistic Psychiatrists Win Acclaim for State Hospitals. The Sunday Sun. Baltimore. December.

Miller, Robert
1983 Turnabout in Maryland State Hospital Employment. Clinical Psychiatry News 11.

Morrissey, Joseph P., Howard H. Goldman and Lorraine V. Klerman
1980 Approaches to the Study of Institutional Reform. In The Enduring Asylum: Cycles of Institutional Reform at Worcester State Hospital. Joseph P. Morrissey, Howard H. Goldman and Lorraine V. Klerman (eds.). New York: Grune and Stratton.

Patai, Raphael
1983 The Arab Mind. New York: Scribners.

Psychiatric News
1984 Cooperation Needed Between Universities, State Institutions 20:1. July 6.

Romano, John
1975 Keynote Address. American Psychiatry: Past, Present, and Future. In American Psychiatry: Past, Present, and Future. George Kriegman, Robert D. Gardner and Wilfred Abse (eds.). Charlottesville: University Press of Virginia.

Russell, Christine
1983 Young Psychiatrists Revolutionize Maryland Institutions. Washington Post. June 26.

Sarbin, Theodore R. and Joseph B. Juhasz
1982 The Concept of Mental Illness: A Historical Perspective. In Culture and Psychopathology. Ihsan Al-Issa (ed.). Baltimore: University Park Press.

Sergeant, Marilyn
1983 The Maryland Plan, Revolution in Mental Health Care. Alcohol, Drug Abuse and Mental Health 9:1. June 24.

Stanton, Alfred and Morris S. Schwartz
1954 The Mental Hospital. New York: Basic Books.

Starr, Paul
1982 The Social Transformation of American Medicine. New York: Basic Books.

Talbott, John, ed.
1980 State Mental Hospitals: Problems and Prospects. New York: Human Sciences.

Thompson, J. W. et al.
1983 The Decline of State Mental Hospitals as Training Sites for Psychiatric Residents. American Journal of Psychiatry 140.

Varma, S. C.
1984 Problems in State Hospitals Versus University Training. American Journal of Psychiatry 139:1036–1039.

Weber, Max
1968 (1922) Economy and Society: An Outline of Interpretive Sociology. G. Roth and W. Ilick (eds.). E. Fischoff, trans. New York: Bedminster Press.

15

Georg Groddeck's Integrative Massage and Psychotherapy Treatment in Germany

Thomas W. Maretzki

Introduction: Groddeck's Medical Conservation and Innovations

"Healing," "curing," and "doctoring" are descriptive terms for the multiple activities and functions of specialized cultural agents providing health care. The restoration of health involves changes of states in human awareness and functioning. This process defies a clear delineation and it is therefore subject to multiple cultural explanations which resonate with the social context in which these processes occur. Healing is the most general of these terms which allows for effects of self-help as well as those of other agents. Only doctoring as a term refers to a more specific process of health restoration in which an expert, specialized in medical curing, applies existing knowledge and associated skills.

In the Western world, and increasingly in most other parts of the world, forms of allopathic medicine, with specific traditions of medical curing and doctoring, have become dominant (e.g., German, French, American biomedicines) and not without a variety of struggles that are specific to the particular nation, e.g., United States (Brown 1979), Germany (Maretzki 1988, 1989; Rothschuh 1983).

It appears to be taken for granted by growing numbers of people that allopathic Western curing principles exceed all others in efficacy. Allopathic medicine implies a preference for the utilization of chemically synthesized pharmaceutical substances to act curatively on cell structures and organ systems. This is done, according to theory, in order to achieve a reversal of detrimental processes.

Such methods contrast with a diverse range of other principles involved in the restoration of health. Some of these "alternatives" involve healing through assumptions or recognitions of events which can not be explained by simple reductionism and are, therefore, often referred to as "natural." The exploration and understanding of these different principles, their culturally created meaning, and their social context lead to a meeting ground of medical anthropologists with medical historians and philosophers of science and medicine. The ethnomedical analyst ventures furthest into comparisons of knowledge systems whose ontological basis and order of complexity enlarges the frames of other philosophical examinations.

Although the knowledge of allopathic medicine is laid down and constantly modified in standard books—the medical texts—physicians are the living carriers of this medical knowledge as well as the responsibles in its application. Through professionalization of health care, the maintenance of normative standards is established and monitored. Professionalization only indirectly standardizes the clinical activities of physicians. Once trained and licensed, physicians are free to deviate from normative curing practices of their profession. Increasingly—at least in the United States—deviance from "community" standards of medical practice invokes the risk of judicial censure. Though physicians who apply a range of health restoration principles that is broader than that taught in medical schools are always in a minority, they have, in the past, played significant roles in society; the same may be said of some "alternative" physicians at present. How much leeway physicians feel is allowed to their doctoring approach varies with national medical systems.

The present chapter begins the illumination of the ways that one Western European physician displayed an independence of medical thought and action within the context of professionalizing and standardizing forces. Georg Groddeck's clinical domain was not then, but is now, classified— especially in North America—as *psychiatric care*, and, more broadly, as *psychotherapy*.

In each culture, the specialist or professional therapist, intentionally or unintentionally, defines and redefines the body of knowledge created and received pertaining to illness interpretation (diagnosis) and intervention (clinical/therapeutic action). Professionals should not be seen as passive recipients of medical education and as blank slates before training. For example, Gaines (1979) has shown how the psychiatrist-in-training holds individualized explanatory models of illness and treatment acquired as members of the wider culture (or an evangelical Christian subculture [1982, 1985]) before undertaking professional training. These conceptions may only partially correspond to the formal and abstracted system(s) of knowledge presented, i.e., the explicit orientation/ideology, in the program of medical education.

The ideology and the role of the medical (in a broad sense) specialist in any culture may, therefore, be seen as constituted from different levels of knowledge. These levels appear as idiosyncratic models or as ethno- or "folk" theories of and in medical practice in the interpretive medical anthropological literature (e.g., Bosk 1979; Gaines and Hahn 1982; Hahn and Gaines 1985; Lock and Gordon 1988).

One challenge for physicians of allopathic medicine, examined and reexamined by medical, social science and popular literature, concerns the transposing of some illness complaints from the reductionist model of the natural sciences to other levels. In the West, this medical task involves—broadly speaking—psychological processes, including the abstraction and interpretation of symbolic constructs. In historical traditions of the West or other cultures parallel illness phenomena were resolved through more integrated interpretations and treatments of equilibrium-based or "holistic" medical practice.

The bifurcation of body and mind in current or "modern" thinking leaves to the individual practitioner (as a conforming or nonconforming professional) the challenge of applying suitable interpretations that do justice at all levels of significance. Kleinman's (1988) discussion of somatization and depression as historically and cross-culturally changing conceptualizations draws attention to the need for an ethnomedical perspective.

Recent discussions centering on historical and cross-cultural ontological conceptualizations of somatization and depression reveal the unresolved philosophical problems to be found in attempts to translate ethnomedical perspectives of the realities of human afflictions into universal parameters (Kleinman and Good 1985; Kleinman 1986, 1988; Shweder 1988).

The conceptual problems we encounter here, and in so many writings, were created through a dominant medical belief system, that of biomedicine, which Young (1976) has characterized as being "internalizing" in its etiological hypotheses, as opposed to the "externalizing" tendencies of traditional medicines. Even if this typology appears too simple, it reaffirms that Western specialists have had to struggle for some time to conceptually integrate phenomena which appear together only through the language use of hyphenation or by other devices (e.g., "metonymic metaphors" [Shweder 1988:489]). These devices are employed to attempt to overcome the conceptual distinctions, which often yet remain (e.g., mind/body).

Georg Groddeck of Germany, whose patients presented their complaints primarily through somatized symptoms, offers an example of a physician sensitive to the complexity of illnesses, complexities which cannot be resolved through reductionism. He developed and maintained a role structured around personal insights and convictions suitable to his cultural context. His individualized clinical experiences and treatments coincide with the innovation of psychosomatic medicine as a new medical category claiming universal clinical relevance. Its validity remains a source for continued arguments and insights.

Some anthropologists have replicated the Western division into soma and psyche by referring to processes of healing and curing as overall dimensions of medical intervention. These distinctions are meaningful only if their referents are made clear by differentiating intended results of actions from the unintended byproducts (Moerman 1979).

We find parallels in Western medical history about etiologies which are marked or masked by language concepts connoting divergent philosophical bases. In such studies, "holistic medicine" as a linguistic label reflects generalized and vague conceptions and responses of more traditional values integrating natural processes in contrast to "psychosomatic medicine," a biomedical specialization which likewise defies a clear definition (Lipowski 1984).

Long before the seventeenth-century philosophical division of body and mind, the phenomena perceived as interfering with human functioning, to which these medical approaches refer, were known and addressed by Hippocratic medicine (Ackerknecht 1982). In the modern allopathic medical context, the distinction reflects the organization of biomedical knowledge. Where holistic medicine strives more eclectically and informally towards simplicity, clarity of problem conceptualization and therapy strategies, psychosomatic medicine is a modernized, systematized, and organized body of knowledge and practice of a biomedical specialization (Uexküll and Wesiack 1979, 1988).

The process of differentiation within biomedicine is gradual. The spread of Freudian psychoanalysis provided a basis which, combined with neurophysiological knowledge, established this specialization over the last five or six decades. Georg Groddeck is often named as one of the earliest physicians practicing psychosomatic medicine. In his philosophy of medicine and in his medical practice are reflected integrated techniques of an earlier period, coupled with diverse etiological and therapeutic approaches encountered in contemporary biomedical practice. The justification for presenting Groddeck's medical philosophy and his role at a critical period of transition lies in the possibilities of gaining further insights into issues entailed by the terms "curing" and "healing" and by the continued bifurcation of human problems in biomedicine.

Groddeck as Medical Practitioner

Groddeck's practice illustrates, as have examples of other ethnomedical studies, that even in a professionalized Western medical system, the construction of clinical reality is as much a product of personal healer philosophy and style of interaction as it is the abstractions of traditional or codified medical theory. Groddeck used time-honored medical practice in a context of biomedical professionalization and institutionalization. The style of this physician, a professional maverick, a nonconforming individual who reintroduced traditional techniques as innovative or deviant professional approaches, illustrates, moreover, how the labels of *holism* or *psychosomatic* medicine viewed as models of clinical practice, are idealized abstractions.

As a physician, Groddeck was not an independent agent who could apply any dazzling healing technique or theory without constraints; he was a member of an organized profession and his activities projected levels of both professional and individual theoretical knowledge construction (also see Gaines [1982, 1985] on Christian psychiatry and DelVecchio Good [1985] on competence discourse). But Groddeck adhered only marginally to normative professional conventions, linkages and contrasts between historical conceptions in medicine and an emerging specialty's body of knowledge, that of psychoanalysis. His deliberate adherence to traditions is particularly noteworthy. The case I present here is based on the literature, his own writings and those of others, and on Groddeck's biography by Herbert Will (1984), not upon personal acquaintance or interviews.

Groddeck's writings offer a mostly restrained and reflexive dialectical role of the therapist, not the treatises of a proselytizing theoretician (e.g., 1966, 1984a, b, 1985). They are expressions of his living and guiding philosophy, partly directed towards those he treated. Groddeck's prolific writings have recently been republished with comments by H. Siefert (1986). Groddeck had a small, very devoted following of patients as well as readers, and the two groups overlapped. He also was respected by some renowned persons of his time as well as some critical or even depreciating comments from his peers. In retrospect, Groddeck stands out as one among a small group of German (or West European) physicians who practiced their own idiosynchratic version of allopathic medicine, coupled with other approaches in a small private hospital, still called—as in Groddeck's days—a *sanatorium*.

Details of Groddeck's medical practice are reflected in his numerous writings and in a few reminiscences by former staff members and patients. One example is that of Magda Knoch, a nurse and the long-time head of the small staff. Her title was *Leiterin* (director) of the sanatorium. She describes some of her early impressions and experiences (1985).

Staff and patients (referred to as "guests") formed a close relationship in the small clinic. Many of the sufferers returned periodically. Patients appeared to present with the range of complaints typical of a general practitioner's or internist's practice. For each guest a separate regimen was prescribed by Groddeck and administered by the staff under his strict supervision. Meals were taken individually in the guest's room, not communally in a dining hall. The sanatorium otherwise reflected a spirit of community which Groddeck fostered through his regular in-house lectures as well as other events. Members of the wider community of Baden-Baden were invited to these along with the sanatorium's own guests.

The sanatorium was a little community in which the doctor was the center of attention and reverence, though every effort was directed towards each patient's individual welfare and healing needs. Groddeck cultivated his role of authority as part of his therapeutic strategy. Some of the descriptions of his activities reflect a very German style of interaction, reminding one of those described for certain Japanese therapies and styles of interaction with physicians typical for hospitals treating *shinkieshitsu* (Reynolds 1980). (See also Nomura, this volume.)

Fifty years after Groddeck's death in Baden-Baden, the significance of his contributions was resurrected when a small, very diverse group of professional and lay persons honored him in a commemorative ceremony. This event, and the republication of his work in paperback editions, testifies to the lasting qualities of this physician (Jagersberg 1984). Georg Groddeck insisted that he was no more than a general practitioner serving people who suffered and needed help. That the group of admirers today is described as "followers, fans and researchers" (Siefert et al. 1986) strengthens an impression of the physician Groddeck as a kind of folk hero, not a popularist, but a therapist who deeply draws on cultural traditions of his social milieu. This practitioner was not the charitable physician of the poor, although he was socially minded. He was a physician of the middle class who commands a renewed interest today as this social level has broadened in Western populations, defining much of medical clinical problem formulation and therapy orientation. Above all, his current appeal is explained as the charisma of an unusual humanist physician.

Georg Groddeck was born in 1866 during the formative years of biomedicine. The son of a spa physician (*Badearzt*) in Thuringia, he began his medical studies in 1885. His clinical activities ended in 1934 with his death. From 1900, when he was thirty-four years old, he owned a small, fifteen-room sanatorium in Baden-Baden, the well-known South German spa area. From his early days of practice, his renown grew throughout Europe and beyond. My interpretation of Groddeck's role as a medical innovator combines an historical and cultural orientation.

A Cultural Philosophical Context

Medical anthropology's worldwide comparisons lead from cultural analyses back to fundamental philosophical questions about the sources of knowledge and action in human health and illness. These issues, buried in the positivism of the social sciences, were also familiar to social anthropologists studying non-Western religions. They also occupied some philosophers and physicians in Europe and continue to do so (Gordon 1988; Lock 1988; Uexküll and Wesiack 1988).

That in their modern (as against classical) form these philosophical issues in medicine of the West date back at least to the eighteenth century in Europe is not usually a part of the received knowledge in North American medical anthropology. European philosophy and medicine had a remarkable interaction during the formation of both fields as formal disciplines. In the Germany of Hegel and Schelling, explanations about illness were part of their naturalistic philosophies (Risse 1976).

A philosophical anthropology of that time which considered explorations into human nature and human suffering as essential knowledge for medical practice remained relevant as empirical knowledge in the treatment of the sick and through metaphysical arguments. These humanistic involvements linked the work of medically trained and otherwise well educated scholars until the first quarter of the nineteenth century, when knowledge systematization and controlled experiments in the natural sciences assumed a dominant role in medical knowledge. Later, studies by physicians and in the new field of psychology extended also to non-Western societies. Once culture emerged—at least in North America—as a central organizing concept for comparative studies, metaphysical and other philosophical explorations receded to obscure corners of the academy and its libraries. Western medicine took up the study of diseases in different societies, following a natural science model. Anthropologists took a long circuitous route *via* non-Western cultures to return to Western medicine as a cultural system.

Once this happened, one observer (Kleinman 1973) wrote that in the study of medicine, the "symbolic realm of ideas and actions becomes a fundamental problem with considerable practical and theoretical importance." North American medical anthropology, just then assuming a distinct profile within social anthropology, was returning to philosophy. In central Europe ethnomedicine developed as an interest within medicine which until recently did not produce cultural analyses. But an awareness of philosophical traditions relevant to medical practice was never lost in Europe among individual practitioners. Groddeck falls into this tradition of German medicine where philosophical and reflexively innovative writing by physicians is not uncommon.

In one sense, every physician faced with individualized illness must act as a therapeutic innovator. Medical therapy requires individual decisions beginning in diagnosis and leading to a therapeutic regimen for which even the most bureaucratized, rationalized medical system has no uniform prescriptions. Usually, our analysis of biomedical decisions is more relevant if it concentrates on the uniform aspects, the professional culture explaining actions, than on deliberate independence from a narrow therapeutic spectrum. In Germany, to this day, there is greater professional tolerance for therapeutic variations within biomedicine than in North America where the term "alternative therapies" is more appropriate. (See Oths, this volume.)

Groddeck represents an unusual example, even for his era, not only because of his deliberate unorthodoxy but because his therapies implicitly recognized the fact that the body speaks its own language of suffering in signs which can be read with approaches other than standard diagnostic examinations and laboratory tests (see Csordas, this volume; Ots 1990). How much this deliberateness stemmed from a coherent ideology whose historical and cultural traces can be identified, and to what extent it is due to the spontaneity of a devoted physician concerned with diverse patient problems, is the question I raise but must leave suspended for further contemplation and comparison.

In his introduction to Groddeck's biography, Will (1984) emphasizes that Freud, Fromm, and others acknowledge and frequently mention Groddeck as the originator of psychosomatic medicine, but this was not the view he had of himself. That he worked directly and creatively at the interface of natural science in medicine and its complimentary, but philosophically distinct, aspects of psychosomatic and psychotherapeutic directions, is unquestioned.

The Healer Role of a Humanistic Physician

Groddeck's medical role began under his major teacher, Ernst Schweninger, a professor at the University of Berlin. Appointed to this post through the influence of Chancellor Bismarck, whose personal physician he was, Schweninger had an explicit naturopathic medical orientation. This tolerance of a monolithic German academic biomedicine of an ideological outsider was not unique. There are other examples. Schweninger's impact was particularly noticeable because of Bismarck, whose multiple health complaints—later called psychosomatic—he managed to keep under control. His considerable influence on Bismarck's significant social legislation dealing with health is still indicated by the continuation into the present of the insurance-backed spa system. This system is now a part of rehabilitation medicine in Germany (Maretzki and Seidler 1985; Maretzki 1989).

The traditions of German romantic medicine lead in a relatively straight line to Schweninger's period when Groddeck was his student and medical assistant. Among these influential historical traditions were not only naturopathic therapies. Psychologically oriented treatments, based on suggestions, likewise have a history in medicine, at least since Mesmer's magnetism therapy (Schott 1985), later followed by Freud's interests in hypnotism. The latter led to the psychotherapeutic era. In the modernizing world, this period experienced a shift in major health problems from infectious to social and psychologically linked diseases associated with individual and group stresses and psychosomatics.

Groddeck followed his training with a short period in military service, then acted briefly as Chief of Medicine in Schweninger's Berlin sanatorium before he opened his own. The combination of hot baths, massage, and dietetic cures, known to him since childhood, and learned through Schweninger, now became a central element for Groddeck. His personal emphasis of an indispensable part of therapy was the therapeutic discourse with each patient.

Each part of therapy was carried out with a deliberate, almost compulsive, stress on the patient's involvement and the drudgery associated with tolerating the manipulations and treatments. Massage, so Groddeck said, offers a significant linkage between soma and psyche which affects all aspects of the human system, especially what he calls the "nervous system."

Important for an understanding of Groddeck's fundamental approach is the integrative nature of his treatment. Massage is necessary for diagnostics as well as for therapy. Massage sharpens the perception (Groddeck said the "eye") of the physician. It amplifies the channels by which a physician "senses" the patient's complaints along a total range of loci. Groddeck's procedures have a feedback value for the patient who is given a chance to focus on his illness and finds that massage channels it in directions which have personal significance or meaning. The sensations, even severely felt pains associated with massage, combined with Groddeck's elicitation of patients' feelings and associations, permitted him to carry out an in-depth analysis of symbolic, psychological and organic interconnections. Diagnosis and therapy merge into a unique, comprehensive analysis which only later Groddeck realized paralleled Freudian psychoanalysis, though it was applied to general somatic complaints.

Therapy is originally associated with serving (*dienen*), he writes (author's translations), "not with treatment (*behandeln*)." He continues, "Whoever serves, acknowledges those he serves as a master..." and, "it is the fate of the physician to serve and to treat (*zu dienen und zu behandeln*); his activity is ambivalent" (1966:224).

Groddeck defined what is now accepted in psychotherapy; the reciprocal relationship of physician and patient. While this relationship has been part of Western medical ideology since Hippocratic medicine, in psychotherapy there is special stress on the psychological dimensions of the doctor-patient relationship (*transference*). Groddeck continues the tradition in which the physicians serves entirely the patient's interests. But he stresses a new element which he abstracts independently of Freud through his organic treatment, i.e., the patient's resistances associated with unconscious emotional dynamics.

The physician's interpretation resolves pains and other symptoms for these patients. There was no formal theory for Groddeck until he began to read Freud and other psychoanalytic writings. But, as Freud later defended Groddeck's contributions against the criticism of others, Groddeck emerged as a unique and creative medical thinker and therapist who tried to systematize clinical experiences. His style proved that the physician's role need not be passive or restrained.

In 1913 Groddeck published a popular book entitled *Nasamecu* (*Natura sanat, medicus curat*) (1985), in which he reviewed his philosophy of illness and healing. Written for the benefit of his then-present and potential patients, the book is also a testimony to the Schweninger philosophy and treatment. It reveals his social philosophy as a citizen, his concerns with lifestyle reforms and organizations. Going beyond this social-minded-ness, Groddeck writes that psychological treatment is not only required with nervous patients, it is the beginning of all medical treatment. He spec-ulates further on the dynamics or those forces linking mind and body which he calls the *Es* (It). This term was later adopted, modified and adapted to his systematic theory by Freud as *Es* (Id).

This first reflexive, speculative book preceded Groddeck's actual knowledge of Freud's growing psychoanalytic theory. In fact, he still thought of the new psychoanalytic movement, known to him only through hearsay, as a dangerous way to split body and mind. He began to read Freud only after *Nasamecu* appeared.

A short book, *Psychological Causes and Psychoanalytic Treatment of Organic Problems*, written and published in 1917, was based on Groddeck's self-analysis (Schott 1986) and was reprinted with a number of his other early essays (1984a). It opens with a description of a personal experience which began with swallowing difficulties and a throat inflammation. The experience was analyzed in terms of unconscious processes going back to earlier experiences in his life. Though now influenced by knowledge of Freud's theory, Groddeck's self-analysis is an autonomous development through which he introduces his own ideas about predispositions to general, organic illnesses. His somewhat rambling thoughts and references to his clin-ical experiences with patients reflect the basics of psychosomatic interests.

Finding parallels in Freud's work with his own ideas, but developed through clinical therapies of a different kind with neurotic patients, Grod-deck wrote to Freud. His letter triggered an intensive correspondence between Freud and Groddeck which lasted many years. During this period, through participating in meetings of the organized group of psychoanalysts around Freud, he was variously accepted or labeled as outsider. Through it all, Groddeck kept a professional, even an intellectual, distance. He wished to remain independent; he did not want to be swallowed by the dogmatism of a professional movement or specialty. Groddeck, the empirical general medicine practitioner, saw as his major task the basic healing work of a physician, not the scientific development of a theory for therapy. He remained a maverick, though one who was widely appreciated.

Groddeck's *Das Buch Vom Es* (The Book About the "Es") with the (translated) subtitle: Psychoanalytic Letters to a Lady Friend (1984b), may have added to the public confusion about his medical ideology or profes-sional identity. It his been suggested that his choice of a subtitle was part of his general parabolic style, just as the term "letters" were not an objective representation of the writings. Groddeck, influenced by philosophy of nature such as the writings of Goethe and Spinoza, initially chose the con-cept 'Es' as a heuristic abstraction for the unknown forces involved with ill-ness phenomena which avoided a split of body and mind. The 'Es' was the object of the physician's medical work and of pursuit of knowledge about illnesses; it was vegetative and psychic existence.

Unlike Freud, Groddeck was neither theoretical nor systematic about defining and anchoring this concept in a structural model. This difference, in fact, led to a temporary cooling of the correspondence relationship between Freud and Groddeck which had developed since 1913 and had stimulated Groddeck's work and activities. Groddeck remained the independent practitioner for whom analysis means something different than to Freud. He wrote:

> Freud's book (*Das Ich und das Es*) is wonderful, as only he could write it. I do not share his views about the Es and the Ich, but it is a pleasure to read what he has to say. Otherwise it is a secondary question which has little to do with analysis whether the Ich (I) is derived from the external world, or whether it is a creation of the Es (id). I believe the different conceptualizations are explained by the different spheres in which we do our work. (From Will 1984:133; author's translation)

Discussion

Was Groddeck an innovator or was he a physician who trained in a medical counterculture with a historical tradition which he tried to continue in but is now threatened by a paradigmatic change in medicine? Furthermore, was he simply led by events to an obvious need arising from a shift in illness phenomena, the need to respond to psychological predispositions (as he referred to symptom expressions) in illnesses? What does he convey to us about the relative relationship of healing which does not claim a scientific basis, and curing, which combines science with empiricism and insightful creativity?

Groddeck appears innovative in a paradoxical sense; he adhered to a medical tradition reflected in naturopathy while simultaneously elaborating on its role in curing through an integrated in-depth analysis of the forces balancing health and illness. He was traditional also in believing in intensive communication with the patient, for treatment of the whole person, to avoid a body and mind dualism. But this empiricism and emphasis on a traditional method of healing could only succeed because of Groddeck's intellectual curiosity.

His inquisitive nature led him to insights which paralleled psychoanalysis to the extent that they were independent ideas and responses to psychoanalytic ideas recast in his own favored way of symbolic abstractions and clinical practice. Only later in his career did his analysis merge with formal psychoanalytic interpretation. Groddeck was driven by professional commitment, enthusiasm, clinical creativity, and a deep humanistic concern for patients. He was a physician who translated traditional ideas and ideology into modern practice and was in every respect a conscientious biomedical practitioner. His appearance and success was possible, perhaps, only in a cultural and intellectual climate of tolerance for physician autonomy.

Groddeck's work and writing in today's world of medicine reveal much about contemporary psychosomatic medicine as a medical specialty. Groddeck could not become more than a burr under the saddle of modern biomedicine as it took its familiar course into more and more divided subfields. He was basically atheoretical, he did not try to establish any "school," nor did he try to modify that of the psychoanalysts with whom he exchanged many ideas. He was a loner who had gained respect, even if slightly bemused, from contemporaries, with Freud foremost among them. He was a socially minded, yet entrepreneurial, individualistic physician, very much a cultural product of his European origins and traditions.

In terms of a cultural approach to history and theory of knowledge, Groddeck's example raises questions about the role in solving medical challenges through individualized innovative empiricism as against systematized, theory-backed knowledge resulting in its organization and specialization. Freud's primary role was that of a careful and systematic scientist. The psychoanalytic movement developed around intensification of its theory and its application to highly specialized patient therapy. It was eventually merged into biomedicine.

The question of empiricism against systematic knowledge and specialization becomes significant for medicine because systematization occurs within a relatively narrow natural science paradigm, poorly equipped to handle psychosomatic illnesses. Groddeck did not flaunt biomedicine, he elaborated on it. But his innovations were outside the biomedical paradigm, they defied constraints of physicians with consequences in the structure and organization of the modern biomedical clinic. Groddeck's example is instructive for an understanding of healing effectiveness within biomedical systems dynamics, seemingly limiting the development of effective solutions of psychosomatic illness problems.

Parallels exist elsewhere (e.g., Gaines 1982, 1985). These suggest that intensive, individualized unstandardized patient-oriented healing can presently develop not only outside or at the fringes of biomedicines but firmly within them. The case of chiropractic in the United States plays such a role (Coulehan 1985a, b; Oths, this volume). As Coulehan (1985a) points out, its basic premise is "the faith that heals." But neither this paradigm nor the necessary organization of clinical practice fit into U.S. biomedicine. If a basic treatment orientation similar to Groddeck's is to be developed within biomedicine, the existing German *Kur* system could be an appropriate setting, perhaps the only such setting, among the modern biomedicines (see Maretzki and Seidler 1985; Maretzki 1989).

Anthropologists have abandoned explorations of what they once called cultural innovations, and of those individuals modifying culture, the innovators (e.g., Wallace 1972). The never-ending challenges of defining the nature of illness, their sources and the responses expected from specialized cultural agents recall interpretations of cultural processes, innovation, acceptance, rejection, integration and other dynamics which once were common to the anthropological, especially psychological anthropological, orientation. If culture contact is still a useful concept in today's world of continuous cultural interaction, an innovative figure such as Georg Groddeck leads us to examine medical practice at the intersection of the individual, historical cultural traditions, professional culture, and the popular cultural context, i.e., the modern space of managed communications in which medicine is practiced every day.

Acknowledgments

My indebtedness is gratefully acknowedge to Prof. Helmut Siefert, who first stimulated me to examine Georg Groddeck's work, and to Prof. Heinz Schott, who generously shared his insights on Groddeck and related topics. I thank also Prof. Atwood Gaines for his many colleagial encouragements and his continued support of, comments on, and patience with the prepartation of this chapter.

References

Ackerknecht, Erwin
1982 The History of Psychosomatic Medicine. Psychological Medicine 12:107–137.

Bosk, Charles
1979 Forgive and Remember: Managing Medical Failure. Chicago: University of Chicago Press.

Brown, E. Richard
1979 Rockefeller Medicine Men. Berkeley: University of California Press.

Coulehan, John
1985a Adjustment, the Hands, and Healing. Culture, Medicine and Psychiatry 9(4):353–382.
1985b Chiropractic and the Clinical Art. Social Science and Medicine 21:383–390.

Gaines, Atwood D.
1979 Definitions and Diagnoses: Cultural Implications of Psychiatric Help-Seeking and Psychiatrists' Definitions of the Situation in Psychiatric Emergencies. Culture, Medicine and Psychiatry 3(4):381–418.
1982 The Twice-Born: 'Christian Psychiatry' and Christian Psychiatrists. In Physicians of Western Medicine: Five Cultural Studies. Atwood D. Gaines and Robert A. Hahn (eds.). Culture, Medicine and Psychiatry Special Issue 6(3):305–324.
1985 The Once- and the Twice-Born: Self and Practice Among Psychiatrists and Christian Psychiatrists. In Physicians of Western Medicine: Anthropological

Approaches to Theory and Practice. Robert A. Hahn and Atwood D. Gaines
(eds.). Dordrecht, Holland: D. Reidel Publishing Company.

Gaines, Atwood D. and Robert A. Hahn, eds.
1982 Physicians of Western Medicine: Five Cultural Studies. Atwood D. Gaines and
Robert A. Hahn (eds.). Culture, Medicine and Psychiatry Special Issue 6(3).

Good, Mary-Jo DelVecchio
1985 Discourses on Physician Competence. In Physicians of Western Medicine:
Anthropological Approaches to Theory and Practice. Robert A. Hahn and
Atwood D. Gaines (eds.). Dordrecht: D. Reidel.

Gordon, Deborah
1988 Clinical Science and Clinical Expertise: Changing Boundaries Between Art
and Science in Medicine. In Biomedicine Examined. M. Lock and D. Gordon
(eds.). Dordrecht: Kluwer Academic Publishers.

Groddeck, Georg
1966 Psychoanalytische Schriften zur Psychosomatik. Gunther Clausner (ed.).
Wiesbaden: Liemes Verlag.
1984a Krankheit als Symbol, Schriften zur Psychosomatik. H. Siefert (ed.). Frank-
furt/M.: Fischer Taschenbuch Verlag.
1984b Das Buch vom Es. Psychoanalytische Briefe an eine Freundin. H. Siefert
(ed.). Frankfurt /M.: Fischer Taschenbuch Verlag.
1985 Die Natur Heilt. Die Entdeckung der Psychosomatik. Frankfurt/M.: Fischer
Taschenbuch Verlag. (originally published as Nasamecu (Natura sanat,
medicus curat): Der Gesunde und Kranke Mensch Gemeinverstandlich
Dargestellt. Wiesbaden: Limat Verlag, 1913.)

Hahn, Robert A. and Atwood D. Gaines, eds.
1985 Physicians of Western Medicine: Anthropological Approaches to Theory and
Practice. Dordrecht: D. Reidel.

Jagersberg, Otto, ed.
1984 Georg Groddeck. Der Wilde Analytiker, Es-Deuter, Schriftsteller, Sozialre-
former und Arzt aus Baden-Baden: Dokumente und Schriften. Buhl-Moos:
Elster Verlag.

Kleinman, Arthur
1973 Medicine's Symbolic Reality. Inquiry 16:206–213.
1986 Social Origins of Distress and Disease: Depression, Neurasthenia, and Pain in
Modern China. New Haven: Yale University Press.
1988 Response to Review Article by Richard Shweder. Culture, Medicine and Psychiatry 14(4):499–502.

Kleinman, Arthur and Byron Good, eds.
1985 Culture and Depression: Studies in the Anthropology and Cross-Cultural
Psychiatry of Affect and Disorder. Berkeley: University of California Press.

Knoch, Magda
1985 Wenn Er Nur das Verzwickte Schriftstellern Lassen Wollte. In Georg Groddeck. Otto Jagersberg (ed.). Moos: Elster Verlag.

Lipowski, Z. J.
1984 What Does the Word "Psychosomatic" Really Mean? A Historical and Semantic Inquiry. Psychosomatic Medicine 46:153–171.

Lock, Margaret
1988 Introduction. In Biomedicine Examined. Margaret Lock and Deborah Gordon (eds.). Dordrecht: Kluwer Academic Publishers.

Lock, Margaret and Deborah Gordon, eds.
1988 Biomedicine Examined. Dordrecht: Kluwer Academic Publishers.

Maretzki, Thomas
1988 Cultural Studies of Medical Institutions, Hierarchies and Training Practice: Therapy Spectrum and Cultural Traditions: Choices for Cures. A Reflexive Report. Paper presented at the Conference, The Medical Anthropologies of Western Europe and North America. University of Hamburg. Hamburg, Germany, December 4–8.
1989 Cultural Variation in Biomedicine: The Kur in West Germany. Medical Anthropology Quarterly *(n.s.)* 3(1):22–35.

Maretzki, Thomas and Eduard Seidler
1985 Biomedicine and Naturopathic Healing in West Germany: A History of a Stormy Relationship. Culture, Medicine and Psychiatry 9(4):383–427.

Moerman, Daniel
1979 Anthropology of Symbolic Healing. Current Anthropology 20(1):59–80.

Ots, Thomas
1990 The Angry Liver, the Anxious Heart and the Melancholy Spleen: the Phenomenology of Perceptions in Chinese Culture. Culture, Medicine and Psychiatry 14(1):21–58.

Reynolds, David
1980 The Quiet Therapies. Honolulu: University of Hawaii Press.

Risse, Guenther B.
1976 Philosophical Medicine in Nineteenth Century Germany. An Episode in the Relations Between Philosophy and Medicine. Journal of Medicine and Philosophy 1(1):72–90.

Rothschuh, Karl E.
1983 Naturheilbewegung, Reformbewegung, Alternativbewegung. Stuttgart: Hippokrates Verlag.

Schott, Heinz, ed.
1985 Franz Anton Mesmer und die Geschichte des Mesmerismus. Stuttgart: Steiner Verlag.
1986 Groddeck's Selbstanalyse. In Groddeck Almanach. H. Siefert et al. (eds.). Basel: Stroemfeld/Roter Stern.

Shweder, Richard
1988 Review of Arthur Kleinman's, Social Origins of Distress and Diseases. Culture, Medicine and Psychiatry 12(4):479–498.

Siefert, Helmut et al., eds.
1986 Groddeck Almanach. Basel: Stroemfeld/Roter Stern.

Uexküll Thure von and W. Wesiack
1979 Psychosomatiche Leiden als Erkrankungen der Individuellen Wirklichkeit. In Lehrbuch der Psychosomatischen Medizin. Th. von Uexkull et al. (eds.). München: Urban und Schwarzenberg.

1988 Theorie der Humanmedizin. Grundlagen des Arztlichen Denkens and Handelns. München: Urban und Schwarzenberg.

Wallace, Anthony F. C.
1972 The Death and Rebirth of the Seneca. New York: Vintage Books.

Will, Herbert.
1984 Die Geburt der Psychosomatik. Georg Groddeck der Mensch und Wissenschaftler. München: Urban und Schwarzenberg.

Young, Allan
1976 Internalizing and Externalizing Medical Belief Systems. Social Science and Medicine 10(1):147–156.

Section IV

Sources and Resources

16

The Ethnopsychiatric Répertoire: A Review and Overview of Ethnopsychiatric Studies

Amy V. Blue and Atwood D. Gaines

Introduction

This concluding chapter provides an overview of the field of ethnopsychiatry. While extensive, the overview cannot be exhaustive. Such an enterprise would itself consume this, and perhaps another, volume. Studies can be reviewed but briefly, even those of some import. We hope to provide the reader familiar with the material a geographic overview while simultaneously furnishing the uninitiated with considerable background and a sense of the breadth of the field. This lengthy chapter covers much ground and gives a comparative base and context to the ethnopsychiatric studies found in the preceding chapters. It may be read in conjunction with chapter 1, especially that chapter's section on the future of the new ethnopsychiatry. Little of that discussion is duplicated in the present chapter.

In this review/overview, all ethnopsychiatric knowledge and practice are considered as cultural. No theory is given priority over another. As a consequence, the theories of biological psychiatry, for example, are presented as forms of theory found in a Western ethnopsychiatry and treated as forms of folk theory (Gaines 1979) in a professional ethnopsychiatry (Kleinman 1988). Its popular basis is shown in its folk biology of social categories of research and practice, its topics of research (e.g., the "biology" of ethnic groups, Lin Poland and Lesser [1986]) and its biased interpretations of findings, rather than in its (often) sophisticated research technologies.[1] Our presentation is divided into two sections. The first presents central ethnopsychiatric issues. The second reviews the ethnopsychiatrically germane literature for most of the world's regions.

In the first section, we consider two disorders, *depression* and *schizophrenia*. These entities are seen as having a worldwide distribution. They are two of only five disorders for which an even vaguely substantive claim of universality can be made given the current status and knowledge in cultural psychiatry (for which see Bibeau 1986/7; Littlewood 1990) and the new ethnopsychiatry. Because of space constraints we cannot here discuss the others, i.e., manic-depressive psychosis, organic brain disorders (Kleinman 1988:16) and some anxiety disorders (for which see Good and KIeinman's review [1985]). We take a closer look at depression and schizophrenia here precisely because they are seen as psychiatry's best cases for disorders that are largely biological. Our consideration of the cultural construction of disorders thought to be real in the West is intended to push further the boundaries of cultural understandings of mental disorders and to deconstruct the biological scientism of biomedicine. We practice the principal of the new ethnopsychiatry; its topics of study are professional as well as popular ethnopsychiatries without the privileging of either form. We thus suggest erasing the vantage point from which judgements of "culture-bound" disorders can be made (Hahn 1985). More consideration needs to be paid to the cultural communicative aspects of illness, themselves seen as cultural productions, encompassing their theatrical and ludic aspects (e.g., Handelman 1979; Kapferer 1982; Karp 1985), without overlooking the communicative nature of healers and healing (e.g., Atkinson 1989) or their cultural psychology (Laderman 1991).

   A number of excellent review articles regarding affective disorders are available for depression (see Marsella 1980; Boyd and Weissman 1981; Bebbington 1978; Murphy, Wittkower and Chance 1964) and schizophrenia (Jablensky and Sartorius 1975; Sartorius et al. 1983, 1986). Because of their ready availability, we will limit the discussion of these central disorders to avoid repetition. The final, lengthy section considers studies of and/or from most culture areas of the world. These are presented as a resource for students in the field. A review of the mental health literature published before 1974, earlier than most works cited here, can be found in Favazza and Oman (1977).

I. Key Ethnopsychiatric Issues
Depression and Schizophrenia: Universal or Culture-Specific?

Depression

   Psychologist Marsella has discussed the epidemiology of depression in cross-cultural settings in his comprehensive review of depressive experience and showed central differences in self and person conceptions across cultures (1980). This signal work clearly implicated person conceptions in the cultural construction of the experience and manifestation(s) of depressive illness and was widely influential. Other reviews of the epidemiology of affective disorders are those of Boyd and Weissman (1981) and Bebbington (1978). Kleinman and Good's collection of essays, *Culture and Depression* (1985), is to be considered the landmark volume in the cross-cultural study of depression and dysphoric affect. The contributions to the volume demonstrate the interrelation of cultural context, history, and power relations in the construction of depressive experience as well as the problematics of Western constructions of emotion, cognition, and depressive disease. Gaines (1987a) provides a detailed review of this important volume, and Gaines and Farmer's account (1986) of the patterning of dysphoric affect and social cynosures in the Mediterranean tradition is an analogue and extension of the selections in the final section of *Culture and Depression*. It is in that section where authors seek to integrate history, social and cultural context, cultural meaning, and experience in the understanding of sickness realities and experiences.

Normal research on depression across cultures is hampered by a number of factors. One is the conceptualization of depression. This psychiatric construct is variously defined as a mood, a symptom, or a syndrome. Another is the tremendous variation in the expression of depression (for example, see Marsella et al. 1973). Expressed feelings of guilt and self-deprecation may be rare, as in the Middle East and elsewhere in the Mediterranean (Good, Good and Moradi 1985; Racy 1980), or common as in Africa (Edgerton 1980; Leighton et al. 1963; Orley and Wing 1979).

Somatic complaints may be the normal cultural expression of what elsewhere may be seen as an intrapsychic problem of depression (Kleinman 1980b; Racy 1980). This is clearly the case in the Mediterranean culture area (Gaines and Farmer 1986; Good, Good and Moradi 1985; Van Moffaert and Vereecken 1989) as well as among many ethnic groups in the United States, e.g., Hispanic and Southern. (The latter tradition includes African-American ethnics as has been noted in anthropology [Gaines 1985a, b, 1992] and recently by the compilers of the *Encyclopedia of Southern Culture* at the University of Mississippi.)

Cultures may not have equivalent conceptions or words for depression at all (Marsella 1980), raising the question if the disorder exists in these contexts. The distinctions between emotional states may differ from those of the West, but for cultural, certainly not "evolutionary," reasons (e.g, Leff 1973). Lutz, in an important article (1985) shows that the distinction between cognition and affect drawn in the West, and which is central to the differentiation of psychiatric disease entities, is a cultural construction; the two are not naturally distinct but culturally created as such (Lutz 1985). While a primary distinction in Western scientific, medical, and lay conceptions of the mind, this presumed natural dichotomy appears certainly to be a cultural creation (Briggs 1970; Gordon 1988; Lutz 1985).

Assessment methods of depression (and other disorders) are often highly ethnocentric (Obeyesekere 1985; O'Nell 1989). Some cultures, such as the Buddhist and the Hispanic and its ancestral tradition, the Mediterranean, have been shown to positively value the experience and expression of dysphoric affect (see Gaines and Farmer 1986; Good, Good and Moradi

1985; Obeyesekere 1985). The recognition of the culturally positive value of dysphoria and its positive cultural meaning lead me (ADG) to coin the term "eudysphoria" as appropriate for these traditions (Gaines 1987a). The need for the term suggests that the use of "dysphoric affect," while intended to be *neutral and descriptive* in line with DSM-III, is actually *diagnostic* and carries with it considerable cultural baggage in the guise of an "objective" label. The implicit notion in psychiatric formulations of depression and of dysphoric affect is their assumed ego-dystonic character. However, the research on Buddhist and Mediterranean cultures noted above suggests otherwise. The very definition of certain feelings as problematic (dystonic) and in need of alteration or remediation (i.e., treatment) is now questionable.

Research has also demonstrated that professional psychiatrists from different nations have different tendencies in diagnosing depression (Kleinman 1988, 1991; Kleinman and Good 1985; Talbot 1980). Rates of depression vary with reports that the rates for non-Western countries is much lower (Marsella 1978). In general, no definitive statement regarding prevalence, incidence or even the form of depressive manifestation across cultures can be given although a variety of assessment techniques have been employed. These include hypothetically universally applicable techniques, e.g., the Zung Self-Rating Depression Scale (1965), the Beck Depression Inventory (Beck 1973, 1976), and "culturally relative" instruments such as the *AIDS* (American Indian Depression Scale-Hopi version) (Manson, Shore and Bloom 1985). The Zung has been shown to produce false positives in the French and Mediterranean context as do the Feighner and DSM-III criteria (Gaines and Farmer 1986). Feelings of guilt, loss of self-esteem, and mood disturbances may constitute a culture-bound syndrome (and perhaps all are) in one Western culture because of its emphasis on stable cognitive functioning and on an ideal of a constant, nonfluctuating and positive affective organization (Gaines 1992; Geertz 1973).

While Beck and others stress a cognitive notion of disorder (Beck 1973) and, indeed, have developed demonstratively efficacious cognitive therapies (Beck 1976), and while social causes are suggested (e.g., Brown and Harris 1978), probably the largest area of current research of affective disorders focuses on the biological parameters (Kleinman 1988). Here as elsewhere (Gaines 1987a, this volume), such a view is seen as a cultural (medical) construction, not as the reflection of a natural, biological reality. Kleinman (1988) has suggested that psychiatrists tend to misconstrue social and cultural data and interpret them as having biological implications or significance. Such interpretations appear to be expressions of a professional "thought model" (Devereux 1978a), a folk theory of "biological essentialism" (Gaines 1992) as well as organicist training (Devereux 1980a).

Most biological hypotheses of affective disorders rely on the assumption that a genetic factor is involved in abnormal brain (biochemical) functioning. Such a dysfunction may exist but not express itself until other events (either endogenous such as hormonal changes, or exogenous, such as stress) expose its vulnerability (Gerner and Burney 1986). However, this sort of vulnerability is purely a *post hoc* form of explanation. It cannot be tested, confirmed, or refuted. Any incidence of illness is said to show the biological predisposition and an absence of illness is said demonstrate the lack of vulnerability. A biological hypothesis held up as explaining all, in fact, explains nothing.

A number of hypotheses exist regarding specifics of the biochemical process at work in affective disorders. These include; altered levels of neurotransmitters such as acetylcholine, catecholamine, dopamine, serotonin, biogenic amine metabolic enzymes; neurotransmitter receptor function; brain peptides; and biorhythms. Gerner and Burney (1986) write that it is unlikely that any current single hypothesis will explain all of the biological abnormalities in affective disorders or their etiology. Beeman (1985) offers a linguistic scheme of the etiology and means of maintenance of dysphoric disorders in terms of their means and modes of communication. And, a recent review of the cross-cultural literature on depression is that by Jenkins, Kleinman and Good (1990). However, the central problem remains; clinical depression is said to be an affective disorder. However, affect distinct from cognition is a cultural construction.

Schizophrenia

Jablensky and Sartorius (1975) and Sartorius et al. (1986) have reviewed schizophrenia in a cross-cultural perspective, its incidence and prevalence, symptomatology, course and outcome, and the historical perspective applied to cultural research of schizophrenia. Research in this field is hampered by of a lack of consistent clarity of the definition of schizophrenia, particularly its boundaries. They conclude that existing data on the prevalence and incidence of schizophrenia in different cultures "tend to support" the notion that there are "broad" similarities. However, they do so only by ignoring considerable evidence to the contrary as Kleinman (1988) ably shows, and by assuming universality of syndromes (Obeyesekere 1985).

Similarities and differences with regard to clinical manifestations of symptomatology have been reported, for example between Irish and Italian schizophrenics in the United States (Opler 1959) and Italian and American schizophrenics (Parsons 1969). Jablensky and Sartorius (1975) note that rare symptoms of schizophrenia in European patients, such as olfactory or haptic hallucinations, seem to be frequent in patients from developing countries. Visual hallucinations, seldom a characteristic symptom of schizophrenia, are more common among some schizophrenics in certain ethnic groups in Africa. Demonstrable organic disease, such as trypanosomiasis in its early stages, may mimic the Western stereotypes of deteriorating schizophrenia and this, some say, is the reason for differential outcomes (see below).

Day et al. (1987) also with the World Health Organization (WHO) study, considered stressful life events. These were seen to often precede the onset of schizophrenic episodes and thereby act as a demonstration or expression of vulnerability. Major differences in the course and outcome of schizophrenia between cultures have been reported (Jablensky and Sartorius 1975; Sartorius et al. 1978; Waxler 1979). Sartorius et al. (1983, 1986), reporting from the International Pilot Study of Schizophrenia, state that schizophrenic patients who had similar symptoms on initial evaluation and whose disorders met strict diagnostic criteria, showed a marked variability of two-year course and outcome, both within and across centers. Those patients in developing countries had a *more* favorable course and outcome than those in developed countries.

Waxler's (1979) work in Sri Lanka explains the better prognosis and outcome of what in the West is chronic mental illness by invoking the social labeling theory. A society labels the person whose primary symptoms it decides to term mental illness. Once a person is given the label, family members and healers respond to the sick person in culturally approved ways. The sick person begins to comply with the expectations of those around him (see Scheff 1966). Thus, society molds the mentally ill person into a socially accepted, albeit deviant, role. In Sri Lanka, people's beliefs and practices reflect a conception of a short term, rather than a chronic illness of schizophrenia. Also implicated in better outcomes are high social support for and tolerance of problematic behaviors in various groups (Jenkins, this volume; Kleinman 1991).

Scheper-Hughes (1979) looked at schizophrenia and the cultural patterns of rural Irish life, including the quality of village and family dynamics. A double bind is said to be at work. However, the double bind etiological theory of the genesis of schizophrenia is not widely held in psychiatry or anthropology, though it stems from anthropologist Gregory Bateson. The work also ascribes results (schizophrenia) from one area to rearing patterns of another and does not consider the social, rather than medical, function of hospital labeling (e.g., increase in stay and benefits for patients). The work recognizes the role of culture in the genesis of mental illness, a subject also considered extensively by Devereux in a different form.

Devereux's work on schizophrenia (1980b) in the 1960s anticipated and very well explains the epidemiological findings noted above. Devereux (1980b) argued cogently that schizophrenia is an "ethnic psychosis." An ethnic psychosis is defined as any disturbance, neurotic or psychotic, in which:

1. The underlying conflict of the patient is present in the majority of other people in the society. The conflict is simply more intense in the patient who hence is different than others only in the degree of the intensity of the conflict.
2. The symptoms are not created by the patient himself, but are provided by his cultural milieu. The society informs the patient in which manner to act insane. If the person deviates from this prescribed manner, he will be considered something else, such as a criminal, a witch, etc.

Schizophrenia is structured by Western society; people are "*taught* to be schizoid outside the psychiatric hospital and therefore to be schizophrenics within it" (p. 222). The most characteristic schizophrenic aspects of the society are: 1) withdrawal, aloofness, and hyporeactivity; 2) absence of affectivity in sexuality; 3) segmentalism and partial involvement; 4) dereism, involving a distortion of reality to make it fit an imaginary model; 5) the blurring of the frontier between reality and the imaginary; 6) infantilism; 7) fixation and regression; and 8) depersonalization.

What makes schizophrenia nearly incurable, according to Devereux, is not only that some of its basic symptoms are encouraged by our society, but that the psychiatrist(s) providing therapy *also* reflect these cultural values and exhibit cultural versions of the symptomatology. Thus, chronicity is culturally constructed, as is the disorder itself.

Devereux, in line with his theory of complementarism (see Swartz, this volume), also argues that the disorder is precipitated by sociological characteristics especially found in the United States. These include widespread mobility coupled with regional and local social and cultural variations. As individuals move, they are expected to make adjustments to new mores, styles, interactional assumptions, even laws. These changes place stress on the individual in requiring him or her to constantly adapt to new situations and subcultural expectations. Some few, however, are unable to make the, potentially large, numbers of necessary adjustments over the life course. These individuals will develop schizophrenia (Devereux 1980b).

In contrast, Warner (1985) suggests a political economic view of schizophrenia. Changes in economy are seen as affecting the epidemiology of schizophrenia. Nonetheless, he accepts that there is a reality, a disease, being caused by something. Another theory, or set of theories, regarding schizophrenia similar in epistemology to Warner are the biological hypotheses. We refer the reader to Davidson et al. (1986) in the Second Edition of the *American Handbook of Psychiatry*, who thoroughly review the literature on this topic. We will mention that research in this field has been based on a view that schizophrenia is a physical illness originating in the central nervous system. Epidemiological, familial, twin, and adoption studies are interpreted to suggest a genetic factor is involved in the disease.

Davidson et al. write that whatever genetic factors exist in this disease must be expressed by proteins perhaps involved in maintaining the structural integrity of the Central Nervous System (CNS), or in the functional control of neurotransmission. However, no genetic link is demonstrable or implicated in the vast majority of cases.

Studies of the biology of schizophrenia have discovered many findings of CNS dysfunction, but none is specific and none is shared by all who have the diagnosis. Further damaging to the biological hypotheses is the fact that no symptom of schizophrenia is unique to it (Malik et al. 1990). And, while studies suggest that schizophrenia is inherited, the specific forms appear not to be. Even more problematic is the fact that there is as yet no specific definition of schizophrenia (O'Grady 1990; Malik et al. 1990; Tsuang et al. 1990; Trimble 1990). (See Gilman [1988a] on the construction of this disease entity.)

Diagnostic Issues

Having briefly discussed the general findings in the literature regarding certain psychiatric key diagnostic entities cross-culturally, we turn attention to the process of diagnosis itself. One problem in this area is that researchers have too often implicitly (if not explicitly) accepted a Western concept of a particular mental disorder as universal, both in terms of its existence and its manifestation. Researchers then look cross-culturally for any evidence of the disorder they have, implicitly, assumed to be universal (Kleinman and Good 1985; Obeyesekere 1985). Some argue for an invariant biology with distinctive cultural expression (Fábrega 1982; Simons and Hughes 1985; Kleinman and Good 1985), while others suggest that invariant biology is arguable (Gaines 1986a, 1987a, this volume; Kleinman 1988).

Even researchers who attempt to understand cultural variations may suggest changing the basic diagnostic criteria to make a locally occurring illness reality fit the preconceived entity. Manson, Shore and Bloom's (1985) study of indigenous mental illnesses among the Hopi Indians and their relationship to depression as *per* the DSM-III is a case in point. They wisely first did a study of local disorders. Among those identified by the Hopi, the researchers looked for those that appeared to be depression, in their terms (i.e., DSM-III criteria). However, the failure to find any indigenous illness that fit DSM-III criteria lead them to suggest not that depression did not exist among the Hopi, but rather to suggest "its" symptoms are different, i.e., of very short duration. The problem here is that the duration of the only disorder meeting a number of criteria for depression is so short that Western psychiatry would be unable to employ its touted pharmacological interventions; the amounts of time required to build up to blood concentrations perceived to be therapeutically efficacious are longer than the Hopi-defined indigenous disorders (less than two weeks).

In an example of universalist thinking, Murphy (1976) concluded that similar types of disturbed behavior are labeled abnormal in different cultures, specifically the Yupik-speaking Eskimos, the Egba Yoruba, Gambia, Sudan, and South Vietnam. She contended illnesses exist independently of labels. It is merely classificatory differences that account for the lack of a classification of *neurotic* among the Yoruba in regards to indigenously described disturbances, such as unrest of mind which prevents sleep, being terrified at night. According to Murphy, these Yoruba disorders would fall into the category of neurotic. However *neurotic* was a construction of Western psychiatry (Menninger 1963), and, in fact, it is not to be found in DSM-III-R (or III). That is, it has been professionally *deconstructed* and no longer exists. One should also note that aside from emic deconstructions there are also reconstructions in professional psychiatry. An example is CFS, *Chronic Fatigue Syndrome*. This appears to be the reconstruction of the long defunct United States psychiatric disorder *neuresthenia* (Kleinman 1991), a disorder itself said to occur widely in contemporary China according to Chinese professional psychiatry (Kleinman 1986; Lin 1989). This construction and deconstruction within psychiatry suggests that external disease realities do not exist simply awaiting the diagnostic and classificatory gaze of one professional psychiatry or another.

Another diagnostic problem is the evidence of a number of studies indicating differences in diagnosis among clinicians of different nationalities. Research with U.S. and British clinicians has repeatedly demonstrated that the former have a broader concept of schizophrenia than do the latter. The U.S. concept embraces not only what the British would regard as depressive illness, but manic illness, neurotic illness, and personality disorder as well. The reorganization leading to DSM-III (APA 1980) had, as one of its intentions, the bringing into line of U.S. psychiatric diagnostic tendencies with those of the British (Talbot 1980). This fact clearly shows the ability of classifications to manipulate the presence or absence of particular mental disorders.

Eker's (1985) research with Turkish and U.S. clinicians showed significant diagnostic differences between these groups, particularly in regards to rating severity of symptoms. Another recent study with results indicating different diagnostic patterns of psychiatrists across cultures is that of Tseng et al. (1986). They examined the diagnosis of neuroses in China, Japan, and the United States. Disorders characterized by a decline in mental function (memory, concentration, and thinking ability) and complaints of mental and physical fatigue were diagnosed as neurasthenic disorder by the Chinese clinicians and as adjustment, anxiety, and depressive disorder by the Japanese and Americans. If trained psychiatrists are diagnosing a uniform phenomenon differently, the question must be raised as to how uniform this phenomenon truly is.

Another issue regarding diagnosis is that of misdiagnosis in certain ethnic groups. Adembimpe (1981) has reviewed this issue with respects to African-Americans. Katz, Cole and Lowery (1969) have considered cultural factors affecting diagnosis. Good and Good (1982) analyzed problems of diagnosis in a multicultural client population in California. And, Rosenhahn's (1973) study of eight pseudopatients complaining of auditory hallucinations admitted to psychiatric hospitals argued that these normal individuals were not detected as sane by mental health professionals. This was to show that the sane could not be told apart from the insane in the context of the antipsychiatry of the 1960s (e.g., Scheff 1966; Szasz 1961). However, because all were released in one to two weeks, it is clear that they were not perceived as regular patients.

Work regarding the development of culture specific mental illness scales has been reported by Ebigbo (1982) and Kinzie et al. (1982), Beiser (1985), Guarnaccia, Rubio-Stipec and Canino (1989), and Manson, Shore and Bloom (1985). In light of the frequency with which Nigerian mental patients complain of various somatic problems, Ebigbo developed a screening scale of somatic complaints indicating psychiatric disturbance. Because of the difficulty in detecting depression in the Vietnamese (immigrants in the United States) due to a cultural tradition which does not emphasize discussing personal feelings openly with others, Kinzie et al. (1982) developed a Vietnamese-Language Depression rating scale containing culturally consistent items describing the thoughts, feelings, and behaviors of depressed individuals.

Reports regarding the appropriateness of DSM-III in cross-cultural settings are provided by Ben-Tovim (1985) and Alarcon (1983). Writing from Botswana, Ben-Tovim concluded that the existing DSM-III criteria could be applied in the everyday practice in this developing country. From Latin America, Alarcon notes the cultural insensitivity in the DSM-III. For example, the antisocial personality has elements which may be adopted by some portions of the Latin American population in order to survive in unstable regimes. One might also recognize the fact of state supported terror in these areas and the attempts to cope with such situations. Farmer (this volume) shows us Haitian psychiatrists' problems with DSM-III's nosology. While these authors see a relative standard, Devereux (1978c) argued for an absolute standard. Adjustment is not a criterion of sanity, for adjustment to an insane society (e.g., Nazi Germany), he argued, is insane.

An excellent study exploring folk criteria for the diagnosis of mental disorder was done by Westermeyer and Wintrob (1979) in rural Laos. The primary focus is a socially dysfunctional behavior rather than disturbances in thought or affect which are so strongly emphasized in Western professional diagnoses.

The system of classification itself has been and is a topic of discussion. The present system (DSM-III-R, APA 1987) was seen as a document based as much on culture as on an external world early on in its career (Farmer 1980). Biological views of psychiatric classification have been advanced (Prince and Tcheng-Laroche 1987; Simons and Hughes 1985) and critiqued (Lock 1987). The classificatory system as a whole has recently received treatment from a bioethical perspective (Post 1992) and has been deconstructed from a cultural constructivist perspective (Gaines 1992). Others have commented on the cultural bases of Western professional ethnopsychiatric classifications (Gilman 1988a; Kirmayer 1988). Particular disorders long have attracted critical examination (e.g., Marsella 1980; Kleinman and Good 1985; Nuckolls 1992; Young 1991). Wig provides perspectives on the DSMs from the Third World 1990.

In summary, the process of psychiatric diagnosis is itself problematic. Although many researchers assume a universalist position, report of the lack of cultural appropriateness of certain nosologies raises important questions regarding their validity. The diagnostic criteria of other cultures assign different priorities to aspects of human thought and behavior than is found in the West. It is the Western, specifically U.S. and Northern European, construction of the human mind, developmental process and behavioral norms which govern the professional psychiatric care and research. This leads to problems when applied to or in other cultures.

Devereux has argued that diagnosis, literally the "telling apart," is a process in which presenting problems are fitted to pre-existing cultural models of abnormality. Problems are not judged and evaluated in terms of absolute standards or deviations from normality (1978a, 1980a), although he himself believed that such standards did exist. In this vein, Gaines (1979), using an interactionist and interpretive perspective, found that emergency psychiatric diagnosis in America was based on psychiatric residents' definitions of mental illness, definitions that existed prior to their psychiatric training. Also noted was the diversity of views held in the same program (also see Light [1976] on therapeutic stances, and Lazare [1973]). The fact that the psychiatric theories of residents predate their training is another reason suggesting the appropriateness of the term ethnopsychiatry for professional U.S. psychiatry.

Epidemiology

The meeting ground in research for problems in diagnosis and classification is epidemiology. The psychiatric version of this enterprise seeks to assess the distribution of psychiatric disorders in a population and to discern the causes for the distribution(s) so discerned. While core schizophrenic symptoms can be said to be found in a large number of societies

(Sartorius and Jablensky 1976), the same can be said of few others. Depression and other disorders vary tremendously across cultures. Kleinman and Lin (1981) found that depression was generally unreported in the epidemiological surveys in China prior to 1981. Writers on Africa, India and elsewhere traditionally minimized the experience of guilt in depression because of a Eurocentric, evolutionist, and not infrequently racist, stance. Thus, their studies 'told us less about them and more about us' (Edgerton 1980; Kleinman 1986). As the critiques of Western nosologies become more powerful, epidemiological work will be increasingly difficult to conduct and interpret even when well-financed and rigorous, such as the five-site Epidemiological Catchment Area Program of N.I.M.H. (e.g., Blazer et al. 1985; Robins and Regier 1991). An important epidemiological effort with considerable anthropological attention has been the Stirling County Study conducted by Leighton (e.g., 1984a), work which still continues 40 years after its start. Recently, women have been the subject of a special supplement of the British Journal of Psychiatry (Women and Mental Health International Conference Committee 1991) which considers the variety of specific problems women encounter world-wide.

    Obeyesekere (1985) very well explodes the validity of the methodology of Western psychiatric epidemiology by positing a study of *semen loss*. The symptoms are well-known in Ayurvedic medicine. So, one simply looks about the world for evidence of these symptoms. Upon finding them, and find them we would in all societies, according to the logic of psychiatric epidemiology, we would have "established" the presence of *semen loss* cross-culturally. We would discover that other cultures would have other names for the historically known disease, or they "mistakenly" assume the symptoms are related to another or other disorders. With this simple thought experiment, Obeyesekere puts into question the logic and the validity of Western psychiatric epidemiology.

Culture-Bound Syndromes

    Culture-bound syndromes are psychiatric illnesses which seem to occur only in a particular culture and no other. Variously termed "atypical, culture-bound psychoses," "culture-bound reactive syndromes" (Yap 1951, 1965) and "ethnic psychoses" (Devereux 1980b), disorders so classified have been of immense interest to, and a virtual stock-in-trade of, ethnopsychiatric research. Are all illnesses culture-bound or are none? (Hahn 1985). Authors argue whether the core of a mental illness is relative to a specific culture or is universal, but merely manifested in a culturally specific manner. They also serve as a sort of proving ground for the validity of particular psychiatric nosological entities.

    Simons and Hughes (1985) published a fairly comprehensive collection of essays, many previously published elsewhere, discussing various culture-bound syndromes. They have attempted to place each culture-bound syndrome within the DSM-III nosology (APA 1980) using what they felt was an empirical behavioral characteristic of the disorders (assault, running, etc.). However, particular characteristic features are not unique to specific culture-bound disorders (e.g., running or assault appear in several). This fact highlights the subjective, rather than objective, basis for the classifications.

At times the editors struggled with their classification of disorders, relying very heavily upon DSM-III's ambiguous categories of "atypical" disorders. Hughes does much work to classify each disorder discussed. However, the most frequent term used is atypical. This rubric in reality serves as no more than a convenient categorical dumping ground with no real classificatory or explanatory power. To say something is atypical is not to classify it. The category exists in order that one can pretend to classify, but in fact avoid classifying, the unclassifiable. It is through this process of self-deception provided by the classificatory system that Western psychiatry maintains the illusion of the validity of the nosology. The extensive use of atypical, then, is a clear indication to the reader that the classificatory enterprise has failed.

More importantly, the assumption that the DSM III is the only plausible psychiatric nosology is highly debatable and is the result only of historical circumstances. Had Japan won the Second World War, we can be sure that the psychiatric and other ostensibly natural diseases in the U.S. would conform to Japanese nosologies and treatments (for which see Lock 1982, 1988; Reynolds 1976, 1980). Below, the more well-known culture-bound disorders discussed in Hughes and Simons and others not found there are briefly described.

A special section of *Social Science and Medicine* in 1985 was titled "New Approaches to Culture-Bound Mental Disorders." Contributions from many of the contributors are noted below where appropriate. Our treatment here will be cursory because the disorders are familiar and have generated a wide literature. We simply call them to mind here. We would point out that since all illnesses become noted, labeled (or not labeled but duly noted), experienced, treated, and acquire significance and social existence in particular cultural contexts, all disorders may be seen as culture-bound (see also Hahn 1985). As a consequence, the distinction between illness and disease, one personal, the other medical, may be seen as two versions of cultural medical theories. Therefore, the distinction is here held to be of little future utility, though the distinction was of immense value for medical anthropological theory, research, and practice, and in medical education for over a decade. However, it may be useful yet in the latter context.

Ethnopsychiatry, which can dispute the validity of all but a handful of disorders, certainly suggests the cultural derivation of culture-bound disorders; they are merely those behaviors/ideation seen by some Western observer as unusual or strange (Hahn 1985). We may assert with some confidence that mental illnesses in the West are culturally constructed, even in the face of, and with the objective methods of an established scientific enterprise focally concerned with finding causes and consequences, therefore, there can be little doubt of the cultural salience and particularity of disorders. As newer forms of research delve into the relationship of language and discourse, emotion/cognition and self (e.g., Good, Good and Fischer 1988; Lutz 1985; Watson-Gegeo and White 1990), the medical imperialist and ethnocentric nature of the category of culture-bound syndromes becomes clearer. (But see Hahn [1985] who warns against a "xenocentric" position.) One may take the position, then, that either all or none of the noted folk and professional ethnopsychiatric entities are culture-bound. Traditionally, perhaps the most widely discussed CBS include *latah*, *amok*, *pibloktoq*, *nervios* and *susto*. (Yap included *koro* in his original outline.) A few of the many studies considering each are noted below. The reader will find many others noted in discussions of the various ethnic or national groups.

Latah

Although both sexes are affected, most *latahs* are women of low status and the syndrome begins in middle age. Once *latah* begins, it continues throughout life. *Latahs* may often become (unfortunate) sources of village entertainment (Murphy 1973, 1976; Simons and Hughes 1985). Kenny (1985) attempts to resolve an apparent paradox regarding *latah*—that it is found in other cultures, not just in the Malay-Indonesian region. Following Geertz, he argues the condition is related to Malayo-Indonesian culture and is a strangely appropriate manner of communicating marginality. Kenny rejects the disease model. The condition is *not* considered a disease by the people among whom it is found, a point first noted by Kenny (1978) but discounted by Simons and H.B.M. Murphy and others. This tends to pathologize the local behavior pattern by stripping it of its local cultural meanings, though Murphy's notion of transcultural psychiatry was to use other cultures as natural tests for psychiatric formulations (Corin 1988) (e.g., Murphy 1974, 1978).

Amok

Amok is another culture-bound syndrome found in Malaysia, Papua, and New Guinea. It is defined as an acute outburst of uncontrollable violence associated with homicidal attack, following a period of brooding and terminating with exhaustion and amnesia (Burton-Bradley 1977; Carr 1978). Carr has provided an "ethno-behavioral" model of *amok* and relates it to depression (1978; with Vitaliano 1985). Psychiatrist Westermeyer looks at the epidemicity of *amok* violence and how the instruments of violence change over time (1973).

Pibloktoq

This is a disease in which a faulty neurotransmitter causes "no single and recurring symptoms to be found in each case" (Gussow 1985:271). The term has become the designation for a group of "hysterical" symptoms which may appear in adult Eskimo men and women at any time (Foulks 1985). There is a seizure in which loss or disturbance of consciousness occurs and any of the following may be involved: tearing off clothing, glossolalia and related phenomena, fleeing, nude or clothed, rolling in snow, performing bizarre but harmless acts, i.e., throwing things around, performing mimetic acts, and coprolalia (Gussow 1985). Biological explanations were offered some time ago by Wallace (1961) while more recently Foulks has seen transformations of Arctic Hysteria in traditional Inuit behaviors and conflicts and their expression in alcohol problems (1985).

Nerves

There are now a host of studies considering *nerves* in a number of ethnic contexts. The disorder, a gloss for a wide variety of problems as locally constructed, appears in Mediterranean, and its daughter cultures in the New World as in Costa Rica, Brazil, Mexico, Puerto Ricans in the U.S., among Greek immigrants in Canada, and so forth (as *Nervios* [Sp], *Nervos* [Port.], *Nevra* [Grk]) (e.g., Blue 1991; Guarnaccia and Farias 1988; Jenkins 1988a, b; Lock 1991; Low 1981, 1988; Scheper-Hughes 1988). Low (1985) provides a review of *nervios* in several societies and looks for their commonalties. She suggests that *nerves* be considered a culturally interpreted symptom (or syndrome?) rather than as a culture-bound disorder. Its use as a gloss for a variety of problems recognized by biomedicine, such as depression and schizophrenia, is also seen in the literature (see Jenkins, this volume).

Susto

Susto, a widely studied folk disorder widely found in Latin American societies, has been extensively reported on by Rubel (e.g., 1977). Rubel et al. (1984) write that the folk interpretation of *susto* is based upon the notion that a person is comprised of two elements, one spiritual and the other organic. The spiritual element is able to detach itself from the organic. Social contexts and meanings of *susto* have been explored among Mexican-Americans (Clark 1959; Madsen 1964).

A host of other culture-bound syndromes is also known and includes disorders discussed here and in other chapters of the present volume, i.e., *tristitia, fatigué* and *triste tout le temps*, *hwa-byung, indisposition, colerina, taijin kyofusho, ode ori, malgri, grisi-siknis, spasmophilie, pena, saladera, falling-out, brain fag syndrome, fright illness*, and others. These are discussed below in sections on specific ethnic groups or geographical regions. It should be noted that U.S. psychiatry and medicine are ever on the move, developing and constructing new diseases. New disorders in U.S. professional ethnopsychiatry include Premenstrual Syndrome (PMS), Chronic Fatigue Syndrome (CFS) (HMSHL 1989), among others (see chapters 1 and 6). The culture-specific nature of "established" disorders, schizophrenia and depression, have been noted above. Some disorders newly seen in a cultural light include *anorexia* (Cathébras, Fayard and Rousset 1991; Prince 1985).

As anthropology comes to understand the Other better, the number of culture-bound disorders will increase as new ones are discovered. So-called culture-bound disorders have a logic within and connection to other ethnopsychological conceptions and assumptions. For this reason, the more we learn of other cultures, the more we will see is different, and difference (from implicit Eurocentric models) is the basis for the notion of culture-bound syndromes. Simultaneously, as is suggested in this volume, we will broaden our understanding of the limits of relevance of Western categories and forms of disorder.

The Self in Ethnopsychiatry

As noted in chapter 1, the ethnopsychological notion of self is key to an understanding of ethnopsychiatry systems, including their notions of disease and appropriate therapy. We find that Weidman (1969) was one of the earliest to discuss the self in the context of ethnopsychiatry (popular). She considered the psychological defense mechanism of projection in the context of Burmese cultural values. Her formulations recall Hallowell's notion of basic orientations provided by cultures (1967) and his innovative works on the self (from 1955). Important was psychologist Marsella's convincing presentation of the role of self conceptions in the experience of depression (1980).

Anthropological discussions of the self in the context of the theory and practice of professional ethnopsychiatry were initiated in the late 1970s (Gaines 1979, 1982a). Illustrated were how concepts of self and styles of self-presentation, e.g., "the rhetoric of complaint," influenced psychiatric theory, therapy, symptom presentation, and meaning (Gaines 1982b,c, 1985a; Gaines and Farmer 1986). Also contrasted were theories of self and definitions of psychiatric disease among Christian and secular psychiatrists as part of a larger formulation of self in Western cultures and their implications for psychiatry (Gaines 1982c, 1985a; see also Shweder and Bourne 1982; Fábrega 1985, and chapter 1).

Good, Good and Moradi's (1985) excellent presentation of Iranian depressive illness also illustrates the significance of cultural conceptions of self in the patterning of dysphoric affect and the cultural means through which experience is constructed and interpreted. Transformation of the self through therapy has been discussed by Kapferer (1979) for Sinhalese exorcist rituals, by Connor (1982) in Balinese healing ceremonies, and by Lebra (1982) for Japanese religious cults. Wikan (1990) has looked at illness from fright and soul loss among the Balinese. Conner, Asch and Asch (1986) have written on and filmed a Balinese healer. The understanding of indigenous concepts of personhood is central to any understanding of psychiatric therapies, illness or theories (Fábrega 1985; Kirmayer 1989; Marsella 1980). These and other works continue to show the connections among religion, ethnopsychology and ethnopsychiatric illness (see Atkinson 1989; Laderman 1991; Csordas, this volume.).

Ethnopsychiatries[2]

Collections by Opler (1959), Kiev (1964), Kiev and Rao (1982), Caudill and Lin (1969), Lebra (1976), Marsella and White (1982) and Westermeyer and Wintrob (1979) all describe aspects of various traditional, usually non-Western, ethnopsychiatric systems. Thorough monographs exhaustively covering a single system, such as Devereux's thorough classic *Mohave Ethnopsychiatry* (1969) are relatively few in number. Crapanzano (1973) has written about an aspect of Moroccan ethnopsychiatry of the religious brotherhoods and the late journalist Clifford has given us an account of Tibetan Buddhist Psychiatry and medicine (1984). And Fábrega and Silver's (1973) account of shamanism in a Mexican community is most thorough. Gaines (1987b) points up the fact that specialization appears not to be a distinction of "modern" medicine and is commonly found in shamanic practice. Prince has examined the biochemical bases for shamanic efficacy (1988).

Ethnopsychiatry within the context of an ethnomedicine (the Zulu's) is presented by Ngubane (1977) in an excellent monograph. In another account from Africa, Prince (1964) presents the West African Yoruba's classificatory and diagnostic systems, giving an overview of both. Kleinman's classic in medical anthropology, *Patients and Healers,* is larger in scope and shows the variety of ethnopsychiatric resources in urban Taiwan including *tang-ki's* and *chien* readers.

Kiev has written the well-known, albeit problematic, account of *curanderismo* among Mexican-Americans (1968a). The system of Puerto Rican Spiritism has been fairly extensively covered by Harwood (1977) and

Garrison (1977). Reynolds (1976, 1980, 1983) has extensively described indigenous Japanese psychotherapies along with Murase (1982), Suzuki and Suzuki (1977), and others. His accounts come from a participant, observer and practitioner. These therapies, and the problems they treat, blend the positions of the continuum of folk and professional ethnopsychiatries more so than one usually finds in a complex society. An excellent, new, and poetic account of shamanic aspects of the ethnomedical/ethnopsychiatric system among Malays is that by Carol Laderman (1991). Laderman wisely allows her voice to recede to leave room for the shamans' own voices.

In general, there has been a considerable amount of work undertaken in developing, or non-Western, societies to describe indigenous conceptions of mental illness and therapy. Overviews of Western systems tend to come from Marxist oriented writers (Castel, Castel and Lovell 1982; Navarro 1976; Waitzkin 1983) who attribute problems to capitalism, confounding it with technological changes, industrialization, and urban living among other things. Reports of folk models of mental illness from Western Europe are relatively few. The examination of the models from this area need much further work such as Townsend's studies of German and U.S. folk and professional ethnopsychiatric knowledge (Townsend 1975, 1978, 1979, also noted below). His work does not attempt a thorough account of all aspects of the systems. A few studies have empirically related etiological conceptions of mental disorders to help-seeking behavior between Western and traditional sources (El-Islam and Ahmed 1971; Finkler 1985a; Kleinman 1980; Weiss et al. 1986).

Ethnopsychiatric studies tend to be largely descriptive in nature and portray aspects of indigenous conceptions of mental health and their relation to overall cultural values. Below, we group traditional and professional conceptions of mental disorder and practices into region. The literature is uneven and consistency of regional reports often lacking. Due to time and space constraints, we can provide the reader with only a sampling of the work in each area.

II. Regional Studies
Subsaharan Africa

Traditional/Folk Ethnopsychiatry

Orley (1970), a psychiatrist, has written a rather thorough, and very readable monograph about the categories of thought related to mental illness among the rural Baganda in Uganda. His data were collected, apart from informal contacts, through a semi-structured interview with both patients and their relatives and nonpatients. Wing and Orley investigated depression in two African villages finding high levels of guilt in those afflicted with depression (Orley and Wing 1979). This and other work (e.g., Leighton et al. 1963) contrasts with "Eurocentric and racist work" (Edgerton 1980) that asserts guilt does not appear in depression in Africa for putatively biological reasons (e.g., Carothers 1953). In such work, there is also manifested the studied inability to recognize that a study in one African group is not generalizable to all others (see Swartz, this volume). Some classic studies will be mentioned here rather than under a specific country or region.

Edgerton (1966) investigated the conception of psychosis in four East African tribes (Sebei, Pokot, Kamba, and Hehe). Despite reports that Africans view mental illness as caused by sorcery or witchcraft, his results found that the Sebei and Pokot tend to attribute psychosis to physical causes. The Pokot also see psychosis as an unspecifiable disorder of the brain while the Hehe and Kamba view witchcraft or sorcery as the cause of psychosis. Edgerton concludes that their conception of psychotic behavior is not greatly different from that of Western symptomatology, especially for *schizophrenia*.

Two classic case studies of African native doctors are those by Turner (1964) and Edgerton (1977). Turner describes an Ndembu doctor, stating that, in the treatment of disease, the Ndembu recognize symptoms and distinguish between diagnosis and therapy. However, they do not know of natural causes for diseases; punitive shades of envious sorcerers afflict them. Diagnosis is thus divination. Edgerton (1977) writes of a Hehe psychiatric practitioner, Abedi. The doctor believes in supernatural causes of illness. At the same time he also recognizes natural causes of illness and seeks medication that will cure these. His pharmacopoeia is extensive and he is a serious empiricist regarding his medications. Edgerton states that Abedi is striking for his secular approach to medicine and his attempts to go beyond the supernatural beliefs of his culture by formulating principles of natural causation and by empirically discovering chemical cures.

MALI

Koumare, Coudray and Miguel-Garcia (1989) describe therapeutic villages where patients live with traditional healers. The healers are part of an integrated network of psychiatric care. The therapeutic village plays a roll as a transitional place on the path to patient resocialization (p.149).

NIGERIA

Psychiatric practices among the Yoruba have been discussed by Canadian psychiatrist Prince (1964), based upon a study of healers and the assessment of diagnosis and efficacy of treatment. Prince details other features of the nomenclature, noting that Yoruba healers do not make a clear distinction between physical disease and the *psychoneuroses*. Among the Yoruba, ancestral to many U.S. African-Americans and Latin Americans, diseases may be caused by natural, preternatural and supernatural forces. Prince concludes that therapy is frequently effective, a point confirmed by other writers (Edgerton 1980; Ademuwagen et al. 1979).

An interesting *depressive anxiety state* found in West African settings is the *brain fag* syndrome. This condition is seen often in school children (German 1972; Prince 1960, 1985). A southern U.S. belief, which is perhaps historical related, is that "too much" study or thinking can cause brain injury, i.e., "hurt" or "wear out" the brain (Gaines 1989). Ebigbo and Anyaegbuna (1989) present case studies of possession by water spirits in a Mermaid Cult in a Nigerian secondary school. They dismiss the beliefs as "obnoxious" "superstition" to be ignored in treatment. Makanjuola finds *ode ori*, a culture-bound disorder in Nigerian patients which presents with extensive somatic complaints (1987).

GHANA

Traditional and spiritualist therapy systems for mental illness in urban Ghana have been analyzed by Mullings (1984) through a Marxist framework. She concludes that traditional healing is more sociotherapy, while spiritualist healing falls more toward psychotherapy. Also examined are the healing roles of Christian churches.

EASTERN AFRICA

Studies of spirit possession in *zar* cults in the Sudan (Boddy 1988) and among schoolgirls in Madagascar (Sharp 1990) have been recent foci of analysis by writers who see these in terms of gender roles and conflicts. Young (1975) also considered *zar* possession among the Amhara in Ethiopia. Kortmann (1990) discusses problems of psychiatric case finding in Ethiopia. And Petros and Schier (1989) discuss popular attitudes and beliefs about mental illness and their classification. Spirit possession is again shown as a major etiological theory as it is in many societies (see Crapanzano and Garrison's collection of essays on spirit possession [1977]). Schulsinger and Jablensky (1991) report on establishment of state-wide services in Tanzania with assistance from anthropologists.

Professional Ethnopsychiatry

Carother's (1953) monograph detailed various physical and mental aspects of some African people. A major problem with the book is the author's racialist generalization of his subject, i.e., the "African." The only distinction made among "Black" people is that drawn between "Blacks" in Africa and those in the United States, ironically a distinction that United

States medicine often does not make even today. Carothers did recognize the significant role of infectious disease and malnutrition in psychiatric problems of this region, something now thought by WHO researchers to cloud psychiatric epidemiological diagnoses (Day, personal communication; Weiss 1985).

CAMEROON

Boroffka (1988) presents epidemiological and case study material. He argues for the continuing need of the latter. Also presented is "therapy by letters," an often successful writing therapy joined with pharmaco- and psychotherapy for acute and chronic psychotic problems.

SOUTH AFRICA

A recent description of the relation of psychiatric practice in South Africa to *apartheid* is by Dommisse (1987). In this country, infectious diseases and malnutrition are still a main cause of psychiatric symptoms. Dommisse notes that a therapist's attempts to help improve a black patient's assertiveness, sense of identity or ego are absurd in the South African context because in the real world, such behavior is negatively sanctioned. This recalls Alarcon's points with respect to Latin America and living under authoritarian regimes. Clinical psychologist with anthropological training, Leslie Swartz (1985, 1986, 1987, this volume), discusses the political restraints of psychiatric practice in South Africa because of *apartheid* and the racism on which it is built.

Jegede et al. (1985) look at modern psychiatric care and its brief history and T.A. Lambo's role in its development. The role of the Christian churches in healing for mental illness and that of the extended family is also considered. Ademuwagun et al. (1979) examine a large number of issues in the ethnopsychiatry of Africa. Many of the book's contributions focus on the Yoruba. The role of traditional practitioners as well as the reality of illness and therapy are also reviewed, among other topics (see Edgerton 1980 for an in-depth review).

KENYA

Ndetei (1980) writes that Western psychiatric services commenced in Kenya in 1912 with the establishment of a smallpox isolation center which soon became a psychiatric unit where mentally ill persons were locked up, primarily to remove them from society. A custodial approach to care of the mentally ill developed, removing the traditional custom of familial care for the disturbed individual. The author notes the paucity of trained psychiatrists in the area. In this context, Mitchell et al. (1987) have studied depressive and anxiety symptoms among secondary school students from the Kikuyu group.

China

Traditional/Folk Ethnopsychiatry

Tseng (1974) and Kleinman (1980b) have described well traditional psychiatric care in Taiwan. Shamanism, as a religious form of healing practice, is an important source of treatment in most of the rural areas. Tseng writes that analyses of the problems presented to a *dang-gi* by clients indicate that more than one-fifth of them are psychiatric in nature. Kleinman (1980b) gives an excellent account of the range of health care providers and their services in his account of Taiwan including *tang-ki's* (Tseng's *dang-gi's*) and *chien* readers.

Hsu (1976) has analyzed the content of the divination messages (*chien*) and discusses the psychotherapeutic elements of this practice. (Also see Kleinman 1980 on this). Another form of folk counseling in Taiwan is fortune telling. Not only does he interpret the problems, the fortune teller suggests how to deal with them (Kleinman 1980b; Tseng 1975). Psychiatrist Cheung looks at popular understandings of psychiatric illness and help-seeking behaviors among contemporary Chinese in Hong Kong and beyond, as well as at community mental health programs (e.g., 1982, 1987, with Snowden 1990). She also considers somatization, a major topic of research with indigenous and immigrant Asian populations (Cheung, Lau and Waldman 1981; Kleinman 1980; T.-Y. Lin 1989; E. Lin, Carter and Kleinman 1985).

The *koro* syndrome originating in Southern China involves genital retraction. A consequential fear, if the retraction continues, is death. Those afflicted, in their anxiety, use any means to prevent the retraction (Leng 1985; Yap 1965). There have been large epidemics of *koro* (Tseng, personal communication). Among the Chinese, we note, there exists a folk belief that the dead do not have genitalia; it is believed they retract into the body upon death.

Conceptions of Mental Illness in Traditional Chinese Medicine

Wu (1982) writes that a basic principal of classical Chinese medicine was an emphasis on the psychological etiology of disease. He discusses the very psychological approach of Chinese medicine often seen by others as lacking. In Zhang Zhongjing's own works, a number of herbal drugs were suggested for psychiatric illnesses. Some of these, such as *Ganmaidaza-otang*, are used today (Liu 1981). Liu also considers the development of nosologies and etiological theories. Tseng (1974) writes that the invasion of evil wind into the positive pole of the body was thought to cause "wind insanity." In Chinese medicine, concepts were not all modified throughout the centuries, thus even today some traditional practitioners refer to these earlier notions of psychiatric disorders (Liu 1981). Liu also explains the preliminary examinations that precede diagnosing a psychiatric illness in a Chinese patient. Wen (1990) recently has chronicled the development in Taiwan of an indigenous asylum for chronic mental patients. Such institutions were virtually unknown in traditional China. The heavy task of providing care has been traditionally borne by the family of the afflicted (Lin and Lin 1981).

Kleinman et al. (1975) and Kleinman and Lin (1981) extensively cover a variety of Chinese medical cultures in the past and present. For Tibet, Clifford (1984) has provided an account of Tibetan ethnopsychiatry. She located this ethnopsychiatry within Tibetan medicine and Buddhism and expresses the unity of medicine and religion there.

Professional Ethnopsychiatry

There have been a number of reports regarding psychiatric practice in China, many from brief trips to the People's Republic of China. Two reports from Chinese psychiatrists are provided by Young (1980) and Young and Chang (1983). Kleinman (1986) has written about Chinese psychiatric practice with specific attention paid to the illness *neurasthenia* and has provided an overview of the development of Chinese ethnopsychiatry (also see Koran 1972). Walls et al. (1975) note sociopolitical factors have been considered greatly influential in mental illness. Sidel (1973) describes how the concept of revolution influenced mental health care after the Cultural Revolution. Contemporary treatment combines both Western methods and Chinese traditional medical techniques. Many schizophrenic patients are treated with acupuncture (Bloomingdale 1980), herbal medicines (Walls et al., 1975), and drugs not yet allowed in the United States have been in use for a number of years (e.g., clozapine). Young and Chang (1983) write that psychoanalysis is not recognized as a treatment technique because it is based on the "subjective rather than the objective" factors (also in Kleinman 1986).

Tung (1984) contrasts the Chinese therapeutic approach with those of the U.S., commenting that the former is pragmatic, rational, public, community, conforming, and dependent, while the latter is theoretical, psychodynamic, confidential, private, individualistic, and independent. She then relates these contrasts to the cultural beliefs of the East and West. Bloomingdale (1980) looks at lack of standardization of the nomenclature. *Neurasthenia* comprises approximately 80 percent of the diagnoses given for all *neurosis* (Young and Chang 1983). Kleinman (1986; Kleinman and Kleinman 1985) provides the most extensive discussion of *neurasthenia* in China. They relate it to personal, social and political factors. Chronicity is understood as constructed in terms of personal, and both the local and wider external socio-political, pressures.

Epidemiological data about mental illness in China are generally scarce. According to Kleinman and Mechanic (1979), psychiatric epidemiological studies conducted in other Chinese communities indicate about the same amount of psychiatric morbidity with respect to the major psychoses as in Western societies. (See Young and Chang [1983] for prevalence rates from the Department of Psychiatry at the Medical College in Hunan.) T. - Y. Lin and Leon Eisenberg (1985) have produced proposals for providing mental health care for China's huge population.

Japan

Traditional/Folk Ethnopsychiatry

Japan has witnessed the development of a variety of indigenous professional psychotherapeutic forms, such as Naikan and Morita therapies. These combine traditional ideas (Lock 1982; Ohnuki-Tierney 1984) with some aspects of modern biomedicine and psychiatry and are thus not purely one thing or another. These therapies have been described by Reynolds (1976, 1980, 1983), Kondo (1976) and Murase (1976). Morita therapy is very effective with a Japanese condition called *shinkeishitsu*. Murase (1982) has discussed the relation of the Japanese value system, expressed by the word *sunao*, to the goals of both Naikan and Morita psychotherapy. Implying a harmonious and natural state of mind vis-à-vis oneself and others, *sunao* is a particularly important value in Japanese culture.

Japanese religious cults have been described by Takie Lebra (1976, 1982) as a psychotherapeutic form. The cult named the Salvation Cult, or *Gedatsukai*, "a society for deliverance," is a cult which focuses upon reconstruction of the self. Lebra's (1976) discussion of this cult concluded that role gratification, through the spirit possession, brings relief from suffering. In a later publication (1982), various aspects of the cult and their relation to wider Japanese culture are discussed.

Professional Ethnopsychiatry

Caudill (1959) conducted the first study of a psychiatric hospital in a non-Western culture, studying psychiatric practice in Japan (see Nomura, this volume). Noting the influence of Western training on the psychiatrists and their use of physical and organic therapies, with very little emphasis on psychoanalysis and psychotherapy. His classic work also considered the social structure and organization of the hospital. The hospital organization reflects the Japanese family model (see Dwyer, this volume; Nomura, this volume, 1987).

Munakata (1986) discusses the low hospitalization rate in psychiatric hospitals and the long periods of hospitalization in Japan; the hospital comes to be regarded as home by the patient (also see Nomura, this volume). Anderson (1985) reports recent advances in Japanese psychiatric hospitals to give patients rights to communicate with the outside world. Nomura (1987, this volume) analyzed the nature of relationships in Japanese psychiatric institutions and found that they replicated the hierarchical social relationships which obtain in Japanese schools. Caudill (1958, 1961) also discussed a distinctly Japanese nursing form, the *tsukisoi*. With the patient twenty-four hours a day, the relationship between the *tsukisoi* and a patient may become very close.

Japanese psychiatry possesses culture-specific diagnostic label, *taijin kyofusho*, meaning "social phobia" or "anthrophobia." *Shinkeishitsu* glosses *neurasthenia, anxiety neurosis,* and *obsessive-compulsive reactions,* recalling archaic uses in U.S. psychiatry but the phenomenology of distress and the therapy are not comparable. *Taijin kyofusho,* a subcategory of *shinkeishitsu,* first appeared as a diagnostic label in the 1920s. It is a distinctly Japanese label but other psychiatric labels are direct translations from the Kraepelinian classificatory system (Kirmayer 1989; Kitamura et al. 1989; Tanaka-Matsumi 1979). Kirmayer shows that the disorder *taijin kyofusho* presents a challenge to the notion of a universally valid DSM psychiatric nosology (1989). Western writers generally try to subsume the disorder under "anxiety disorders" (Liebowietz, Fyer and Klein 1985).

Tanaka-Matsumi (1979) designed a study to examine whether or not U.S. mental health professionals could diagnose Japanese case descriptions of *taijin kyofusho* and what kind of labels they would apply to these cases. U.S. judges placed the Japanese cases of *taijin kyofusho* into a number of heterogeneous categories, such as *schizophrenia, paranoid personality, simple schizophrenia, anxiety neurosis,* and *phobic neurosis.* What the Japanese see as unity, U.S. clinicians see as disparate entities (see also Kirmayer 1990). Lock has noted the development in Japan of several new psychiatric problems that are being assimilated into professional Japanese psychiatry. These include *school refusal* and *housewife* syndromes (Lock 1987, 1988).

Korea

Traditional/Folk Ethnopsychiatry

For Korea, we have several studies of shamans. Research thus far has tended to emphasize female shamans. This work, first by the late anthropologist Kim Harvey (e.g., 1976) is continued by anthropologist Laurel Kendall (1985). Both have also provided detailed biographical accounts of shamans (Harvey 1982: Kendall 1988). Writers have also noted that the disorder found in Japan and noted above, *taijin kyofusho,* is also found in Korea (Kirmayer 1989; Tanaka-Matsumi 1979). *Hwa-byung,* a local disorder which Prince (1985:201) suggests would be cases of *anxiety-depression*, is also noted in the literature (K.-M. Lin 1983).

The Mediterranean: Middle East and North Africa

Traditional/Folk Ethnopsychiatry

The Arabic word for insanity is *junun*, and for the insane, *majnun*, derivative of *jinn* or evil spirit. Distinguished from *junun* are the conditions *alasaab* (nerves) and *wahm* (imagination), which refer to mental and emotional disturbances not as serious as insanity. Causes of mental disorders are considered by a number of authors for various countries in the area. Folk and religious treatments are considered by Racy (1970). And Ozturk (1964) has described folk treatment of locally defined mental disorders in Turkey. Recently, institutionalized drug use has been considered in the area (Kennedy 1987).

El-Islam (1982) mentions the tombs of highly revered dead sheikhs as a source of therapeutic activities. A local "neurotic" disorder has been found among the women of Qatar (El-Islam 1975). The *zar* cult is another indigenous therapeutic form (Kennedy 1967, Fakhouri 1968, Racy 1970, El-Islam 1982). Kennedy (1967) writes that the term *zar*, referring to both a ceremony and a class of spirits, is usually associated with Ethiopia. However, it is also found around the Nile. He examined the *zar* cult in its Egyptian Nubian context in terms of its therapeutic effectiveness.

Morsy has provided an excellent account of the affliction of *'uzr'* among women of an Egyptian village. As part of her analysis, this Egyptian anthropologist deftly exposes the cultural biases of Western feminist writers considering women and affliction. She goes on to show the meaning of affliction, healing and action in terms of the meaning worlds of Egyptian women.

Crapanzano's (1973) account of the Hamadsha describes this Moroccan religious brotherhood that engages in healing rituals. A study in ethnopsychiatry, he analyzes how the Hamadsha therapy system operates on social, psychological and physiological levels for the members of this brotherhood.

El-Islam and Ahmed (1971) studied patients at the outpatient clinic of Cairo regarding their beliefs about traditional illness and found plural belief systems. (See also the description of Islamic psychiatry discussed below in the Malaysian context.) The Goods have provided a number of accounts of folk illness, their diagnosis and treatment, and their generative cultural contexts. Their populations have included Turkic speakers in Iran, and Iranian immigrants in the United States. Illnesses discussed have included *Narahati*, *Fright Illness* and *Heart Distress* (e.g., Good 1977; Good and Good 1982; Good, Good and Moradi 1985). This work represents some of the most articulate examples of interpretive scholarship and has of late focused on situated discourse as the royal road to interpreting affliction and suffering (Good, Good and Fischer 1988).

Professional Ethnopsychiatry

ISRAEL

Minuchin-Itsigsohn et al. (1984) discuss how illness beliefs and knowledge influence therapeutic encounters in Israeli with Moroccan, Persian, and Ashkenazi Jews. Social or economic problems are viewed by Moroccans as the root of their difficulties. (The same notion is found among African-Americans and Hispanics with respect to alcoholism when and if such problems were seen as distinct from the person him- or herself [Frankel et al. 1978]). In another report from Israel, Gorkin (1986) discusses countertransference in the Jewish therapist and Arab patient (also see Basker and Domínguez [1984] for other problems of therapists in this area, and Good, Herrera, Good and Cooper [1985] for a study of countertransference in another context).

Bilu (1979) and associates (1990) have looked at local etiological beliefs and idioms of distress in Israel and have demonstrated through successful psychotherapy the usefulness of merging and recasting professional understandings with local understandings. (See also Abel et al. [1987], Littlewood and Lipsedge [1987] and Devereux [1951] for discussions of psychotherapy across cultures.) Pliskin's account of medical practice in Israel (1987) shows us a conflictual situation in which Israeli general physicians are confronted with Arabic and Persian speakers' ethnopsychiatric somatized conditions which the physicians cannot interpret, resulting in stereotyping and poor care. Basker and Domínguez (1984) consider the limits of therapists' abilities when they are immigrants to Israel.

ARAB EAST

Racy (1970) provides a thorough review of psychiatry in the Arab East, though it now may be somewhat outdated. A more general, though more up-to-date report is given by El-Islam (1982). He writes that emotional and behavioral disorders may not be perceived as mental illness in this region because, 1) they may be explained and thereby normalized by invocation of local cultural beliefs, 2) patient's tolerance of emotional suffering (see also Good, Good and Moradi 1985, Gaines and Farmer 1986), and 3) relative's tolerance of their behavioral disturbances. The family plays an important role in mental health care decision-making and often tries to manage psychiatric illnesses of adolescents and young adult females at home. Regarding modern treatment, Arab patients may insist on somatic treatments, trusting injections more than pills, paid medical service more than free service, and may not accept talking (psychotherapy) as a treatment which can replace drugs. Many Arabs do not accept the notion of rehabilitation and of adaptation to residual disability, thus going from one practitioner to another in search of an ultimate cure as is found in the South in the U.S.

SAUDI ARABIA

Discussing psychiatric practice in Saudi Arabia, Dubovsky (1983) comments that concepts of feminine modesty may prevent a woman from unveiling with a psychiatrist (even at the insistence of her husband), making intimate disclosures impossible. Another problem is created by a widespread tendency to overemphasize points. A very difficult element in psychiatric practice is the pervasive belief known as *in'shallah* (as God wills), in which events and their outcomes, including if one gets well, are in God's hands. Similar beliefs are found in U.S. folk psychiatry and among Christian psychiatrists (their tradition is ultimately Mediterranean) (Gaines 1982c)

Rakawy (1979), an Egyptian psychiatrist, writes that psychiatric practice in Egypt generally follows the Anglo-Saxon model. No particular discipline dominates the practice as a whole and the predominant theory is "no theory" (p.23). He discusses the various inclinations of existing institutions. Non-medical healers, such as religious healers, are also important sources for psychiatric care. In an earlier article (1978) Rakawy discussed the Egyptian nosology, the *Diagnostic Manual of Psychiatric Disorders* and provides some epidemiological material based upon the DMPD.

LEBANON

An historical account of psychiatry in Lebanon is given by Katchadourian (1980). Langsley et al. (1983) report that there were about 100 psychiatrists in the country (population 35 million)—half of them trained in the United States, England, or Germany. Western methods of care were used in hospitals, with biological explanations for, and treatment of, mental illness favored. Since the revolution, the 1975–1978 community mental health innovations have been largely dismantled.

Italy

Traditional/Folk Ethnopsychiatry

As in the case of Greece, in Italy we note the presence of the notion of the *evil eye*, indeed as it is found throughout the Mediterranean (Maloney 1976). The notion of spirit possession as a cause of unusual mental states has a long history and is a belief found in many places. In the many ethnographies of the country, witches are also implicated as causes of mental disorders. Quite widespread in the Mediterranean are the sad conditions such as *triste/fatigué tout le temps, narahati, tristitia, nevra, nervios* and others. The cultural patterning and rhetoric of sadness are clearly important features of the ethnopsychology and ethnopsychiatry of the Mediterranean.

Professional Ethnopsychiatry

One of the most discussed mental health care systems in recent years is that of Italy, and the "radical" reforms of Franco Basaglia. His philosophy stemmed from a conviction that the psychiatric institution itself impedes the therapeutic process and that psychiatry is politics. Lovell, with Scheper-Hughes (1987), translated a collection of writings of Basaglia. Papeschi (1985) and Mosher (1982) critically review some of Basaglia's work and writings. Jones and Poletti (1986) suggest that the changes have been more apparent than real. Crepet (1990) provides epidemiological data and an overview of the changes in Italy's psychiatric system which he suggest is in a transitional state.

Pandolfi, combining philosophy, psychoanalysis and anthropology, looks at how Southern Italian village women author themselves (1987, 1988). They embody themselves, physically or through narration, and their being-in-the-world to hide and reveal their particular identities. The accounts suggests another dimension of the "rhetoric of complaint," the interactional means of presenting a valorized self (Gaines 1982b), and "eudysphoria" (Gaines 1987a), the positive cultural value placed on displays, and the experience of, dysphoria in the Mediterranean tradition; and, hence, the cultural salience of illness discourse and illness itself (see Good, Good and Fischer 1988).

France (and Spain)

Traditional/Folk Ethnopsychiatry

Folk ethnopsychiatric beliefs in France have been considered by Audibert (1983), Gaines and Farmer (1986), Gaines (this volume), Helman (1990), and Payer (1990) and include *fatigué/triste tout le temps, fatigué,* and *spasmophilie.* Also considered were conceptions of self and self presentation and the social cynosure of the visible saint (contemporary community resident) who, as an exemplary sufferer, serves as a model of and for life viewed as tragic (Gaines 1982a, b, c; Gaines and Farmer 1986). French sociologist Dodier (1985) considers the moral appropriateness of *fatigué* in the workplace. And, a few rural ethnopsychiatric studies have been conducted. Among these is Agnes Audibert et al.'s (1983) study of ethnopsychiatric beliefs and practices in rural Britanny.

Central aspects of the history of French medicine and psychiatry have been ably handled by Foucault. He has had an influence on the study of ethnopsychiatry far outside of France (e.g, Fábrega n.d.; Rhodes, this volume; Scheper-Hughes and Lock 1988; Turner 1987). Foucault was concerned to show the relationship between aspects of discourses in medicine and the exercise of power and authority ("knowledge/power") in society. This reflected Foucault's interest in what he saw as the changing forms of surveillance of people in society effected by means of control over their bodies (1973, 1975, 1979, 1980).

However, writers often see Foucault's work as if it had general applicability rather than locating it within the space of French history and culture (e.g, Fábrega n.d.; Turner 1987). For many centuries France has been an extremely highly centralized state. This makes many of his comments problematic in their application to the United States, for example, because of its fragmented and decentralized governmental structure. Many levels of authority (city, county, region, state) supplant federal authority at a given level. As a consequence, only a few crimes are federal, most others have locally determined punishments, rules of evidence, legal procedures, and so forth. Perhaps this is why Foucault confuses metaphors of confinement with the actuality of it, as Gilman has noted (1988a:275; also see Skultans 1979).

Other relevant historical works include Castel's (1988) on the development of psychiatric institutions and the change in legal and social status that was entailed for people judged insane. Also of interest is Goldstein's study of the history of French psychiatry (1987). The reform of asylums in France led to the development of a specialty, the medical *alienist* (because their charges were referred to in France as *aliénés* and the asylum, *asile d'aliénés*). It was here asylum reforms developed and diffused to other lands and where psychiatry became medicalized (Gilman 1988b; Goldstein 1987).

Turkle (1978) has analyzed the changes in attitude toward Freudian psychoanalysis which have occurred in the last twenty years. Freudian psychoanalysis was initially rejected in France, but since the revolutionary spirit of 1968, it has become a central theme in French intellectual life, including the French women's movement. The contemporary French style of psychoanalytic theorizing is Lacanian, after Jacques Lacan, and emphasizes psychoanalysis as an interpretive science in which images of analytic "listening" (*écouter*) and analytic understanding are more salient than promises of analytic "cure" (p.7). (Also see Lacan 1968, 1977.) This is a contrast to U.S. beliefs, found in popular and psychoanalytic ethnopsychology, that people can and do change themselves. The lack of emphasis on change of the person in French psychoanalysis relates to the Mediterranean culture tradition in which the life course is not seen in terms of progressive improvement, though self presentation may vary with circumstance (Gaines 1985a).

Another form of "ethnopsychoanalysis" (Devereux 1978b) is that of Mendel (1972). He has argued for the development of a "sociopsychoanalytic anthropology." His configuration appears not unrelated to the work of Devereux. Nathan (1986) is one of Devereux's students who is developing a

Devereuxian form of an anthropological psychoanalysis based on work with immigrants in France.

Lovell (n.d.) has discussed bioenergetics, a French psychotherapeutic movement found in both psychiatric hospital and nonhospital settings. Although diverse in actual practice, the core of bioenergetics is a series of techniques and therapeutic systems emphasizing the corporeality of an individual. Psychoanalysis provides the etiological explanation and physiological analysis explains the manner in which the pathology functions. In therapy there is a "reading" of the body and stress exercises are performed. This appears as an ethnomedical system which takes the notion of embodiment of illness seriously (see Csordas [1991] on embodiment). There is resonance here with Groddeck's work in Germany, discussed by Maretzki (this volume) and with the very old French *vitalist* tradition (see Florkin 1971). For Spain, we have little to report. An overview of sociocultural studies of mental illness for the whole peninsula is provided by Seva-Diaz et al. (1985).

Greece

Traditional/Folk Ethnopsychiatry

No specific study of Greek folk concepts of mental illness and healing have yet been published (see Blue 1991, this volume). However, it is common for histories of psychiatry to start with classical examples which are interpreted as examples of contemporary disease entities (e.g, Simon 1978), as in the case of schizophrenia (Gilman 1988a). Work by Blum and Blum (1965, 1970) regarding Greek rural health and healing reveals cultural notions about mental illness. Mental illness may be caused by a variety of supernatural agents: demons, spirits, and preternatural agents, such as the *evil eye*. Local folk healers, either male or female, and the priest may be sought for diagnosis of the *evil eye*. In cases where some form of spirit possession may be involved, the priest may also act in the role of healer.

Danforth (1979, 1983) has analyzed an annual folk celebration, the Anastenaria as a ritual system of psychotherapy. Foci of concern are unusual, obsessive or deviant behavior particularly of a religious nature or involving fire; persistent dreams or visions concerning the Anastenaria; periods of unconsciousness, paralysis or involuntary and uncontrolled activity; or states of depression or anxiety characterized by general malaise and an inability to work, eat or sleep.

Danforth attributes women's participation in the Anastenaria as an opportunity to act with an authority which is generally denied them due to traditional notions of gender roles. Dunk (1985) and Lock (1988, 1991) have reported beliefs about *nevra* amongst Greek immigrants in Montréal. *Nevra* was reported to be the major health problem in the community, especially among women. *Nevra*, supernatural beliefs, psychiatric institutions and the rise of professional Greek psychiatry, only a little over a decade old, have been recently explored by Blue (1991, this volume). Also discussed are *stenohorias,* popular disorders in Greece to be distinguished from *nevra* (Blue 1991).

Latin America

As in the case of Native North America, there are a large number of studies that are relevant to this review of studies in and of the field of ethnopsychiatry. Generally not mentioned here are the many studies of folk healers which were conducted not as parts of medical anthropology, but as part of the anthropology of religion, including studies of ritual (e.g., Kroeber, Lévi-Strauss, LaBarre). In both North and South America, there are also many, many studies of acculturation involving mental difficulties and substance abuse (e.g., Adair, Kunitz, Spindler). Then, there are the numerous works on shamanism which considered their normality or abnormality, recruitment and characteristics (e.g., Devereux, Spiro, Linton, Lewis, Aberle, LaBarre, Lowie, among others). These are generally omitted from the present discussion.

Traditional/Folk Ethnopsychiatry

Beliefs about traditional mental disorders among the Caribe, a West Indian tribe in Costa Rica, were investigated by Hill and Cottrell (1986). *Nervios* the folk illness is reported to exist in a number of Latin American communities (Low 1988; Rubel et al. 1984; Scheper-Hughes 1988), Mexican-American communities (Jenkins, n.d., 1988a, b) as well as in the Mediterranean, as among Greeks as noted above. Low (1988) reports a variety of somatic complaints, such as headache, lack of appetite, and depression, fears, and anger in patients complaining of *nervios.*

Fábrega and Silver (1973) studied shamanism and illness in Zinacantan, Mexico combining an ethnomedical study with some of the older issues of psychological anthropology such as the normality and or abnormality of the shaman. In Zinacantan, illness is moral; it concerns the relationships to self, society and the gods, and shamans treat illness of the mind and body, former often responsible for the latter. Scheper-Hughes (1988) suggests a biological explanation for the Portuguese term for *nervios, nervos,* by arguing that it is a gloss employed by Brazilian biomedicine for hunger used in order to conceal a potentially revolutionary reality. This view of illness as potentially revolutionary has been voiced by others, concerning physical illness, including Waitzkin (1983). In contrast, Low writes with a recognition of the culture history of the disorder and shows it to have a complex set of meanings that are involved in its presentation and interpretation. It is shown that the multiple meanings are shared and understood by both lay persons and biomedical practitioners (1988), much as the notion of *fatigué* is known, shared and interpreted by French physicians and lay persons (see Gaines 1986a, this volume). Also in Brazil, Krippner assesses *multiple personality disorder* in the context of Brazilian *Spiritism* (1987).

Stevenson (1977) describes *colerina*, a convulsive illness found in the central Andes of Peru. All of the attacks occur in adults and are more frequent in females than males. *Pena*, an emotional state caused by pent up negative sentiments, is cited by locals as giving rise to *colerina*. (See Tousignant [1984] for a discussion of *pena* in Ecuador.)

Another folk illness in Peru is *saladera*, described by Dobkin de Rios (1985). The patients complaining of *saladera* were highly anxious, frequently bursting into tears, unable to perform normal work duties, unable to concentrate and fearful of the future. *Saladera* is thought to result from bewitchment or the use of magic potions. Dobkin de Rios writes that *saladera* differs from another illness, *dano*, in that the latter is caused by the evil willing of others who harbor malice toward a patient. Citing the difficulties of rapid acculturation among Third World urbanizing peasantry, the author concludes that the illness is a response to the stress of modernization in a society where witchcraft beliefs may be invoked to explain the appearance of illness. The ahistorical views of contemporary forces are not infrequently invoked to explain very ancient popular sickness realities.

Grisi siknis (Dennis 1985) is found among the Miskitos along the Atlantic coast of Nicaragua and Honduras. An attack of *grisi siknis* begins when the devil arrives to take his victim away. Prodromal symptoms are sharp, stabbing headaches, dizziness (*bla*), general anxiety and fear.

The Caribbean

Fisher (1985) has analyzed psychiatric problems on Barbados. He attributes them to the destructive influence of the earlier colonial arrangements. Philipe and Romain (1979) have done research on *indisposition*, a folk disorder in Haïti. Saint-Gérrard (1984) has considered the role of poverty in the development and incidence of mental disorders in Haïti. (See Farmer, this volume for more on professional psychiatry in Haïti.)

Ethnic Groups in North America

As noted above, many references which could be cited here have been omitted. These relate to the hundreds, if not thousands, of studies which, while now classifiable under the rubric of ethnopsychiatry, were originally conducted as studies in the anthropology of religion, studies of ritual, acculturation, racism, stress, internal colonialism, urbanization, psychological anthropology, and/or public health. Here we will briefly look at immigrant and native groups in the U.S. and Canada, with an emphasis on the U.S due to our own limitations.

Traditional/Folk Ethnopsychiatries

PUERTO RICAN-AMERICANS

Harwood (1981) writes that Puerto Ricans make a clear distinction between the concepts *locura* (insanity) and *nervios* ("nerves"), the subject of research of a number of authors. *Locura* refers to unpredictable behavior, often violent. *Nervios* may include such symptoms as chronic agitation, inability to concentrate or pacing, and crying or silent brooding. Garrison has extensively considered healing among this group on the East Coast of the United States (1977a). Earlier called the "Puerto Rican Syndrome" (Garrison 1977b), *Ataque de nervios* has been considered by a number of people recently including Guarnaccia et al. (1989). As noted below, the disorder has been studied in the context of Mexican-Americans. Guarnaccia, Good and Kleinman (1990) have critiqued epidemiological studies of mental illness among Puerto Ricans from a cultural standpoint.

Gaviria and Wintrob (1976) examined folk beliefs about mental illness among Puerto Ricans. Two broad categories of mental disorder were described, as in the case of Harwood above, i.e., *loco* (crazy) behaved aggressively or bizarrely, including homicidal or suicidal tendencies and *nervios*. Gaviria and Arana (1987) consider a range of problems, services and needs of Puerto Rican and other Latinos.

A Puerto Rican folk psychotherapy is provided by a spiritist (*espiritista*). Spiritists work together in a group headed by the medium believed to have the strongest powers (Garrison 1977a, b; Harwood 1981; Rogler and Hollingshead 1961). Harwood (1981) writes that surveys indicate approximately one-third of all Puerto Rican adults seek help from a spiritist at some time in their lives (and not necessarily for a mental or emotional problem). Oths (this volume) compares spiritism with biomedical and chiropractic theory and practice. Earlier, Garrison compared Puerto Rican *espiritismo* to psychiatry (1977b) finding marked commonalties between it and analytic forms of psychiatric practice. Finkler provides us with excellent accounts of spiritism in Mexico (1985a, b). She has considered gender differences in help-seeking and symptom expression.

AFRICAN-AMERICANS

Already noted has been the problem of misdiagnosis in certain ethnic groups, such as African-Americans (Adebimpe 1981). Dressler has done considerable work on stress, depression and status conflicts among Southern African-Americans (1985 a, b, 1986; Dressler and Badger 1985). Garrison (1977) has considered spiritualist help-seeking and healing among African-Americans involved in Puerto-Rican spiritism. Snow (1977) provides an account of the ethnopsychiatric beliefs in the context of the ethnomedicine and of various healer's roles. Baer's critical medical view of "black" healers discounts culture to favor of a form of deprivation theory (1981) to explain enthusiastic religion.

Weidman's magisterial work on the Miami area shows us the ethnomedical and ethnopsychiatric systems of a number of groups in the American South (Weidman et al. 1978). She has also discussed *falling-out*, a folk disorder among African-Americans, Haitians, Anglos, and other Southern ethnic groups (Weidman et al., 1978, 1979). Kuna (1977) argues that *hoodoo* is the principal form of black ethnopsychiatry and ethnomedicine.

Cases concerning the intersection of psychiatry, medicine, and folk beliefs of southern African-Americans have been conducted by psychiatrists with anthropological interests and skills (Hillard and Rockwell 1978; Lyles and Hillard 1982). These studies have focused on problems caused by hexes from witchcraft. McNally, Casiday and Calamari (1990) report a case of *taijin kyofusho* in an African-American woman.

Frankel et al. (1978), Borker, Herd and Hembry (1980) and Gaines (1985b) have considered cultural conceptions of alcohol use, abuse, and problem behavior among urban "blacks"; (the latter also critiques the validity of the topical social category itself). Up to 1980, Maltz (1980) had compiled the most complete and extensive bibliography on African-Americans and drinking practices and problems.

The culture of a U.S. state's alcohol research division, its problematic assumptions and system of social classification related to African-Americans have also has come under study (Gaines 1981). Recently, chronic illness has been taken up as a topic of research. Alzheimer's disease is beginning to receive some attention among African-Americans (Gaines 1989) and Hispanics (see below).

MEXICANS IN NORTH AMERICA

Madsen (1964) has described the role of the *curandero* in southern Texas. The *curandero* serves as a folk therapist for Mexican-Americans in this region and others in the United States and Mexico. *Mal ojo*, evil eye, is a manifestation of envy and may provoke mental illness in those who are admired. The conception is widely found in the Mediterranean and among Latin Americans (Maloney 1976). Witchcraft and witches are likewise causes mental disorders as is found widely in the world. *Espanto* (fright) is caused by seeing a ghost or demon while *susto* (fright) can be caused by natural fright. *Bilis* (bile) is a disease caused by an emotional upset, quite often the result of anger which stimulates yellow bile production and causes an imbalance of humors (also see Clark 1959; Kay 1977; Rubel et al. 1984).

Both *susto* and *bilis*, though emotional in origin, are classified as "natural diseases." Their etiologies are conceived as natural imbalances, while other ailments like *mal ojo* are thought to be supernatural in origin

(Kay 1977). The *curandero* is viewed as one with a gift from God who brings disordered bodies and souls back to normal conditions (Kiev 1968a). Distinguished from the witch (*bruja*), the *curandero's* power is derived from God, while the former's is from Satan.

Because the *curanderos* are familiar with the nature of the value conflicts in Mexican-American society and those arising from contact with the wider Anglo culture, they are frequently successful in healing (Madsen 1964). Rubel (1977), as noted, has analyzed the epidemiology of susto, locating its etiology in social situations of stress or conflict. In 1984, Rubel et al. gave a thorough, comprehensive evaluation of *susto* and research findings on it.

Nervios has also been found to gloss what psychiatrists define as *schizophrenia* (Jenkins 1988a, b; Guarnaccia and Farias 1988). Work suggests the family context of that condition among Mexican-Americans is centrally important to its understanding (Jenkins, this volume). The determination of the nature of the problem is generally made within that context (Jenkins 1988a).

Good et al. (1985) have considered countertransference in a multidisciplinary psychotherapeutic clinic case with a Mexican-American woman in Northern California. Keefe, Padilla and Carlos (1979) have considered the social support system provided by Mexican-American families, related to the sort of "over-support" or locally perceived pathologies of support as found in Jenkins's study (this volume).

Dugan (1988) has discussed *compadrazgo*, the fictive kinship network, and its effect on the lowering of the incidence of *depression* among Mexican-American women at risk. And, Alzheimer's has recently been taken up as a topic with reference to specific ethnic groups. Social Work professor Vallé has been doing research on Alzheimer's and barriers to access and resources for Hispanics (1989). This promises to be an important area of future research.

Another topic of continuing interest is the problem of adjustment of Latino immigrants. Much of this work again points to the role of the family. Of concern are also problems of stress, role conflicts, and acculturation for many Latino groups including Mexican-Americans (Gaviria and Arana 1987; Edgerton and Karno 1971; Keefe, Padilla and Carlos 1979; Rogler, Malgady and Rodriguez 1989). The literature increasingly discusses mental health help-seeking and culture-specific psychiatric services (e.g., Rogler, Malgady and Rodriguez 1989; Westermeyer 1989).

NORTH AMERICAN INDIANS

Among the thousands of potentially relevant studies of North American Indians, there is Devereux's classic (1961) tome which described in detail the Mohave ethnopsychiatric system (see also Devereux 1941). In general, a basic etiological principle is suggested; the concept of disorganized power, due to some type of conflict, which may be externally or internally generated.

Many psychiatric studies of Native Canadians can be found in the *White Cloud Journal* (begun 1980) as well as the *Canadian Psychiatric Association Journal* (begun 1955). Boag considers the general picture of mental health in of peoples of the Arctic (1970) while Jilek (1971) has shown the professional reconceptualization of Native American medicine men from a marginal native to auxiliary psychotherapist. Other descriptions of aspects of North American Indian ethnopsychiatries include Hallowell (1967) on self and illness among the Ojibwa. Wallace's classic on the Iroquois showed us a system that is an ethnopsychoanalytic cthnopsychiatry (1972, also see 1959). The *burnt child reaction* has been analyzed among the Yukon Eskimos (Inuit) (Boyer et al. 1978). Psychiatrist Kirmayer (in press) gives an overview of Inuit mental health among whom he also does field research in Canada.

Kaplan and Johnson (1964) and Kunitz provide insight into Navajo ethnopsychiatry, while Levy, Neutra and Parker (1987) consider a variety of seizure disorders among the Navajo and the indigenous nosology which classifies them. Sandner, a Jungian psychiatrist, considers Navajo healers, healing and myths (1979). Boyer, also a psychiatrist (and honorary shaman), approaches Apaches shamanism from an psychoanalytic perspective (1964), while Jilek (1974) gives us an account of Northwest Coast Indians' traditional ethnopsychiatric therapies. Many other, older studies are notable including those by such scholars as Aberle, Opler, Eggan, Kroeber, Lowie, LaBarre and Parker, among many others.

In a thorough review, Trimble et al. (1984) report on the variety of local conceptions of mental disorders among American Indians. Matchett (1972, in O'Nell 1989) discusses a case of nonpsychotic hallucinations among the Hopi arguing against universalist explanations which pathologize an exceptional, but culturally acceptable, mourning experience of encountering deceased relatives. Markides and Coreil (1988) also consider the phenomenon of mourning hallucinations. Little explored is the fact that this type of behavior is common among both "blacks" and "whites" in the U.S. South as was found by the senior author (ADG), in the course of epidemiological research preliminary to the Epidemiological Catchment Area (ECA) Project at Duke University (1982–83).

For many years, the only complete published account of a psychotherapy was that of Devereux. This was the complete record of a psychotherapy with a plains Indian detailed in his classic *Reality and Dream* (1951). Most recently, O'Nell has ably assessed the literature on psychiatric studies of American Indians including the problems of classification of culture-bound syndromes and universalist interpretations of phenomena. Irigoyen-Rascon (1989) discussed the etiological theories of madness among the Tarahumara Indians of Northern Mexico.

ALASKAN NATIVES

Dinges et al. (1980) and Manson and Trimble (1982) have also written on psychotherapy and counseling with American Indians and Inuit. Psychiatrist Foulks (1985) has long considered *pibloktoq* (arctic hysteria), at times proposing biochemical explanations for it. Gussow (1985) has considered it recently in local ethnopsychiatric terms. Some time ago, Murphy (1964) considered shamans and shamanism among Alaskan Natives. There are as well a host of studies on social problems among the Inuit, many considered in O'Nell's review (1989), such as the pressures on young adults in the process of change (O'Neil 1986).

EUROPEAN NORTH AMERICAN ETHNICS

While there are good ethnographies of religious communities such as the Amish (e.g, Hostetler), generally, as with the psychiatric studies of them, those with psychiatric foci have tested professional theories of mental illness rather than studying the local ethnopsychiatry. Like the default mode of a computer, the thousands of studies of mental illness in the United States and Canada concern European-Americans or Canadians of like origin, though the research is presented as generic. Thus, the cultural context of problems is obscured.

In the so-called "general population," because of deinstitutionalization, there appears to be a greater burden on families as patients are treated in community-based programs and have shorter hospital stays; the afflicted stay or return sooner to their families and, therefore, often with higher levels of distress (Biegel, Sales and Schultz 1991:165). The area of chronic disorders, and their construction and maintenance, would appear to be likely topics for future anthropological research. As well, ethnopsychiatric problems of people caring for the chronically ill, whether the afflicted have what are termed physical or mental disorders, may also be a topic of interest. Katon and associates have considered depression extensively in the context of general medical care (1982a, b, 1987), also the concern of Attkinson and Zich's recent volume (1990).

Physicians Like and Ellison (1981) have considered the folk notion of *sleeping blood* among Portuguese-Americans. They present an interesting case of a cultural construction of a conversion reaction in the context of family medical practice in a North Coast city. Scheper-Hughes (1987) has considered the meaning of mental illness among the Irish of the South Boston area. Foulks et al. (1977) provide us with an example of forensic ethnopsychiatry in their treatment of a case of witchcraft and murder among Italian-Americans.

Janes and Ames (1989) have considered alcohol use among male blue-collar workers on the West Coast who are seen as a subculture sharing values and roles. Blue-collar women also have been investigated (Klee and Ames 1986). Many other ethnic groups, including Polish-, African- and Italian-Americans were considered in the successful cross-cultural compendium on alcohol beliefs and practices edited by Bennet and Ames (1985).

Middle-class suburbanites have been looked at recently as well. McGuire (1988) studied the variety of "New Age" alternate therapies and healing strategies. She finds a plethora of such practices which may also draw from the occult domain of Western culture. Many are now well-known to the public and form the basis for large public fairs and other gatherings (e.g., Lattin 1990).

FILIPINO-AMERICANS

Some groups appear only infrequently in the literature relating to ethnopsychiatry. Davidson and Day (1974), for example, considered the cosmology, diagnostic and healing practices of a Filipina healer on the West Coast. They found that her diagnostic and healing strategies were symbolic statements with referents in her own past traumatic experiences in the context of Filipino Catholicism.

ASIANS IN NORTH AMERICA

The large scale emigration from the Middle East, Asia, South and Southeast Asia has resulted in a large number of immigrants in U.S. urban areas. They bring with them folk disorders such as *Hwa-byung* (Pang 1990) which then become of interest not only to anthropologists, but also to clinicians. Psychologists Sue and Morisima (1982) have considered West Coast Asian and Pacific Islanders, their problems and appropriate therapies. Waxler-Morrison et al. (1990) have just recently provided us with a handbook concerning the mental health idioms of distress and social and psychological needs of South and Southeast Asian immigrants in Western Canada. The Goods have considered treatment problems of Chinese (and Iranian) immigrants in a West Coast U.S. psychiatric practice (e.g., 1982, with Moradi, 1985). Pang has interpreted *Hwa-byung* among elderly Korean women immigrants (1990). And Ying explored popular models of depression and help-seeking among Chinese women immigrants (1990).

Canadian psychiatrist Morton Beiser has been particularly concerned with the mental disorders among Asian refugees (Beiser and Fleming 1986; Beiser 1988, 1989). Also prominent in this field and in work on China is T.-

Y. Lin (see Kleinman and Lin 1989; Lin 1986). H. B. M. Murphy investigated the problems of Asian elites immigrating to Canada (1983), a social stratum rarely studied.

As a nation of immigrants, the United States has, at any given point in history, large numbers of newly arrived peoples. While African-Americans can trace back their North American-born ancestry at least seven generations and as far as thirteen, the vast majority of European-Americans can trace their North American-born ancestry just three generations to the first half of this century. Approximately 2.5 million people now in the U.S. are refugees (Westermeyer 1989:3). It has been said that in fact "America's biggest import is people" (Oxford Analytica 1986; in Westermeyer 1989:3).

Professional Ethnopsychiatry

The Epidemiological Catchment Area Project (ECA) is a noteworthy event in U.S. psychiatric epidemiology. It is the largest psychiatric epidemiological study to be done in this country. Using research universities in five sites, East and West Coast, Northern and Southern, rural and urban, it sought to assess the incidence and prevalence of various disorders in each of the major social categories, African-, European-, Asian- and Hispanic-American. (These groups, while conceptual categories, are clearly not cultural groups or even coherent social groups.) Its results currently are being published (e.g., Biegel, Sales and Schulz [1991]; Blazer et al. 1985; Goldstein [1987]; Kleinman [1988]; Robins and Regier 1991).[3] Its findings will be the basis for most decisions in the U.S. regarding research, care and resource allocation related to mental illness for many decades to come.

Some important epidemiological research in Canada has been done by Alexander Leighton. The famous Stirling County Study was begun some 40 years ago. Dr. Leighton is conducting a 40-year follow-up study looking epidemiologically at, among other things, depression. This work is being done with Jane Murphey. He has remained active and written on the roles of anthropology and epidemiology in the Stirling County study (1984a) and the social, psychological and economic barriers to providing adequate care for the mentally ill (1982, 1984b). Syrotuck and D'Arcy (1981) considered the impact of spousal and social (community) support on the course of mental disorders in Canada.

H. B. M. Murphy looked at differences in symptoms of French and British Canadians (1974) and has also looked at cultural influences on schizophrenia in Canada (1978). Murphy and colleagues compared depression in urban and rural French Canadians (Murphy, Kovess and Tousignant 1987). Bibeau et al. (1989) analyzed mental health research in Province Québec and discerned an often inappropriate Anglo-Saxon bias in the research models employed.

Important to the development of the anthropology of professional ethnopsychiatry in the United States were the critiques of theory and practice from within. Most notable among these are the works by Kleinman, Eisenberg, and Fábrega (Manschreck and Kleinman 1977; Eisenberg 1977; Fábrega 1985, 1987). Though these were not based on ethnographic research, they, and interpretive social cultural anthropology (i.e., Geertz and Turner), inspired the first interpretive ethnographic studies of U.S. professional (Gaines and Wood 1978; Gaines 1979) and other, popular ethnopsychiatries (e.g. Good 1977).

Some early anthropological work on the mentally ill was the innovative work by Jules Henry (1973), who did participant observation of psychotic children and their families in their respective homes (1973, orig. 1963), foreshadowing aspects of Jenkins's research shown in this volume. Also noteworthy and influential was the work of Goffman (1961) on the total institutions. Szasz (1961) with many others, produced the antipsychiatric literature of the 1960s wherein the existence of mental illness was said to be mythical, a metaphor. Gaines (1979) focused on the social interaction of an urban resident of a West Coast city who was afflicted with the "metaphor" of paranoia. Frank's (1961) work on U.S. and other forms of psychotherapy and the nature of efficacy should be mentioned as well as Young's critique of its assumptions (1988b).

Historian Morantz-Sanchez (1985) provides us with a good history of women in the medical profession including psychiatry. She discusses female physicians in psychiatric institutions (by the late 1880s) where it was believed their services were more salutary for patient health than those of male physicians. Menninger (1963) has given us a detailed history of psychiatric classifications, including a compendium of different nosologies from the classical age to the present. He shows that hundreds of distinct nosologies were in use in the U.S. of the early 1960s. Today some 450 distinct named therapeutic orientations exist in United States psychiatry and psychology.

As the reader is doubtless cognizant, Devereux made his mark here as well. He wrote on diagnosis, classification, therapy, the central problem of normality and abnormality, and a host of other issues in relation to psychiatry and its institutions in the U. S. (see 1944, 1949, 1978a, b, 1980a, b, among others). Issues of diagnosis as cultural practices and classifications as cultural artifacts are again very much in evidence (e.g., Farmer 1980; Fábrega 1987; Gaines 1992; Kirmayer 1990; Lock 1987; Nuckolls 1992; Prince and Tcheng-Laroche 1987; Post 1992; Young 1991). This avenue of research promises to provide new insights into psychiatries and their hidden cultural bases of thought and action (also see Littlewood and Lipsedge 1987, but note the views in the *Journal of Abnormal Psychology Special Issue*, August 1991).

Sociologist Light (1976) describes three distinct work styles among East Coast psychiatric residents. Gaines's study (1979) explores psychiatrists' approaches to patients and their definitions of the psychiatric illnesses and their work which revealed the logic of evident diagnostic styles. Self conceptions were suggested (in a footnote) to underlie the entire organization of practice and theory in psychiatry. Subsequent work focused on conceptions of self and person and on ethnographic accounts of theory, practice, and diversity within "secular" and Christian psychiatry (e.g., Gaines 1982b, 1985a).

Townsend compared folk and professional ideology regarding mental disorders in Germany and the United States (1978, 1979). Light's studies of psychiatric education should be mentioned as well (1980). Young (1980) has shown how psychiatry's discourse on stress reproduces conventional cultural knowledge. Ingleby has viewed psychiatry from a critical perspective in several works (1980, 1983).

Family physician-anthropologist Helman (1988) continued his interest in psychosomatic illness (which began as work in England) with a study in the U.S. This is a potentially huge area of ethnopsychiatric interest though little studied (see Maretzki, this volume). Johnson (1985) has considered consultation-liaison psychiatry and shows the marginal relationship of the specialty of psychiatry to other medical specialties. Johnson and Kleinman (1984) provide a more clinical and cultural view of this psychiatric specialty. And McGovern (1985) discusses the social origins of the psychiatric profession in the U.S.

A number of studies on psychiatric institutions have been done, including those by historian Dwyer (1987, this volume), Castel, Castel and Lovell (1982), Rhodes' (1985, 1991, this volume), and Katz (this volume), among many others. Especially noteworthy is the historical work of Foucault (1973), which has contributed to the modern understanding of psychiatric institutions.

A. Young (1988, 1991) has been providing us with excellent accounts of the construction of Post-traumatic Stress Disorder (PTSD) as a psychiatric disease. He considers the production of psychiatric knowledge and the social and moral organization of an institution that treats it. Recently, Young has considered moral conflicts and their modulation involved in the treatment of this disorder, that is, the "topography of ethical judgement" in his psychiatric setting (1990), thereby initiating anthropological research on ethnopsychiatric ethics. Psychiatrists Lidz and Mulvey (1990) also consider ethical questions. They do so in the context of a consideration of institutional fiscal concerns and their influence on psychiatric decision-making with reference to admission and commitment.

Psychologists Oltmanns and Maher (1988) have edited a work incorporating a variety of viewpoints and theories of delusions. Gaines (1988) therein considers the cultural relativity, construction and interpretation of the delusional. The variable nature and locus of traumatic experiences cross-culturally has also been discussed (Gaines 1986b). Anthropologist Rittenberg and psychiatrist Simons (1985) give us an outsider's and an insider's view of the brief initial psychiatric evaluation where the construction of a sensible "story" is sought by the interviewing psychiatrist. Rhodes (1984) interprets metaphors employed in psychiatric institutions for often powerful medicines. Nichter proposes a role for anthropologists in clinical settings, that of therapist facilitator (1985).

India

Traditional/Folk Ethnopsychiatry

Bhattacharyya (1983) writes that beliefs of ghost possession are one paradigm held by Bengalis regarding mental illness. Ghosts are thought to be deceased persons unable to leave this world because they died before their time. A change in a person's personality is the major indicator of ghost possession. Sorcery is another explanatory paradigm. Sorcery can mimic a variety of symptoms of mental illness as well as cause the individual to act against his/her own best interests, such as a married man having an affair. A final paradigm, head disturbance, is derived from Ayurvedic theory. Bengalis acknowledge the three humors (wind, bile, and phlegm) and consider the disease as an imbalance in these three. Mental illness is a hot disease attributed to excess bile which generates heat in the head. Indian notions of mental disorder and their relation to help-seeking were investigated by Weiss et al. (1986). A mixture of conceptual models was found in the patients. There are a large number of studies of possession illnesses in the psychological anthropological literature (e.g., Crapanzano and Garrison 1977). Nichter's (1981) study of folk idioms of distress for particular problems of women is noteworthy as is Shweder and Bourne's (1982) study of Indian self conceptions discussed in the first chapter. Lynch's recent volume (1990) depicts the cultural construction of emotions. The work has direct relevance to those interested in self and illness in India as do the growing number of studies on emotion reviewed in Chapter One.

Professional Ethnopsychiatry

India has two professional medicines (three, if one includes Islamic Galenic or Unnani) and so both will be briefly described.

AYURVEDIC ETHNOPSYCHIATRY

Obeyesekere (1976, 1981) has described Ayurvedic conceptions of the mind. According to classic Ayurveda, the mind has four basic functions, very much like the ego-functions of psychoanalytic theory. Symptoms of

psychopathology are due to the malfunctioning of the mind through physiological factors. The majority of classical theorists maintain that the mind
and self are located in the heart, not the brain. Mental illness arises when
the heart does not function properly, because the ducts and channels that
carry the *dosas* (humors) and *dhatus* (vital elements) to that organ have
failed to function properly. Hence, Obeyesekere writes, the etiology of mental illness is somato-psychic, rather than psychosomatic. The basic principle of treatment is the same in all physical and mental diseases: control and
counteract humoral upset.

WESTERN-STYLE ETHNOPSYCHIATRY

A good overview of the theory and practice of psychiatry in India is
given by Sethi et al. (1977). They discuss briefly the social and cultural
environment of the country. In recent history, the practice of psychiatry
was limited to the few mental hospitals located in suburban areas. These
facilities were inadequately equipped, poorly staffed and fulfilled primarily
custodial functions. By the mid-1970s, the number of psychiatric beds had
significantly increased and postgraduate programs in psychiatry were available in more than a dozen institutions.

The authors provide data regarding the incidence of psychiatric disorders, noting that mental retardation is very prevalent, and suggest that 2
percent of the population is psychiatrically ill (excluding cases of mental
retardation). Freudian psychoanalysis is not popular, attributed by the
authors to the generation of guilt feelings through discussions of sex.
Regarding guidance services, the authors state that prior to 1950, few existed in the country. Currently, more are found and a brief description of such
services is provided. Bennett (1971) discussed the influence of the Indian
family upon the practice of psychiatry. He states there exists a high incidence of depression which is often associated with disruptions of family life.

Southeast Asia: Malaysia and Indonesia

Traditional/Folk Ethnopsychiatry

Concepts of mental illness, among Malays, called *gila*, were assessed by
Resner and Hartog (1970) through unstructured interviews and observations in West Malaysian villages. The authors state that although there is
some overlapping, *gila* is not equivalent to schizophrenia. Other disorders
are also discussed. Hartog (1972) has described the Malaysia system of intervention for mental and social deviants. The family is the first line of intervention, followed by the village headman and the folk healer. Laderman's
recent study deftly combines foci on psychology, aesthetics and medicine in
her study of Malay shamanic performances (1991), showing the artificiality

of our usual disciplinary boundaries. Also of note are Westermeyer and Wintrob (1979) and the many studies of *amok* and *latah*, discussed above.

Provencher (1984) describes in detail a Malaysian folk healer and notes that a Western-trained psychiatrist may not be successful in treating patients because the ritual of Western psychiatry may be meaningless to the patients. Laderman (1991) demonstrates the multicultural history of Malaysian shamanism. Salan and Maretzki (1983) discuss a number of Indonesian folk healers. They conclude that common characteristics of these individuals are: experiences of personal or family suffering during their life and the consequential search and call which result in healing powers. Ong (1988) has discussed possession by young women in factories and sees it in relation to gender symbolism and social boundaries. The view is contrasted with the "corporate" or biomedical view which turns the possessed into patients and thereby obscures their voices.

Professional Ethnopsychiatry

ISLAMIC-STYLE

An Islamic psychiatric institution, *asrama*, in West Java is described by Horikoshi (1980). This rare institution, built in 1952, was operated by a local healer who had learned his curing art from his own father, a religious figure. Generally, curing knowledge is handed down from master, *ulama* (religious figure) to apprentice, *santri*, students. Most *ulama* practice medicine only for family, patron/friends and villagers, and not in clinics. In Islamic psychiatry, religion and medicine are inseparable. Recovery from illness required both medical and religious efforts.

WESTERN-STYLE

Most reports of psychiatry in this region date back to the 1970s (Kinzie et al. 1974; Bennett 1971, 1976; Neki 1973) and are dated. Neki (1973) states that there was a lack of psychiatrists in this region (he considers specifically Burma, Ceylon, India, Indonesia, and Thailand) and those who practice do so mostly in overcrowded asylums. There is an absence of auxiliary personnel; psychiatric nurses are rare and psychiatric social workers even rarer. A large majority of psychiatrists are trained in the West. Salan and Maretzki (1983) provide some recent information regarding Indonesian mental health care. The origin of services derives from the Mental Health Act under Dutch colonial rule in 1882 and the building of a hospital in Bogor. New legislation after independence established a "modern" mental health approach based on Western concepts. A Mental Health Act in 1966 introduced the "open-hospital" style management.

The Second Five Year Development Plan (1974–1979) directed the development of several health centers and one small general hospital in each district. The authors write that the new health care strategies have prompted a shift in the medical thinking of psychiatrists from a biological orientation to a wider, community-oriented, clinical approach. In an earlier paper, Bennett (1971) states that the influence of Dutch psychiatry remains and many doctors have been trained in Holland.

THE PHILIPPINES

Guthrie and Szanton (1976) looked specifically at folk diagnosis and therapy in the Philippines. Griffiths (1988), while providing an ethnography of a Philippine village, also provides much data on evil spirits implicated in ethnopsychiatric illness. Lieban's fine study looks at healing and malign magic in the Philippines focusing on some indigenous healers of local renown (1967).

Oceania

Traditional/Folk Ethnopsychiatry

THE MAORI

Ritchie (1976) has discussed the ethnopsychiatry of the Maori. In classic Maori culture, mad persons were called *keka* (deranged) or *kikiki* (idiot) and were believed to be possessed by a *kikokiko*, the ghost of a dead person (or demon), or came in to that condition by *makutu*, the practice of black magic and the casting of spells. Ritchie writes that there were strong elements of seclusion, positively sanctioned withdrawal, special attention and support in the traditional Maori manner of dealing with psychological stress. These elements comprise a traditional form of therapy which he terms "time out."

A range of traditional activities in Oceania, termed "disentangling" (Watson-Gegeo and White 1990) serve to resolve conflicts but also to explore social arrangements and facilitate resolution and change. In the Watson-Gegeo and White volume, a number of Oceanic societies are considered including the Solomon Islands, Fiji, Tuvalu, Hawai'i, and Vanuatu.

HAWAI'I

McDermott et al. (1980) have provided a psychocultural portrait of the people of Hawai'i, including *locals* (local-born and reared, usually of mixed ancestry), Japanese, Hawaiians, Chinese, Portuguese, *kama'inas* (long-term Anglo residents) and *ha'oles* (Anglo foreigners). Gaines (1982a) presents psychiatric cases involving ethnicity and psychiatric knowledge in Hawai'i while Katz et al. (1969) and Marsella et al. (1973), among others, have considered illness experience and expression among the many ethnic groups of Hawai'i. Ito (1985) and Boggs and Chun (1990) have considered the use of *ho'oponopono*, a traditional native Hawaiian conflict resolution and therapeutic form. Ito specifically shows how this traditional ethnopsychiatric process has been adapted for use as family therapy under agency supervision in modern Hawai'i (1985).

SAMOA AND FIJI

Clement (1982) has described Samoan conceptions of mental illness, relating to them other aspects of the culture and society. Data were collected through traditional ethnographic methods and a variety of ethnosemantic techniques indicating indigenous categories as well as the influence of missionaries on their etiological theories. Duranti (1990) has considered various forms of *fono*, various institutions dealing with "disentangling" conflicts in Samoan society. Some of these have relevance for ethnopsychiatry. Brenneis (1990) studies Indians in Fiji and the therapeutic aspects of *pancayat*.

TAHITI AND TONGA

Psychiatrist-anthropologist Robert Levy has considered mental illness in the course of his highly regarded psychological study of the Tahitians (Levy 1973). He notes Tahitian etiological conceptions, therapies and therapeutic outcomes. While not much is available for this area, we have C. Parsons' fairly recent account of idioms of distress and well as the local conceptions of disorders, some of psychiatric interest, in Tonga (1984).

SOLOMON ISLANDS

White (1990) looks at "disentangling" as emotion talk which serves to certify and or restore a harmony between social relations and personal thoughts/feelings (1990:57). Watson-Gegeo and Gegeo (1990) examine *fa'amanata'anga*, a social context and speech activities among the Kwara'ae of the Solomon Island in which "personal problems and social conflicts are examined and resolved or managed" (p. 161). Among the Kwara'ae, teaching, counseling and conflict resolution are extension of each other by virtue of psychocultural framework underlying local conceptions of self and social relationships.

NEW GUINEA AND AUSTRALIA

Cawte has provided some information on two groups from this area. He has given us an account of beliefs and indigenous illnesses of Aranda people of Australia (1965) and of other tribal groups there (1974). Later, he looked at *malgri*, a culture-bound syndrome, in terms of its folk etiology and treatment (and prevention) (1976). Schieffelin (1985) considers depressive affect among his New Guinea people, the Kaluli, who live near Mount Bosavi. He explores the cultural structure of anger and grief and argues that their structure and the cultural patterning of expression do not allow for the repression of such emotions which might lead to later emotional problems or interpersonal conflicts.

IFALUK

Catherine Lutz has considered the nature of emotion in Ifaluk in Micronesia. In several important articles and a recent book (e.g., 1985, 1988), she has convincingly shown that Western conceptions of emotion, and their putative natural separation from cognition, are culturally constructed. This is important for it shows the cultural basis for a key dichotomy used to classify mental disorders in the West (Gaines 1992) (see Kirmayer 1988; Gordon 1988).

Aspects of professional ethnopsychiatry in the region can be found in McDermott el al. (1980), Ito (1985), and Boggs and Chun (1990).

Eastern Europe

Professional and Folk Ethnopsychiatries

Although historical developments in psychiatric practice vary among the Eastern Block countries, care for the mentally ill during the Middle Ages was generally provided through monasteries. These countries had contact with Western Europe during the nineteenth century. Many well-known psychiatrists there received training in France and Germany, and some worked with Freud and Adler. While the search for organic, social, and psychological elements received emphasis in European psychiatry at this time, in Eastern Europe, dominant theories spoke of diseases of the brain. The European focus on an organic approach to mental illness persists in these countries today, though Pavlov's organic conception of psychiatry has been the most accepted (Kiev 1968b).

EAST GERMANY (FORMER)

Psychiatry did not develop any differently here than it did in West Germany until 1945. The strong tie between psychiatry and neurology was established when W. Griesinger founded the Psychiatric and Neurological Clinic of the University of Berlin Charity Hospital in the late nineteenth century. The treatment of mental illness was placed on the same level with physical illness, discouraging "moralistic" psychiatry. Under Griesinger's influence, it became customary to train in both psychiatry and neurology. During 1933–1945, official doctrine forced many psychiatric patients to undergo mass sterilization, i.e., to prevent growth of putatively hereditary psychiatric diseases. In the second half of the dictatorship, many thousands were systematically killed (Meyer-Lindenberg 1991).

With the division of Germany, psychoanalysis and psychosomatic medicine and existential analysis continued in the West, while the teachings of Pavlov gained prominence in the East. The majority of psychiatrists adhere to a conservative principle based on Kraepelin so neurology and psychiatry are treated as one discipline. Reunification, doubtless, will change its nature.

HUNGARY

Scientific psychiatry began in this country in 1850 when Ferenc Schwartzer opened his private mental hospital. A peculiarly Hungarian endeavor was the so-called "hospitalization movement" which advocated that general hospitals should establish wards for psychotics in the same complex of buildings so that patients would not be labeled and inhibited from returning to society (Nyiro 1968). Nyiro (1968) considers the further development of Hungarian psychiatry in the pre- and post-war periods.

YUGOSLAVIA (FORMER)

Professional psychiatry developed in the second half of the nineteenth century with the establishment of mental hospitals, the first of which was founded in Belgrade, Serbia. A brief history is provided by Jakovljevic (1968). A strict materialistic-organic orientation was established and an antipsychological orientation emerged. However, in 1953 two institutions with psychodynamic orientations were founded. The holistic dynamic orientation predominates more and more, in which an integration of biological, psychological, and social elements occurs (Jakovljevic 1968).

CZECHOSLOVAKIA

The most modern psychiatric facility in Europe in the first half of the nineteenth century was the "New House" built in the garden of the Prague Hospital in 1844. Besides pharmacotherapy (mainly sedative), rehabilitation was through physical therapy, hydrotherapy and the drinking of waters from Karlsbad, occupational therapy, physical training and musicotherapy. The first textbook of psychiatry by Karel Kuffner was published in 1897 and laid the foundations for the Czech scientific psychiatric terminology. It was organistic in its nosological conception and descriptive in its psychological parts (Prokupek et al. 1968). During World War II and almost ten years after, Czech psychiatry was isolated from the rest of the world of psychiatry. It basically still maintains the materialistic conception, based on reflex theory. Emphasis is on outpatient services, which did not begin until after World War II. Neurology was separated from psychiatry in 1955. Hydrotherapy and physiotherapy, used in treatment at spas for neurotics and some psychotics, are highly developed forms of treatment in Czechoslovakia (Prokupek et al. 1968).

POLAND

The first laws recognizing the insane as ill people and free of demonology were the Lithuanian Statutes of 1529. Founded in 1920, the Polish Psychiatric Association exerted a great influence on the development and organization of the mental health services in the country. Frydman (1983) has provided an excellent description of psychiatric practice in Poland. He notes the tremendous impact World War II had upon psychiatric practice in Poland. Prior to World War II, Polish psychiatry was influenced by the German descriptive, organic approach, and to a lesser extent, by the psychodynamic movement from Vienna. However, once the war was over, the Soviet view of mental disorders—mental disturbance could only be attributed to a biologically based psychopathological process within the individual himself—became prominent. After Stalin's death, Polish psychiatry began to attain some professional autonomy. A shift away from the major psychoses toward neurotic and characterological disturbances occurred. (See Aleksandrowicz and Czbala [1982] for a brief description of psychotherapy in Poland.) Diagnosis is based upon the International Classification of Diseases of WHO.

THE (FORMER) SOVIET UNION

Of all regional practices of psychiatry, that of the Soviet Union has received the most attention. Much work on Soviet psychiatry has been done by Field (1960, 1964, 1967, 1968, 1977) and Field and Aronson (1964, 1965). Miller looks at the early asylums for the mentally ill individuals and later developments (1985). Easson (1977) examines the Leninist government following the 1917 revolution and its impact on lay and psychiatric society. A Marxist theory of psychology, a materialist outlook, was sought, and Freud and psychoanalysis were condemned by 1930. Pavlov and his neurophysiological theory became the hallmark of Soviet psychiatry, and Pavlov himself was deemed the founding father of Soviet psychiatry. Genetic, biochemical, neurological, and physiological explanations have been sought for the etiology of psychiatric disorders. Mental illness is conceived to be impairment of "conscious, willful, rationally directed activity" (Miller 1985, p.17). Kline et al. (1961) provide a standardization of Soviet and American Psychiatric Diagnosis. They mention that no category of *paranoia* is used by the Soviets. Field and Aronson (1965) note that according to

Soviet clinical experience, a sharp dislike of work often indicates a subsequent diagnosis of *schizophrenia.*

A Soviet psychiatric disease not recognized in the West is *creeping schizophrenia* which exhibits no symptoms apart from political or religious nonconformity (Rich 1985). Diagnostic criteria have created a barrier to communication, for Soviet psychiatry utilizes a complex system which is rooted in the international classification index used in much of European psychiatry, with varieties of specifically Soviet diagnostic classifications for many disorders (Miller 1985). Segal (1975) provides a fuller discussion of the theoretical bases of Soviet psychotherapy. He concludes that current Soviet psychotherapy lacks a unitary theoretical basis. (See Field and Aronson [1965] for a discussion of work therapy in Soviet psychiatric hospitals). Education, reeducation, guidance and some emotional support are the primary elements of group psychotherapy in the Soviet Union (Ziferstein 1972).

Electroconvulsive therapy is not widely popular and medications are prescribed at much higher dosage levels than recommended in the United States (Easson 1977). Other forms of therapy include narcotherapy, speech therapy, physiotherapy and injections (Field and Aronson 1965). Field (1964) reports the term "psychoanalysis" is used but refers to "rational," i.e. non-Freudian, analysis.

The mental hospital does not occupy a central role in the psychiatric system (Field and Aronson 1964). The tradition of Russian and Soviet psychiatry is more French than German and the orientation more toward the neuropsychiatrists (Field 1960). As a rule, the neuropathologist is more likely to treat neuroses, or what are referred as "nervous diseases," and the psychiatrist the psychoses, referred by the Soviets as "psychic diseases." Miller (1985) discusses psychiatric training and education in the Soviet Union while Chodoff (1985) notes the expected loyalties of the physician (to the state, not the patient).

The Soviet Union resigned from the World Psychiatric Association in January, 1983, pre-empting a motion of exclusion by the World Psychiatric Congress in Vienna the following July. The Cuban, Bulgarian, and Czechoslovak associations also resigned. The motion of expulsion resulted from an increasing body of evidence on the Soviet misuse of psychiatric methods and psychotropic drugs for the repression of political dissidents and religious believers (Rich 1985). Here again, massive changes are on the horizon.

Western Europe

Great Britain

British psychiatry developed out of the reforms of the British insane asylums. It was established as a specialty based on a new and scientistic definition of psychiatry but was marginalized and, literally, isolated in the asylum.

It was a profession of low status (Gilman 1988b). This low status continues today where we find it a rather unpopular medical specialty. Proportionately, Britain has one-third fewer psychiatrists than does the United States (Stevens 1966). The British specialty of today began its development after World War I. And though less popular than elsewhere, British psychiatry has had wide influence. It has been highly successful in getting others to accept its version of psychiatric reality. We note that the architects of DSM-III devised ways to bring U.S. diagnostic practices into line with those of the British, especially as regards manic depression and schizophrenia (Talbot 1980).

As well, it is the British diagnostic criteria which have been largely adopted by the WHO in its pilot and full-scale studies of *Outcome of Severe Mental Disorders* (Day et al. 1987; WHO 1973, 1979). Psychiatrists in the studies, British and non-British, were usually trained there. Brown and Harris's famous study of the social origins of depression was done in Britain (1978).

Skultans (1975, 1979) provides us with histories of both popular and professional notions of mental illness. Urban sociologist Margaret Stacy (1976) gives an account of the sociological dimensions of the National Health Service of which British psychiatry is a part. Jones has done an important history of the system (1972) while Navarro (1978) provides a Marxist interpretation of the same system. Within that system, physician (General Practice) Cecil Helman (1985) has studied help-seeking for a "pseudo-disease," problems whose clinical manifestations are without evidence of organic pathology. He shows that these disorders are often seen as psychogenic and or psychosomatic and that medical clinical explanatory models of them are similar to those of lay persons; they are vague, have blurry boundaries and are susceptible to frequent changes.

More recent interpretive work has begun to focus on the manifestations and the role(s) of racism in psychiatry. Littlewood (1982, 1986; with Cross 1981) has been analyzing racism and discrimination in British psychiatry. He notes "cultural psychiatry" is concerned exclusively with ethnic minorities and tends to relate psychiatric problems to an ethnic (i.e., biological) background (1986). Chen, Harrison and Standen exemplify the English cultural psychiatry with their study of Afro-Caribbean psychotic patients (1991). Racism is a topic that has been considered relatively recently from more interpretive anthropological points of view for U.S. psychiatry and public health (Brandt 1978, 1985; Gaines 1982b, 1992; Hahn 1990; and see Adembimpe 1981, for a professional view).

The Netherlands

Breemerter et al. (1986) have discussed the structure of the mental health care in the Netherlands. The current structure and functioning of the health care system dates back to a series of laws from 1865. Founded upon a political philosophy of liberalism, these laws advocated that the state refrain as much as possible from intervening in social and economic life. The authors describe the history of the system, including the resistance to changes and the resulting efforts in integrating the entire Dutch mental health care system. The famous community asylum, Geel, has been considered of late in the literature. Roosens (1979), for example, has studied the nature of the integration of mental patients into the social life of the town. The notion of a therapeutic community is also found as an indigenous form in parts of Africa.

Germany

The German influence on DSMs in the United States has been noted by Young (1991). Gaines (1992) has argued that the biological explanations in German psychiatry, and borrowed by U.S. psychiatry through Griesinger, Kraepelin, Schneider and others, is actually a German folk theory regarding the nature of self-identity. Gilman (1988b) has shown the racists roots of German biology and psychiatry and its influence on the development of psychoanalysis (also see Verwey 1985). The apotheosis of that racism is noted in Meyer-Lindenberg's analysis of the Holocaust and German psychiatry (1991).

In Austria and Germany, psychiatry developed as an applied specialty in control of asylums. But by the 1850s, neurology (pure medical science influenced by French biology [Lesch 1984]) and psychiatry had come to share certain assumptions grounded in racist ideology. This ideology was first articulated by Kant (1760s). Griesinger's dictum, "mind illness is brain illness" came to dominate German psychiatry in the 1850s, partly due to its replication of popular ideology wrapped in scientific guise. This was to be preferred by modernists to what was regarded as "moralist," "natural philosophic" and even psychoanalytic views, as Kraepelin himself argued (Gilman 1988b).

Townsend (1978) states that German psychiatry distinguishes mental disorders that are environmentally caused, and therefore transitory and curable, and those that are endogenous, and therefore chronic and incurable. Townsend notes that this is significant in that in Germany, neurology is given more attention in the psychiatric curriculum than is training in psychotherapeutic methods.

Maretzki (this volume) has discussed the psychotherapeutic philosophy of the German physician, Georg Groddeck. This appears to have some similarity to the description of Islamic psychiatry by Horikoshi (1980) noted above. Maretzki (1988) has also provided us with a useful comparative study of German and United States medicine. Gilman's work on U.S.

and German psychiatry and literature represents a major contribution to our understanding of the cultural bases of professional ideology (e.g., Gilman 1985, 1988a, b, c). A recent concern in German ethnopsychiatric circles has been the mental health problems and service needs of immigrant worker populations. Especially noted in the literature are problems of Turkish workers in Germany (Kroeger and Pfeiffer 1986; Pfleiderer 1991).

Summary

In the foregoing, we have considered briefly a large number of studies of ethnopsychiatric interest. These represent many, but not all, of the studies in and of the field. Our intent was to be fairly extensive, but we could not hope also to be exhaustive. And, the extensive coverage necessarily reduces the depth of the review. The articles in the present volume may be seen as complementing this review and overview and as providing in-depth accounts of a variety of popular and professional ethnopsychiatries. They serve as amplifications, challenges, and exemplifications of some of the perspectives noted in this review.

Notes

1. For overviews representing both sides, local beliefs and Western conceptions applied to others, see Murphy and Leighton (1965), Kiev and Rao (1982), Kennedy (1974), Tseng and McDermott (1981), Mezzich and Berganza (1984), among others.

2. Many studies by key figures in the then-psychological anthropology are noted here as relevant but are largely uncited in this chapter. These include work by the Leightons, Leighton and Murphy, Kluckhohn, Wallace, DeVos, Carstairs, Schwartz and Parker, among others. See White (1982) for a review of the methodologies employed in mental health research.

3. The senior author (ADG) worked on the ECA while at Duke University helping to pretest portions of the instruments and developing a glossary of Southern cultural terms to assist interviewers conducting field interviews.

Acknowledgments

The senior author thanks Allan Young for support while updating this chapter, and Laurence Kirmayer for help locating references.

References

Abel, T., R. Métraux and S. Roll
1987 Psychotherapy and Culture. Albuquerque, NM: University of New Mexico.
Adembimpe, V.
1981 Overview: White Norms and Psychiatric Diagnosis of Black Patients. American Journal of Psychiatry 138:279–285.

Ademuwagun, Z. A., J. A. Ayoade, Ira Harrison and D. M. Warrn, eds.
1979 African Therapeutic Systems. Waltham, MA: Crossroads Press.

Alarcon, Renato D.
1983 A Latin American Perspective on DSM-III. American Journal of Psychiatry 140(1):102–105.

Aleksandrowicz, J. W. and J. C. Czbala
1982 Psychotherapy in Poland. American Journal of Psychiatry 139(8):1051–1054.

American Psychiatric Association
1980 Diagnostic and Statistical Manual III (DSM-III). Washington, D.C.: American Psychiatric Association.
1987 Diagnostic and Statistical Manual III-Revised (DSM-III-R). Washington, D.C.: American Psychiatric Association.

Anderson, A.
1985 Japanese Psychiatry Hospital Reforms Under Way. Nature 318:8.

Atkinson, Jane Monnig
1989 The Art and Politics of Wana Shamanship. Berkeley: University of California Press.

Attkinson, C. C. and J. M. Zich, eds.
1990 Depression in Primary Care: Screening and Detection. New York: Routledge.

Audibert, Agnes, et al.
1983 Rencontre de Cultures et Pathologie Mentale en Bretagne. CICB, #1. Rennes: Institut Culturel de Bretagne.

Baer, Hans
1981 Prophets and Advisors in Black Spiritual Churches: Therapy, Palliative, or Opiate? Culture, Medicine and Psychiatry 5(2):145–170.

Basker, Eileen and Virginia Domínguez
1984 Limits to Cultural Awareness: The Immigrant as Therapist. Human Relations 37(9):693–719.

Bebbington, P. E.
1978 The Epidemiology of Depressive Disorder. Culture, Medicine and Psychiatry 2(4):297–341.

Beck, A.
1973 The Development of Depression: A Cognitive Model. In The Psychology of Depression. R. Friedman and M. Katz (eds.). New York: Winston-Wiley.
1976 Cognitive Therapy and the Emotional Disorders. New York: International Universities Press.

Beeman, William
1985 Dimensions of Dysphoria: The View from Linguistic Anthropology. In Culture and Depression. A. Kleinman and B. Good (eds.). Berkeley: University of California Press.

Beiser, Morton
1985 A Study of Depression Among Traditional Africans, Urban North Americans and Southeast Asian Refugees. In Culture and Depression. A. Kleinman and B. Good (eds.). Berkeley: University of California Press.

1988 The Mental Health of Immigrants and Refugees in Canada. Santé, Culture, Health 5(2):177–214.

1989 Migration and Mental Health. Annals of the Royal College of Physicians and Surgeons 22(1):21–25.

Beiser, M. and J. Fleming

1986 Measuring Psychiatric Disorder Among Southeast Asian Refugees. Psychological Medicine 16:627–639.

Bennet, A. E.

1971 Some Impressions of Psychiatric Facilities in the Orient. Hospital and Community Psychiatry May:153–155.

1976 Impressions of Psychiatry in Singapore, Malayasia, Thailand, and Taiwan. Biological Psychiatry 11(3):345–353.

Bennett, Linda and Genevieve Ames, eds.

1985 The American Experience with Alcohol. New York: Plenum Press.

Ben-Tovim, David I.

1985 DSM-III in Botswana: A Field Trial in a Developing Country. American Journal of Psychiatry 142(3):342–345.

Bhattacharyya, Deborah

1983 Psychiatric Pluralism in Bengal, India. Social Science and Medicine 17(14):947–956.

Bibeau, Gilles

1986/7 Nouvelles Directions dans l'anthropologie Medico-Psychiatrique Nord Américain. Santé, Culture, Health 4:10–20.

Bibeau, Gilles, C. Sabtier, E. Corin, M. Tousignant and J. F. Saucier

1989 La Recherche Sociale Ango-Saxonne. Santé Mentale au Québec 14(1):103–120.

Biegel, David E., E. Sales and R. Schulz

1991 Family Caregiving in Chronic Illness. Newbury Park, CA: Sage.

Bilu, Yoram

1979 Demonic Explanations of Disease Among Moroccan Jews in Israel. Culture, Medicine and Psychiatry 3(4):363–380.

Bilu, Yoram, Eliezer Witztum and Onno Van Der Hart

1990 Paradise Regained: "Miraculous Healing" in an Israeli Psychiatric Clinic. Culture, Medicine and Psychiatry 14(1):105–127.

Blazer, Dan G. et al.

1985 Psychatric Disorders: A Rural/Urban Comparison. Archives of General Psychiatry 41:971–978.

Bloomingdale, Lewis M.

1980 Chinese Psychiatry After Mao-Zedong. Psychiatric Annals 10(6):217–224.

Blue, Amy V.

1991 Culture, *Nevra* and Institution. The Making of Greek Professional Psychiatry. Unpublished Ph.D. dissertation in Anthropology. Case Western Reserve University. Cleveland, Ohio.

Blum, Richard and Eva Blum

1965 Health and Healing in Rural Greece. Stanford: Stanford University Press.

1970 The Dangerous Hour: The Lore of Crisis and Mystery in Rural Greece. New York: Scribner.

Boag, T. J.
1970 Mental Health of Native Peoples of the Arctic. Canadian Psychiatric Association Journal 15(2):115–120.

Boddy, Janice
1988 Spirits and Selves in Northern Sudan. American Ethnologist 15(1):4–27.

Boggs, Stephen and Malcolm Chun
1990 *Ho'oponopono:* A Hawaiian Method of Solving Problems. In Disentangling. K. Watson-Gegeo and G. White (eds.). Stanford: Stanford University Press.

Borker, Ruth, Denise Herd and Karen Hembry
1980 Ethnographic Report for the *Black Drinking Practices Study*. 3 Vols. Berkeley, CA: Source, Inc.

Boroffk, Alexander
1988 15 Jahre Beobachtung und Therapie eines Afrikanischen Wahnkranken. Curare 11(3):177–186.

Boyd, J. and M. Weissman
1981 Epidemiology of Affective Disorders. Archives of General Psychiatry 38:1039–1046.

Boyer, L. Bryce
1964 Folk Psychiatry of the Apaches of the Mescalero Indian Reservation. In Magic, Faith and Healing. Ari Kiev (ed.). New York: The Free Press.

Boyer, L. Brice, George DeVos, O. Borders and A. Tani-Borders
1978 The *Burnt Child Reaction* Among the Yukon Eskimo. Journal of Psychological Anthropology 1(1):7–56.

Brandt, Allan
1978 Racism and Research: The Case of the Tuskegee Syphilis Study. The Hastings Center Report, Dec.:21–29.
1985 No Magic Bullet. Cambridge: Harvard University Press.

Breemerter Stege, C. D. C. and P. Van Heugten
1986 Changing Structure of Dutch Mental Health Care. Social Science and Medicine 23(3):283–291.

Brenneis, Donald
1990 Dramatic Gestures: The Fiji Indian *Pancayat* as Therapeutic Event. In Disentangling. K. Watson-Gegeo and G. White (eds.). Stanford: Stanford University Press.

Briggs, Jean
1970 Never in Anger. Cambridge. Harvard University Press.

Brown, G. W. and T. Harris, eds.
1978 Social Origins of Depression: A Study of Psychiatric Disorder in Women. London: Tavistock.

Burton-Bradley, Burton G.
1977 Longlong-Transcultural Psychiatry in Papua Nieuw Guinea. Port Moresby: Public Health Department.

Carothers, J. C.
1953 The African Mind in Health and Disease. WHO Mgr. 17. Geneva: WHO.

Carr, Jack
1978 Ethno-Behaviorism and the Culture-Bound Syndromes. Culture, Medicine and Psychiatry 2:269–293.

Carr, Jack and Peter Vitaliano
1985 Theoretical Implications of Converging Research on Depression and Culture-Bound Syndromes. In Culture and Depression. A. Kleinman and B. Good (eds.). Berkeley: University of California Press.

Castel, Robert
1988 The Regulation of Madness. W.D. Halls, trans. Berkeley: University of California Press.

Castel, Robert, Françoise Castel and Anne Lovell
1982 The Psychiatric Society. A. Goldhammer, trans. New York: Columbia University Press.

Cathébras, P., Fayard, L. and Rousset, H.
1991 L'anorexie Mentale; Est-elle un Désordre Culturel? La Revue de Médecine Interne 12(2):104–110.

Caudill, William
1958 The Psychiatric Hospital as a Small Society. Cambridge: Harvard University.
1959 Observations on the Cultural Context of Japanese Pychiatry. In Culture and Mental Health. Marvin K. Opler (ed.). New York: The Macmillan Co.
1961 Around the Clock Patient Care in Japanese Psychiatric Hospitals: The Role of the *Tsukisoi*. American Sociological Review 26:204–14.

Caudill, William and Tsung-Yi Lin, eds.
1969 Mental Health Research in Asia and the Pacific. Honolulu: University Press of Hawaii.

Caudill, William and Takeo Doi
1963 Interrelations of Psychiatry, Culture and Emotion in Japan. In Man's Image in Medicine and Anthropology. Iago Galdston (ed.). New York: International University Press.

Cawte, J. E.
1965 Ethnopsychiatry in Central Australia. British Journal of Psychiatry 111:1069–1077.
1974 Medicine is the Law. Honolulu: University Press of Hawaii.
1976 *Malgri:* A Culture-Bound Syndrome. In Culture-Bound Syndromes, Alternate Therapies and Ethnopsychiatry. William Lebra (ed.). Honolulu: University Press of Hawaii.

Chen, E., G. Harrison and P. Standen
1991 Management of First Episode Psychotic Illness in Afro-Caribbean Patients. British Journal of Psychiatry 158:517–522.

Cheung, F. M.
1982 Psychological Symptoms Among Chinese in Urban Hong Kong. Social Science and Medicine 16:1339–1344.
1987 Conceptualization of Psychiatric Illness and Help-Seeking Behavior Among Chinese. Culture, Medicine and Psychiatry 11 (1):97–106.

Cheung, F. K. and L. R. Snowden
1990 Community Mental Health and Ethnic Minority Populations. Community Mental Health Journal 26 (3):277–292.

Cheung, F.M., B. W. Lau and E. Waldmann
1981 Somatization Among Chinese Depressives in General Practice. International Journal of Psychiatry in Medicine 10 (4):361–374.

Chodoff, Paul
1985 Ethical Conflicts in Psychiatry: The Soviet Union vs the U.S. Hospital and Community Psychiatry 36(9):925–928.

Clark, Margaret
1959 Health in the Mexican-American Culture. Berkeley: University of California Press.

Clement, Dorothy
1982 Samoan Folk Knowledge of Mental Disorders. In Cultural Conceptions of Mental Health and Therapy. Anthony J. Marsella and Geoffrey M. White (eds.). Dordrecht: D. Reidel.

Clifford, Terry
1984 Tibetan Buddhist Medicine and Psychiatry. York Beach, Maine: Samuel Weiser.

Collins, James L.
1982 Psychiatry in China. Journal of the National Medical Association 74(10): 993–998.

Corin, Ellen
1988 La Culture, Voie Royale vers l'élaboration d'une Psychiatrie Scientifique. Santé, Culture, Health 5(2):157–176.
1990 Facts and Meaning in Psychiatry; An Anthropological Approach to the Life World of Schizophrenics. Culture, Medicine and Psychiatry 14(2):153–188.

Conner, Linda
1982 The Unbounded Self: Balinese Therapy in Theory and Practice. In Cultural Conceptions of Mental Health and Therapy. Anthony J. Marsella and Geoffrey M. White (eds.). Dordrecht: D. Reidel.

Conner, Linda, Patsy Asch and Timothy Asch
1986 Jero Tapakan: Balinese Healer: An Ethnographic Film Monograph. Cambridge: Cambridge University Press.

Crapanzano, Vincent
1973 The Hamadsha: Moroccan Ethnopsychiatry. Berkeley: University of California Press.

Crapanzano, Vincent and Vivian Garrison, eds.
1977 Case Studies in Spirit Possession. New York: John Wiley.

Crepet, Paolo
1990 A Transition Period in Psychiatric Care in Italy Ten Years After the Reform. British Journal of Psychiatry 156:27–36.

Csordas, Thomas
1983 The Rhetoric of Transformation in Ritual Healing. Culture, Medicine and Psychiatry 7(4):333–375.

1988   Elements of Charismatic Persuasion and Healing. Medical Anthropology Quarterly 2(1):121–142.

Danforth, Loring

1979   The Role of Dance in the Ritual Therapy of the Anastenaria. Byzantine and Modern Greek Studies 5:141–163.

1983   Power Through Submission in the Anastenaria. Journal of Modern Greek Studies 1(1):203–224.

Davidson, Michael, Miklos F. Losonczy and Kenneth L. Davis

1986   Biological Hypotheses of Schizophrenia. In American Handbook of Psychiatry. Silvano Arieti (ed.). New York: Basic Books.

Davidson, Ronald and Richard Day

1974   Symbol and Realization. Berkeley: Center for South and Southeast Asia Studies. Research Monograph #12.

Day, Richard, et al.

1987   Stressful Life Events Preceding the Acute Onset of Schizophrenia. Culture, Medicine and Psychiatry 11(2):123–206.

Dennis, G.

1985   *Grisi Siknis* in Miskito Culture. In Culture-Bound Syndromes. R. Simons and C. Hughes (eds.). Dordrecht: D. Reidel.

Devereux, George

1941   Primitive Psychiatry. Bulletin of the History of Medicine 8:1194–1213.

1944   The Social Structure of a Schizophrenic Ward and Its Therapeutic Fitness. Journal of Clinical Psychotherapy 6(2):231–265.

1949   The Social Structure of the Hospital as a Factor in Total Therapy. American Journal of Orthopsychiatry 19(3):492–500.

1951   Reality and Dream. New York: International Universities Press.

1969 (1961) Mohave Ethnopsychiatry. Washington, D.C.: Smithsonian Institution Press.

1978a Cultural Thought Models in Primitive and Modern Psychiatric Theories. In Ethnopsychoanalysis: Psychoanalysis and Anthropology as Complementary Frames of Reference. G. Devereux. Berkeley: University of California Press.

1978b Ethnopsychoanalysis: Psychoanalysis and Anthropology as Complementary Frames of Reference. Berkeley: University of California Press.

1978c Normal and Abnormal: The Key Problem in Psychiatry Anthropology. In Ethnopsychoanalysis: Psychoanalysis and Anthropology as Complementary Frames of Reference. G. Devereux. Berkeley: University of California Press.

1980a Basic Problems of Ethnopsychiatry. Chicago: University of Chicago Press.

1980b Schizophrenia: An Ethnic Psychosis. In Basic Problems of Ethnopsychiatry. G. Devereux. Chicago: University of Chicago Press.

1980c Primitive Psychiatric Diagnosis: A General Theory of the Diagnostic Process. In Basic Problems of Ethnopsychiatry. G. Devereux. Chicago: University of Chicago Press.

Dinges, N. J. Trimble, S. Manson and F. Pasquale

1980   The Social Ecology of Counseling and Psychotherapy with American Indians and Alaskan Natives. In Cross-Cultural Counseling and Psychotherapy. A. Marsella and P. Pedersen (eds.). New York: Pergamon Press.

Dobkin de Rios, M.
1985 *Saladera*—A Culture-Bound Misfortune Syndrome in the Peruvian Amazon. In The Culture-Bound Syndromes. R. Simons and C. Hughes (eds.). Dordrecht: D. Reidel.

Dodier, Nicolas
1985 Social Uses of Illness at the Workplace. N. Mellot, trans. Social Science and Medicine 20(2):123–128.

Doi, Takeo
1962 *Amae:* A Key Concept for Understanding Japanese Personality Structure. In Japanese Culture: Its Development and Characteristics. R.J. Smith and R.K. Beardsley (eds.). Chicago: University of Chicago Press.

Dommisee, John
1987 The State of Psychiatry in South Africa Today. Social Science and Medicine 24(9):749–761.

Dressler, William W.
1985a Extended Family Relationships, Social Support and Mental Health in a Southern Black Community. Journal of Health and Social Behavior 26(1):39–48.
1985b Psychosomatic Symptoms, Stress, and Modernization: A Model. Culture, Medicine and Psychiatry 9:257–286.
1986 Unemployment and Depressive Symptoms in a Southern Black Community. Journal of Nervous and Mental Disease 174:639–645.
1991 Stress and Adaptation in the Context of Culture. Albany: State University of New York Press.

Dressler, William and Lee W. Badger
1985 Epidemiology of Depressive Symptoms in Black Communities: A Comparative Analysis. Journal of Nervous and Mental Disease 173:212–220.

Dubovsky, Steven L.
1983 Psychiatry in Saudi Arabia. American Journal of Psychiatry 140(11): 1455–1459.

Dugan, Anna Baziak,
1988 *Compadrazgo* as a Protective Mechanism in Depression. In Women and Health: Cross-Cultural Perspectives. Patricia Whelehan and Contributors (eds.). Granby, MA: Bergin and Garvey Publishers, Inc.

Dunk, Pamela
1985 Greek Women and Broken Nerves in Montréal. Paper presented at American Anthropological Association Annual Meeting. Washington, D.C. November.

Duranti, Alessandro
1990 Doing Things with Words. In Disentangling. K. Watson-Gegeo and G. White (eds.). Stanford: Stanford University Press.

Dwyer, Ellen
1987 Homes for the Mad. New Brunswick, NJ: Rutgers University Press.

Easson, William M.
1977 Orientations in Psychiatric Diagnosis and Therapy in the Soviet Union. Current Psychiatric Therapies 17:333–337.

Ebigbo, Peter

1982   Development of a Culture-Specific (Nigeria) Screening Scale of Somatic Complaints Indicating Psychiatric Disturbance. Culture, Medicine and Psychiatry 6(1):29–43.

Ebigbo, Peter and B. Anyaegbuna

1989   (1988) The Problem of Student Involvement in the *Mermaid Cult*. Curare 12(3/4):153–160.

Edgerton, Robert

1966   Conceptions of Psychosis in Four African Societies. American Anthropologist 2:408–425.

1971   (1967) The Cloak of Competence: Stigma in the Lives of the Mentally Retarded. Berkeley: University of California Press.

1977   A Traditional African Psychiatrist. In Culture, Disease and Healing. D. Landy (ed.) New York: Macmillan.

1980   Traditional Treatment for Mental Illness in Africa: A Review. Culture, Medicine and Psychiatry 4(2):167–189.

Edgerton, Robert B. and Marvin Karno

1971   Mexican-American Bilingualism and the Perception of Mental Illness. Archives of General Psychiatry 24:286–290.

Eisenberg, Leon

1977   Disease and Illness: Distinctions Between Professional and Popular Ideas of Sickness. Culture, Medicine and Psychiatry 1(1):9–24.

Eker, Dogan

1985   Diagnosis of Mental Disorders Among Turkish and American Clinicians. International Journal of Social Psychiatry 31(2):99–111.

El-Islam, M. F.

1975   Culture Bound Neurosis in Qatari Women. Social Psychatry 10:25–29.

1982   Arabic Cultural Psychiatry. Transcultural Psychiatric Research Review 19:5–24.

El-Islam, M. F. and S. A. Ahmed

1971   Traditional Interpretation and Treatment of Mental Illness. Journal of Cross-Cultural Psychology 2:301–307.

Estroff, Sue

1981   Making It Crazy. Berkeley: University of California Press.

Fábrega, Horacio

1985   Culture and Psychiatric Illness: Biomedical and Ethnomedical Aspects. In Cultural Conceptions of Mental Health and Therapy. A. Marsella and G. White (eds.). Dordrecht: D. Reidel.

1987   Psychiatric Diagnosis: A Cultural Perspective. Journal of Nervous and Mental Diseases 175(7):383–395.

n.d.   The Social Problématique of Anglo-American Psychiatry: A Case Study in Critical Medical Anthropology. In Analysis in Medical Anthropology. Shirley Lindenbaum and Margaret Lock (eds.). ms.

Fábrega, Horacio and Daniel Silver

1973   Illness and Shamanistic Curing in Zinacantan. Stanford: Stanford University Press.

Fakhouri, Hani
1968 The *Zar* Cult in an Egyptian Village. Anthropological Quarterly 41(2):49–56.
Farmer, Paul E.
1980 A New Approach to Psychiatric Diagnosis: Acultural or Anglicized? First Contact 6(2):11–14.
Favazza, Armando and Mary Oman
1977 Anthropological and Cross-Cultural Themes in Mental Health. Columbia: University of Missouri Press.
Field, Mark G.
1960 Approaches to Mental Illness in Soviet Society: Some Comparisons and Conjectures. Social Problems 7(4):277–297.
1964 Soviet and American Approaches to Mental Illness: A Comparative Perspective. Review of Soviet Medical Sciences 1:1–36.
1967 Soviet Psychiatry and Social Structure, Culture and Ideology: A Preliminary Assessment. American Journal of Psychotherapy 21:230–243.
1968 Psychiatry and Ideology: the Official Soviet View of Western Theories and Practices. American Journal of Psychotherapy 22:602–615.
1977 Psychiatry and the Polity: The Soviet Case and Some General Implications. Annals of the New York Academy of Sciences 285:687–697.
Field, Mark G. and Jason Aronson
1964 The Institutional Framework of Soviet Psychiatry. The Journal of Nervous and Mental Disease 138(4):305–322.
1965 Soviet Community Mental Health Services and Work Therapy: A Report of Two Visits. Community Mental Health Journal 1(1):81–90.
Finkler, Kaja
1985 Spiritist Healers in Mexico: Successes and Failures of Alternative Therapeutics. New York: Praeger.
1985b Symptomatic Differences Between the Sexes in Rural Mexico. Culture, Medicine and Psychiatry 9(1):27–57.
Fisher, Lawrence E.
1985 Colonial Madness: Mental Health in a Barbadian Social Order. New Brunswick, NJ: Rutgers University Press.
Florkin, Marcel
1971 Des Force-de-Vie à la Bioénergétique. Revue d'Histoire des Sciences et Leur Application 24(4):289–298.
Foucault, Michel
1973 Madness and Civilization. Richard Howard, trans. New York: Vintage Books.
1975 The Birth of the Clinic: An Archeology of Medical Perception. Alan Sheridan, trans. New York.
1979 Discipline and Punish: The Birth of the Prison. Alan Sheridan, trans. New York: Vintage Books.
1980 Power/Knowledge: Selected Interviews and Other Writings 1972–1977. Colin Gordon (ed.). New York: Pantheon.
Foulks, Edward
1985 The Transformation of Arctic Hysteria. In The Culture-Bound Syndromes. R. Simons and C. Hughes (eds.). Dordrecht: D Reidel.

Foulks, Edward et al.
1977   The Italian Evil Eye. Journal of Operational Psychiatry 8:28–34.

Fox, J. R.
1964   Witchcraft and Clanship in Cochiti. In Magic, Faith and Healing. Ari Kiev
       (ed.). New York: Free Press.

Frank, Jerome
1961   Persuasion and Healing. Baltimore: Johns Hopkins Press.

Frankel, S., A. D. Gaines, J. Reingold and N. Robles
1978   Conceptions of Alcohol Use, Abuse and Problem Behavior in Three Califor-
       nia Counties. Berkeley: School of Public Health, University of California at
       Berkeley. Monograph of the U.C.B. Social Research Group.

Frydman, Louis
1983   Psychiatric Hospitalization in Poland. Social Science and Medicine
       17(10):617–623.

Gaines, Atwood D.
1978   Illness and Interaction: A Case of Paranoia. Kroeber Anthropological Society
       Papers 53–54:71–87.
1979   Definitions and Diagnoses: Cultural Implications of Psychiatric Help-Seeking
       and Psychiatrists' Definitions of the Situation in Psychiatric Emergencies.
       Culture, Medicine and Psychiatry 3(4):381–418.
1981   Hard Contract: Issues and Problems in Contract Social Anthropological
       Research. Kroeber Anthropological Society Papers 59–60:82–91.
1982a Cultural Definitions, Behavior and the Person in American Psychiatry. In
       Cultural Conceptions of Mental Health and Therapy. Anthony Marsella and
       Geoffrey White (eds.). Dordrecht: D. Reidel.
1982b Knowledge and Practice: Anthropological Ideas and Psychiatric Practice. In
       Clinically Applied Anthropology: Anthropologists in Health Science Settings.
       Noel Chrisman and Thomas Maretzki (eds.). Dordrecht: D. Reidel.
1982c The Twice-Born: 'Christian Psychiatry' and Christian Psychiatrists. In
       Physicians of Western Medicine: Five Cultural Studies. Atwood D. Gaines
       and Robert A. Hahn (eds.). Culture, Medicine and Psychiatry Special Issue
       6(3):305–324.
1985a The Once- and the Twice-Born: Self and Practice Among Psychiatrists and
       Christian Psychiatrists. In Physicians of Western Medicine: Anthropological
       Approaches to Theory and Practice. Robert A. Hahn and Atwood D. Gaines
       (eds.). Dordrecht: D. Reidel.
1985b Alcohol: Cultural Conceptions and Social Behavior Among Urban 'Blacks.'
       In The American Experience with Alcohol. Linda Bennett and Genevieve
       Ames (eds.). New York: Plenum.
1986a Culture and Medical Knowledge in France and America. Paper presented at
       American Anthropological Association Meetings. Washington, D.C. Novem-
       ber. (Revision included here as chapter 6.)
1986b Disease, Communalism and Medicine. Culture, Medicine and Psychiatry
       10(3):397–403.
1986c Trauma: Cross-Cultural Issues. In Advances in Psychosomatic Medicine Vol-
       ume 16: Psychiatric Aspects of Trauma. Linda B. Peterson and Gregory
       O'Shanick (eds.). Basel, Switzerland: Karger.

1987a Cultures, Biologies and Dysphorias. Transcultural Psychiatric Research Review 24(1):31–57.
1987b Shamanism and the Shaman: A Plea for the Person-Centered Approach. Anthropology and Humanism Quarterly 12(3 & 4):62–68.
1988 Delusions: Culture, Psychosis and the Problem of Meaning. In Delusions: Interdisciplinary Perspectives. Thomas Oltmanns and Brenden Maher (eds.). New York: John Wiley.
1989 Alzheimer's Disease in the Context of Black (Southern) Culture. Health Matrix 6(4):33–38.
1992 From DSM-I to III-R: Voices of Self, Mastery and the Other: A Cultural Constructivist Reading of United States Psychiatric Classification. In The Cultural Construction of Psychiatric Classification. C. Nuckolls (ed.). Social Science and Medicine Special Issue/Section. (in press)

Gaines, Atwood D. and Paul Farmer
1986 Visible Saints: Social Cynosures and Dysphoria in the Mediterranean Tradition. Culture, Medicine and Psychiatry 10(4):295–330.

Gaines, Atwood D. and Robert A. Hahn, eds.
1982 Physicians of Western Medicine: Five Cultural Studies. Atwood D. Gaines and Robert A. Hahn (eds.). Culture, Medicine and Psychiatry Special Issue 6(3).

Gaines, Atwood and Sandra Trego Wood, organizers
1978 The Anthropology of Psychiatry. Symposium. Southwestern Anthropological Association Meetings. San Francisco, CA.

Garrison, Virginia
1977a Doctor, *Espiritista* or Psychiatrist?: Health-Seeking Behavior in a Puerto Rican Neighborhood of New York City. Medical Anthropology 1(2):65–191.
1977b The "Puerto Rican Syndrome" in Psychiatry and *Espiritismo*. In Case Studies in Spirit Possession. Vincent Crapanzano and Vivian Garrison (eds.). New York: John Wiley.

Gavira, Moises and Ronald M. Wintrob
1976 Supernatural Influence in Psychopathology: Puerto Rican Folk Beliefs About Mental Illness. Canadian Psychiatric Association Journal 21:361–369.

Gaviria, Moises and José Arana
1987 Health and Behavior: Research Agenda for Hispanics. Chicago: University of Illinois at Chicago Press.

Geertz, Clifford
1973 The Interpretation of Cultures. New York: Basic Books.

German, A.
1972 Aspects of Clinical Psychiatry in Sub-Saharan Africa. British Journal of Psychiatry 121:461–470.

Gerner, Robert H. and William E. Burney Jr.
1986 Biological Hypotheses of Affective Disorders. In American Handbook of Psychiatry. Silvano Arieti (ed.) New York: Basic Books.

Gilman, Sander
1985 Difference and Pathology: Stereotypes of Sex, Race and Madness. Ithaca, NY: Cornell University Press.

1988a Constructing Schizophrenia as a Category of Mental Illness. In Disease and Representation: Images of Illness from Madness to AIDS. Sander Gilman. Ithaca, NY: Cornell University Press.

1988b Constructing the Image of the Appropriate Therapist: The Struggle of Psychiatry and Psychoanalysis. In Disease and Representation: Images of Illness from Madness to AIDS. Sander Gilman. Ithaca, NY: Cornell University Press.

1988c Disease and Representation: Images of Illness from Madness to AIDS. Sander Gilman. Ithaca, NY: Cornell University Press.

Goffman, Erving
1961   Asylums. New York: Anchor.

Goldstein, E. G.
1987   Mental Health and Illness. Silver Spring, MD: National Association of Social Workers.

Goldstein, Jan
1987   Console and Classify: The French Psychiatric Profession in the 19th Century. Chicago: University of Chicago Press.

Goleman, Daniel
1989   From Tokyo to Tampa, Different Ideas of Self. New York Times. March 7, 1989. Pp. B1 and B10.

Good, Byron
1977   The Heart of What's the Matter. Culture, Medicine and Psychiatry 1(1):25–58.

Good, Byron and Mary-Jo DelVecchio Good
1982   Toward a Meaning-Centered Analysis of Popular Illness Categories: *Fright Illness* and *Heart Distress* in Iran. In Cultural Conceptions of Mental Health and Therapy. A. Marsella and G. White (eds.). Dordrecht: D. Reidel.

Good, B., H. Herrera, M.-J. DelVecchio Good and J. Cooper
1985   Reflexivity, Countertransference and Clinical Ethnography: A Case from a Psychiatric Cultural Consultation Clinic. In Physicians of Western Medicine: Anthropological Approaches to Theory and Practice. R. Hahn and A. Gaines (eds.). Dordrecht: D. Reidel.

Good, Byron, Mary-Jo DelVecchio Good and Robert Moradi
1985   The Interpretation of Iranian Depressive Illness and Dysphoric Affect. In Culture and Depression. Arthur Kleinman and Byron Good (eds.). Berkeley: University of California Press.

Good, Byron and Arthur Kleinman
1985   Culture and Anxiety. In Anxiety and the Anxiety Disorder. A. Turns and J. Maser (eds.). Hillsdale, N.J.: Lawrence Earlbaum.

Good, Mary-Jo DelVecchio, Byron Good and Michael Fischer, eds.
1988   Emotion, Illness and Healing in Middle Eastern Societies. Culture, Medicine and Psychiatry Special Issue 12(1).

Gordon, Deborah
1988   Tenacious Assumptions in Western Medicine. In Biomedicine Examined. Margaret Lock and Deborah Gordon (eds.). Dordrecht: Kluwer Academic.

Gorkin, Michael
1986 Countertransference in Cross-Cultural Psychotherapy: The Example of Jewish Therapist and Arab Patient. Psychiatry 49:69–79.

Griffiths Stephen
1988 Emigrants, Entrepreneurs, and Evil Spirits. Honolulu: University Press of Hawaii.

Guarnaccia, Peter and P. Farias
1988 The Social Meanings of *Nervios*: A Case Study of a Central American Woman. Social Science and Medicine 26:1223–1232.

Guarnaccia, Peter, Byron Good and Arthur Kleinman
1990 A Critical Review of Epidemiological Studies of Puerto Rican Mental Health. American Journal of Psychiatry 147(11):1449–1456.

Guarnaccia, Peter, Maritza Rubio-Stipec and Glorisa Canino
1989 *Ataques de Nervios* in the Puerto Rican Diagnostic Interview Schedule. Culture, Medicine and Psychiatry 13(3):275–296.

Gussow, Z.
1985 *Pibloktoq* (Hysteria) Among the Polar Eskimo: An Ethnopsychiatric Study. In The Culture-Bound Syndromes. R. Simons and C. Hughes (eds.). Dordrecht: D Reidel.

Guthrie, G. M. and D. L. Szanton
1976 Folk Diagnosis and Treatment of Schizophrenia: Bargaining with the Spirits in the Philippines. In Culture-Bound Syndromes, Ethnopsychiatry and Alternate Therapies. William Lebra (ed.). Honolulu: University Press of Hawaii.

Haafkens, J.,G. Nijhof and E. Vand der Poel
1986 Mental Health Care and the Opposition Movement in the Netherlands. Social Science and Medicine 22(2):185–192.

Hahn, Robert
1985 Culture-Bound Syndromes Unbound. Social Science and Medicine 21(2): 165–171.
1990 Concepts of Race and Ethnicity in Public Health. Paper presented at the American Anthropological Association Meeting. New Orleans, LA. Nov. 28–Dec. 2.

Hahn, Robert A. and Atwood D. Gaines
1982 Physicians of Western Medicine: An Introduction. In Physicians of Western Medicine: Five Cultural Studies. Atwood D. Gaines and Robert A. Hahn (eds.). Culture, Medicine and Psychiatry Special Issue 6(3):215–218.

Hahn, Robert and Atwood D. Gaines, eds.
1985 Physicians of Western Medicine: Anthropological Approaches to Theory and Practice. Dordrecht: D. Reidel.

Hallowell, A. I.
1963 Ojibwa World View and Disease. In Man's Image in Medicine and Anthropology. I. Galdston (ed.). New York: International Universities Press.
1967 [1955] Culture and Experience. New York: Schocken Books.

Handelman, Don
1979   Is Naven Ludic? Paradox and Communication of Identity. Social Analysis
       1(1):15–21.

Hartog, Joel
1972   The Intervention System for Mental and Social Deviants in Malaysia. Social
       Science and Medicine 6:211–220.

Harvey, Y. Kim
1976   The Korean *Mundang* as a Household Therapist. In Culture-Bound Syn-
       dromes, Ethnopsychiatry and Alternate Therapies. William Lebra (ed.).
       Honolulu: University Press of Hawaii.
1982   Six Korean Shaman. Washington, D.C.: American Ethnological Society.

Harwood, Alan, ed.
1981   Ethnicity and Medical Care. Cambridge: Harvard University Press.

Harwood, Alan
1977   *Rx*: Spiritist as Needed. New York: John Wiley.

Helman, Cecil
1985   Disease and Pseudo-Disease: A Case History of Pseudo-Angina. In Physicians
       of Western Medicine: Anthropological Approaches to Theory and Practice. R
       Hahn and A. Gaines (eds.). Dordrecht: D. Reidel.
1988 [1985] Psyche, Soma and Society: The Social Construction of Psychosomatic
       Disorders. In Biomedicine Examined. M. Lock and D. Gordon (eds.). Dor-
       drecht: Kluwer Academic Publishers.
1990   Culture, Health and Illness (2nd ed.). London: Wright.

Henry, Jules
1973 [1963] Pathways to Madness. New York: Vintage Books.

Hill, Carole E. and Lisa Cottrell
1986   Traditional Mental Disorders in a Developing West Indian Community in
       Costa Rica. Anthropological Quarterly 59(1):1–14.

Hillard, James and W. Rockwell
1978   Disesthesia, Witchcraft and Conversion Reaction. Journal of the American
       Medical Association 240:1742–1744.

Horikoshi, Hiroko
1980   *Asrama*: An Islamic Psychiatric Institution in West Java. Social Science and
       Medicine 14B:157–165.

Hsu, Jin
1976   Counseling in the Chinese Temple: a Psychological study of Divination by
       Chien Drawing. In Culture-Bound Syndromes, Ethnopsychiatry and Alter-
       nate Therapies. William Lebra (ed.). Honolulu: University Press of Hawaii.

Ingleby, David, ed.
1980   Critical Psychiatry. New York: Pantheon Books.

Ingleby, David
1983   Mental Health and Social Order. In Social Control and the State: Historical
       and Comparative Essays. S. Cohen and A. Scull (eds.). Oxford: Martin.

Irigoyen-Rascon, Fructuoso
1989 Psychiatric Disorders Among the Tarahumara Indians of Northern Mexico. Curare 12(3/4):169–173.

Ito, Karen L.
1985 *Ho'oponopono*, "To Make Right": Hawaiian Conflict Resolution and Metaphor in the Construction of a Family Therapy. Culture, Medicine and Psychiatry 9(2):201–218.

Jablensky, A. and N. Sartorius
1975 Culture and Schizophrenia. Psychological Medicine 5:113–124.

Jakovljevic, Vladimir
1968 The Development of Psychiatry in Yugoslavia. In Psychiatry in the Communist World. Ari Kiev (ed.). New York: Science House.

Janes, Craig and Genevieve Ames
1989 Men, Blue-Collar Work and Drinking: Alcohol Use in an Industrial Subculture. Culture, Medicine and Psychiatry 13(3):245–274.

Jenkins, Janis Hunter
1988a Ethnopsychiatric Interpretations of Schizophrenic Illness: The Problems of *Nervios* within Mexican-American Families. Culture, Medicine and Psychiatry 12:301–329.
1988b Conceptions of Schizophrenia as a Problem of Nerves: A Cross-Cultural Comparison of Mexican-Americans and Anglo-Americans. Social Science and Medicine 26(12):303–331.

Jenkins, Janis H., Arthur Kleinman and Byron Good
1990 Cross-Cultural Studies of Depression. In Advances in Mood Disorders J. Becker and A. Kleinman (eds.). New York: Earlbaum Press.

Jegede, R. Olukayode, A. O. Williams and A. O. Sijuwola
1985 Recent Developments in the Care, Treatment and Rehabilitation of the Chronically Mentally Ill in Nigeria. Hospital and Community Psychiatry 36(6):658-661.

Jilek, W.
1971 From Crazy Witchdoctor to Auxiliary Psychotherapist: The Changing Image of the Medicine Man. Psychiatrica Clinica 4:200–220.
1974 Indian Healing Power: Indigenous Therapeutic Practice in the Pacific Northwest. Psychiatric Annals 4(9):13–21.

Johnson, Thomas
1985 Consultation-Liaison Psychiatry. In Physicians of Western Medicine: Anthropological Approaches to Theory and Practice. R. Hahn and A. Gaines (eds.). Dordrecht: D. Reidel.

Johnson, Thomas and Arthur Kleinman
1984 Cultural Concerns in Psychiatric Consultation. In Manual of Psychiatric Consultation and Emergency Care. F. Guggenheim and M. Weiner (eds.). New York: Jason Aronson.

Jones, Kathleen
1972 A History of the Mental Health Services. London: Routledge and Kegan Paul.

Jones, Kathleen and Alison Poletti
1986 The 'Italian Experience' Revisited. British Journal of Psychiatry 148:144–150.

Kapferer, Bruce

1979   Mind, Self and Other in Demonic Illness. American Ethnologist 6(1):110–133.

1982   A Celebration of Demons. Bloomington: Indiana University Press.

Kaplan, B. and D. Johnson

1964   The Social Meaning of Navaho Psychopathology and Psychotherapy. In Magic, Faith and Healing. Ari Kiev (ed.). New York: Free Press.

Karp, Ivan

1985   Deconstructing Culture-Bound Syndromes. Social Science and Medicine 21(2):221–228.

Katchadourian, Herant

1980   The Historical Background of Psychiatry in Lebanon. Bulletin of the History of Medicine 54:544–553.

Katon, W.

1987   The Epidemiology of Depression in Medical Care. International Journal of Psychiatry in Medicine 17(1):93–112.

Katon, W., A. Kleinman and G. Rosen

1982   Depression and Somatization: A Review, Part I. American Journal of Medicine 72:127–135.

1982   Depression and Somatization: A Review, Part II. American Journal of Medicine 72:241–247.

Katz, Martin, J. Cole and H. Lowery

1969   Studies of the Diagnostic Process: The Influence of Symptom Perception, Past Experience, and Ethnic Background on Diagnostic Decisions. American Journal of Psychiatry 125:109–119.

Kay, Margarita A.

1977   Health and Illness in a Mexican-American Barrio. In Ethnic Medicine in the Southwest. Edward Spicer (ed.). Tucson: University of Arizona Press.

Keefe, Susan, Amado Padilla and Manuel Carlos

1979   The Mexican-American Family as an Emotional Support System. Human Organization 38:144–52.

Kendall, Laurel

1985   Shamans, Housewives, and Other Restless Spirits. Honolulu: University Press of Hawaii.

1988   The Life and Hard Times of a Korean Shaman. Honolulu: University Press of Hawaii.

Kennedy, John

1967   Nubian *Zar* Ceremonies as Psychotherapy. Human Organization 26(4):185–194.

1974   Cultural Psychiatry. In Handbook of Social and Cultural Anthropology. John Honigmann (ed.). New York: Rand McNally.

1987   The Flower of Paradise: The Institutionalized Use of the Drug *Qat* in North Yemen. Dordrecht: D. Reidel .

Kenny, Michael

1978   *Latah*: The Symbolism of a Putative Mental Disorder. Culture, Medicine and Psychiatry 2:209–231.

1985 Paradox Lost: The *Latah* Problem Revisited. In The Culture-Bound Syndromes. R. Simons and C. Hughes (eds.). Dordrecht: D. Reidel.

Kiev, Ari
1968a *Curanderismo*: Mexican American Folk Psychiatry. New York: Free Press.

Kiev, Ari, ed.
1964 Magic, Faith and Healing. New York: Free Press.
1968b Psychiatry in the Communist World. New York: Science House Publishers.

Kiev, Ari and A. V. Rao, eds.
1982 Readings in Transcultural Psychiatry. Madras: Higgenbothams.

Kinzie, J. D., J. I. Teoh and E. S. Tan
1974 Community Psychiatry in Malaysia. American Journal of Psychiatry 131(5): 573–577.

Kinzie, J. D., et al.
1982 Development and Validation of a Vietnamese Language Depression Rating Scale. American Journal of Psychiatry 139:1276–1281.

Kinzie, J. D., et al.
1990 The Prevalence of Posttraumatic Stress Disorder and Its Clinical Significance Among Southeast Asian Refugees. American Journal of Psychiatry 147(7): 913–917.

Kirmayer, Laurence J.
1988 Mind and Body as Metaphors: Hidden Values in Biomedicine. In Biomedicine Examined. M. Lock and D. Gordon (eds.). Dordrecht: D. Reidel.
1989 Psychotherapy and the Cultural Concept of the Person. Santé, Culture, Health 6(3):241–270.
1990 Culture and International Psychiatric Classification: The Example of *Taijin Kyofusho*. In Psychiatry: A World Perspective. C. N. Stefanis et al. (eds.). Amsterdam: Elsevier Science.
In Press Inuit Mental Health. Transcultural Psychiatric Research Review.

Klee, Linnea and Genevieve Ames
1986 Re-evaluating Risk Factors for Women's Drinking: A Study of Blue-Collar Wives. American Journal of Preventive Medicine 3(1):31–41.

Kleinman, Arthur
1977 Problems and Prospects in Comparative Cross-Cultural Medical and Psychiatric Studies. In Renewal in Psychiatry. Theo Manschreck and Arthur Kleinman (eds.). Washington, D.C.: Hemisphere/Halsted Books.
1980a Major Conceptual and Research Issues for Cultural (Anthropological) Psychiatry. Culture, Medicine and Psychiatry 4(3):3–13.
1980b Patients and Healers in the Context of Culture. Berkeley: University of California Press.
1986 Social Origins of Distress and Disease: Depression, Neurasthenia, and Pain in Modern China. New Haven: Yale University Press.
1988 Rethinking Psychiatry: From Cultural Category to Personal Experience. New York: Free Press.
1991 Cultural Bias in Psychiatry. Grand Rounds in Psychiatry. Department of Psychiatry. Case Western Reserve University School of Medicine. Cleveland, OH. March.

Kleinman, Arthur and Byron Good, eds.
1985 Culture and Depression: Studies in the Anthropology and Cross-Cultural Psychiatry of Affect and Disorder. Berkeley: University of California Press.

Kleinman, Arthur and Joan Kleinman
1985 Somatization: The Interconnections in Chinese Society Among Culture, Depressive Experiences and the Meanings of Pain. In Culture and Depression. A. Kleinman and B. Good (eds.). Berkeley: University of California Press.

Kleinman, Arthur, Peter Kunstadter, E. Russell Alexander and James L. Gale, eds.
1975 Medicine in Chinese Cultures: Comparative Studies of Health Care in Chinese and Other Societies. Washington D.C.: U.S.D.H.E.W. for the Fogerty Center.

Kleinman, Arthur and T.-Y. Lin, eds.
1981 Normal and Abnormal Behavior in Chinese Culture, Dordrecht: D. Reidel.

Kleinman, Arthur and David Mechanic
1979 Some Observations of Mental Illness and its Treatment in the People's Republic of China. The Journal of Nervous and Mental Disease 167(5): 267–274.

Kline, Nathan S., Mark G. Field and Jason Aronson
1961 Soviet Psychiatric Nomenclature. American Journal of Psychiatry 68:178–180.

Kondo, Kyoichi
1976 The Origin of Morita Therapy. In Culture-Bound Syndromes, Ethnopsychiatry and Alternate Therapies. William Lebra (ed.). Honolulu: University Press of Hawaii.

Koran, Lorrin M.
1972 Psychiatry in Mainland China: History and Recent Status. American Journal of Psychiatry 128(8):84–92.

Koumare, B., J. P. Coudray and E. Miguel-Garcia
1989 Der Psychiatrische Dienst in Mali. Curare 12(3/4):145–152.

Kovess, V., H. B. M. Murphy and M. Tousignant
1987 Urban-Rural Comparisons of Depressive Disorders in French Canadians. Journal of Nervous and Mental Diseases 175(8):457–465.

Krippner, S.
1987 Cross-Cultural Approaches to Multiple Personality Disorder: Practices in Brazilian *Spiritism*. Ethos 15(3):273–295.

Kroeger, Axel and Wolfgang Pfeiffer
1986 Kranksein und Migration. Curare Theme Issue 9(2).

Kuna, R. R.
1977 Hoodoo: The Indigenous Medicine and Psychiatry of Black America. Mankind Quarterly 18(2):137–151.

Kunitz, Stephen J.
1989 [1983] Disease Change and the Role of Medicine: The Navajo Experience. Berkeley: University of California Press.

Lacan, Jacques
1968 Language of the Self. Baltimore: Johns Hopkins University Press.
1971 Écrits. A. Sheridan, trans. New York: Norton.

Laderman, Carol
1991 Taming the Wind of Desire: Psychology, Medicine, and Aesthetics in Malay Shamanistic Performance. Berkeley: University of California Press.

Langsley, Donald G., James T. Barter and Ali Amir-Moshiri
1983 Psychiatry in Iran and China. International Journal of Social Psychiatry 29(1):39–47.

Lattin, Don
1990 Goddess Movement Is Big at Coming 'New Era' Expo. San Francisco Chronicle. April 25, 1990:A6.

Lazare, Aaron
1973 Hidden Conceptual Models in Clinical Psychiatry. New England Journal of Medicine 288:345–351.

Lebra, Takie
1976 Taking the Role of Supernatural 'Other': Spirit Possession in a Japanese Healing Cult. In Culture-Bound Syndromes, Ethnopsychiatry and Alternate Therapies. William Lebra (ed.). Honolulu: University Press of Hawaii.
1982 Self-Reconstruction in Japanese Religious Psychotherapy. In Cultural Conceptions of Mental Health and Therapy. A. Marsella and G. White (eds.). Dordrecht: D Reidel.

Lebra, William, ed.
1976 Culture-Bound Syndromes, Ethnopsychiatry, and Alternate Therapies. Honolulu: University Press of Hawaii.

Leff, Julian
1973 Culture and the Differentiation of Emotional States. British Journal of Psychiatry 123:299–306.

Leighton, Alexander
1982 Caring for Mentally Ill People. Cambridge: Cambridge University Press.
1984a Anthropology and Epidemiology in the Stirling County Study. Santé, Culture, Health 2(2):3–9.
1984b Barriers to Adequate Care for Mentally Ill People. Social Science and Medicine 18(3):237–242.

Leighton, Alexander, T. A. Lambo, Charles Hughes, et al.
1963 Psychiatric Disorder Among the Yoruba. Ithaca, New York: Cornell University Press.

Leng, Gwee Ah
1985 *Koro:* A Cultural Disease. In The Culture-Bound Syndromes. Ronald C. Simons and Charles C. Hughes (eds.). Boston: D. Reidel.

Lesch, John
1984 Science and Medicine in France. Cambridge: University of Harvard Press.

Levy, Jerrold, Raymond Neutra and Dennis Parker
1987 Hand Trembling, Frenzy, Witchcraft, and Moth Madness: A Study of Navajo Seizure Disorders. Tucson: University of Arizona Press.

Levy, Robert
1973 Tahitians. Chicago: University of Chicago Press.

Lidz, Charles and Edward Mulvey
1990 Institutional Factors Affecting Psychiatric Admission and Commitment Decisions. In Social Science Perspectives on Medical Ethics. George Weisz (ed.). Dordrecht: Kluwer Academic Publishers.

Lieban, Richard
1967 Cebuano Sorcery. Berkeley: University of California Press.

Lieboweitz, M., J. Gorman, A. Fyer and D. Klein
1985 Social Phobia: Review of a Neglected Anxiety Disorder. Archives of General Psychiatry 42:729–735.

Light, Donald
1976 Work Styles Among American Psychiatric Residents. In Anthropology and Mental Health. Joseph Westermeyer (ed.). The Hague: Mouton.
1980 Becoming Psychiatrists: The Professional Transformation of the Self. New York: W. W. Norton.

Like, Robert and J. Ellison
1981 *Sleeping Blood*, Tremor and Paralysis: A Transcultural Approach to an Unusual Conversion Reaction. Culture, Medicine and Psychiatry 5(1):49–63.

Lin, E. H. B., W. B. Carter and A. Kleinman
1985 An Exploration of Somatization Among Asian Refugees and Immigrants in Primary Care. American Journal of Public Health 75:1080–1084.

Lin, Keh-Ming
1983 *Hwa-byung:* A Culture-Bound Syndrome? American Journal of Psychiatry 140:105–107.

Lin, Keh-Ming, R. E. Poland, and Ira Lesser
1986 Ethnicity and Pharmacology. Culture, Medicine and Psychiatry 10(2):151–167.

Lin, T. -Y.
1986 Multiculturalism and Canadian Psychiatry: Opportunities and Challenges. Canadian Journal of Psychiatry 31:681–690.
1989 Neurasthenia Revisited: Its Place in Modern Psychiatry. Culture, Medicine and Psychiatry 13(2):105–130.
1989 Measuring Depressive Symptomatology in China. Journal of Nervous and Mental Disease 177 (3):121–131.

Lin, T. -Y. and L. Eisenberg, eds.
1985 Mental Health Planning for 1 Billion People: A Chinese Perspective. Vancouver: University of British Columbia Press.

Lin, T. -Y. and M. C. Lin
1981 Love, Denial and Rejection. In Normal and Abnormal Behavior in Chinese Culture. Arthur Kleinman and T. -Y. Lin (eds.). Dordrecht: D. Reidel.

Littlewood, Roland
1982 Aliens and Alienists: Ethnic Minorities and Psychiatry. Harmondsworth: Penguin.
1986 Cultural Psychiatry in Britain Today. Curare 9(1):9–16.

Littlewood, Roland and S. Cross
1981 Ethnic Minorities and Psychiatric Services. Sociology of Health and Illness 2:194–201.

Littlewood, Roland and M. Lipsedge
1987 The Butterfly and the Serpent: Culture, Psychopathology and Biomedicine. Culture, Medicine and Psychiatry 11:289–336.

Liu, Xiehe
1981 Psychiatry in Traditional Chinese Medicine. British Journal of Psychiatry 138:429–433.

Lock, Margaret
1982 Popular Conceptions of Mental Health in Japan. In Cultural Conceptions of Mental Health and Therapy. Anthony J. Marsella and Geoffrey M. White (eds.). Dordrecht: D. Reidel.
1987 Protests of a Good Wife and Wise Mother. In Health and Medical Care in Japan. E. Norbeck and M. Lock (eds.). Honolulu: University Press of Hawaii.
1987 DSM-III as a Culture-Bound Construct. Culture, Medicine and Psychiatry 11(1):35–42.
1988 A Nation at Risk: Interpretations of School Refusal in Japan. In Biomedicine Examined. Margaret Lock and Deborah Gordon (eds.). Dordrecht: Kluwer Academic Publishers.
1991 Nerves and Nostalgia: Greek-Canadian Immigrants and Medical Care in Québec. In Anthropologies of Medicine. Beatrix Pfleiderer and Gilles Bibeau (eds.). Wiesbaden: Vieweg Verlag.

Lock, Margaret and Deborah Gordon, eds.
1988 Biomedicine Examined. Dordrecht: Kluwer Academic Publishers.

Lovell, Anne
n.d. Bioenergetics in France. ms.

Low, Setha
1981 The Meaning of *Nervios*. Culture, Medicine and Psychiatry 3(1):25–47.
1985 Culturally Interpreted Symptoms or Culture-Bound Syndromes: A Cross-Cultural Review of Nerves. Social Science and Medicine 21(2):187–196.
1988 Medical Practice in Response to a Folk Illness. In Biomedicine Examined. Margaret Lock and Deborah Gordon (eds.). Dordrecht: Kluwer Academic Publishers.

Lutz, Catherine
1985 Depression and the Translation of Emotional Worlds. In Culture and Depression. A. Kleinman and B. Good (eds.). Berkeley: University of California Press.
1988 Unnatural Emotions. Chicago: University of Chicago.

Lyles, Michael and James Hillard
1982 Rootwork and the Refusal of Surgery. Psychosomatics 23:1–4.

Lynch, Owen, ed.
1990 Divine Passions. Berkeley: University of California Press.

Madsen, William
1964 The Mexican-Americans of South Texas. New York: Holt, Rinehart and Winston.

Makanjuola, R. O. A.
1987 *Ode Ori*: A Culture-Bound Disorder with Prominent Somatic Features in Yoruba Nigerian Patients. Acta Psychiatric Scandinavia 73.

Malik, S., M. Ahmed, A. Bashir and T. Choudhry
1990 Schneider's First-Rank Symptoms of Schizophrenia: Prevalence and Diagnostic Use: A Study From Pakistan. British Journal of Psychiatry 156:109–111.

Maloney, Clarence, ed
1976 The Evil Eye. New York: Columbia University Press.

Maltz, Daniel
1980 Black Drinking Practices Study Archival Research Report to the Department of Alcohol and Drug Abuse, State of California. Berkeley, CA: Source, Inc.

Manschreck, Theo and Arthur Kleinman, eds.
1977 Renewal in Psychiatry. Washington, D.C.: Hemisphere/Halsted Books.

Manson, Spero, J. Shore and J. Bloom
1985 The Depressive Experience in American Indian Communities: A Challenge for Psychiatric Theory and Diagnosis. In Culture and Depression. A. Kleinman and B. Good (eds.). Berkeley: University of California Press.

Manson, Spero and J. E. Trimble
1982 Mental Health Services to American Indian and Alaska Natives' Communities: Past Research, Future Inquiries. In Reaching the Underserved. L. Snowden (ed.). Beverly Hills: Sage.

Maretzki, Thomas W.
1988 Cultural Studies of Medical Institutions, Hierarchies and Training Practice: Therapy Spectrum and Cultural Traditions: Choices for Cures. A Reflexive Report. Paper Presented at the Conference, Anthropologies of Medicine: Western Europe and North American Perspectives. University of Hamburg. Hamburg, Germany. December 4–8.

Maretzki, Thomas and Eduard Seidler
1985 Biomedicine and Naturopathic Healing in West Germany: A History of a Stormy Relationship. Culture, Medicine and Psychiatry 9(4):383–427.

Markides, K. S. and J. Coreil
1988 The Hopi Indian's Mourning Hallucinations. Journal of Nervous and Mental Diseases 17(6):365–368.

Marsella, Anthony J.
1978 Thoughts on Cross-Cultural Studies on the Epidemiology of Depression. Culture, Medicine and Psychiatry 2:343–357.
1980 Depressive Experience and Disorder Across Cultures. In Handbook of Cross-Cultural Psychology. Vol. 5. Culture and Psychopathology. H. Triandis and J. Draguns (eds.). Boston: Allyn and Bacon.

Marsella, Anthony and Geoffrey White, eds.
1982 Cultural Conceptions of Mental Health and Therapy. Dordrecht: D. Reidel.

Marsella, Anthony, J. D. Kinzie and P. Gordon
1973 Ethnic Variations in the Expression Depression. Journal of Cross-Cultural Psychology 4:435–458.

Matchett, William
1972 Repeated Hallucinatory Experience as Part of the Mourning Process Among Hopi Indian Women. Psychiatry 35:185–194.

McDermott, John, Wen-Shing Tseng and Thomas Maretzki
1980 Peoples and Cultures of Hawai'i: A Psychocultural Perspective. Honolulu: University Press of Hawaii.

McGovern, Constance M.
1985 Masters of Madness: Social Origins of the American Psychiatric Profession. Hanover, NH: University Press of New England.

McGuire, Meredith B. (with the assistance of Debra Kantor)
1988 Ritual Healing in Suburban America. New Brunswick, NJ: Rutgers University Press.

McNally, R. J., R. Casiday and J. Calamari
1990 *Taijin-kyofusho* in a Black American Woman. Journal of Anxiety Disorders 4:83–87.

Mendel, Gérard
1972 Anthropologie Différentielle: Vers une Anthropologie Sociopsychoanalytique. Tome I. Paris: Payot.

Menninger, Karl, with M. Mayman and P. Pruyser
1963 The Vital Balance. New York: Viking.

Meyer-Lindenberg, Johannes
1991 The Holocaust and German Psychiatry. British Journal of Psychiatry 159:7–12.

Mezzich, J. and C. Berganza, eds.
1984 Culture and Psychopathology. New York: Columbia University Press.

Milagros, Bravo, Glorisa Canino, Maritza Rubio-Stipec
and Michal Woodbury Farina
1991 A Cross-Cultural Adaptation of a Psychiatric Epidemiological Instrument: The D.I.S.'s Adaptation in Puerto Rico. Culture, Medicine and Psychiatry 15(1):19–45.

Minuchin-Itzigsohn, S. D. et al.
1984 The Effect of Cultural Conceptions on Therapy: A Comparative Study of Patients in Israeli Psychiatric Clinics. Culture, Medicine and Psychiatry 8(3):229–254.

Miller, Martin A.
1985 The Theory and Practice of Psychiatry in the Soviet Union. Psychiatry 48:13–24.

Morantz-Sanchez, Regina Markell
1985 Sympathy and Science: Women Physicians in American Medicine. New York: Oxford University Press.

Morsy, Soheir
1978 Sex Roles, Power, and Illness in an Egyptian Village. American Ethnologist 5(1):137–150.

Mosher, Loren R.
1982 Italy's Revolutionary Mental Health Law: An Assessment. American Journal
      of Psychiatry 139(2):199–203.

Mullings, Leith
1984 Therapy, Ideology and Social Change. Berkeley: University of California
      Press.

Munakata, Tsunetsugu
1986 Japanese Attitudes Toward Mental Illness and Mental Health Care. In Japan-
      ese Culture and Behavior. T. Lebra and W. Lebra (eds.). Honolulu: Univer-
      sity Press of Hawaii.

Murase, T.
1976 Naikan Therapy. In Culture-Bound Syndromes, Ethnopsychiatry and Alter-
      nate Therapies. William Lebra (ed.). Honolulu: University Press of Hawaii.
1982 *Sunao*: A Central Value in Japanese Psychotherapy. In Cultural Conceptions
      of Mental Health and Therapy. Anthony Marsella and Geoffrey White (eds.).
      Dordrecht: D. Reidel.

Murphy, H. B. M.
1973 History and Evolution of Syndromes: The Striking Case of *Latah* and *Amok*.
      In Psychopathology. M. Hammer, K. Kalzinger and S. Sutton (eds.). New
      York: John Wiley.
1974 Differences Between Mental Disorders of French Canadians and British
      Canadians. Canadian Psychiatric Association Journal 19(3):247–257.
1976 Notes for a Theory on *Latah*. In Culture-Bound Syndromes, Ethnopsychiatry
      and Alternate Therapies. William Lebra (ed.). Honolulu: University Press of
      Hawaii.
1978 Cultural Influences in Incidence, Course and Treatment Response. In The
      Nature of Schizophrenia. L. Wynne, R. Cromwell and S. Mattryse (eds.).
      New York: John Wiley.
1983 Culture, Stress and Health in an Asian Elite. Santé, Culture, Health
      3(1):11–17.

Murphy, H. B. M., E. Wittkower and N. Chance
1964 Cross-Cultural Inquiry into the Symptomatology of Depression. Transcultur-
      al Psychiatric Research Review 1:5–21.

Murphy, Jane
1964 Psychotherapeutic Aspects of Shamanism on St. Lawrence Island, Alaska. In
      Magic, Faith and Healing. A. Kiev (ed.). New York: Free Press.
1976 Psychiatric Labeling in Cross-Cultural Perspective. Science 191:1019–1028.

Murphy, Jane and Alexander Leighton
1965 Approaches to Cross-Cultural Psychiatry. Ithaca: Cornell University Press.

Nathan, Toby
1986 La Folie des Autres. Paris: Dunod.

Navarro, Vincente
1978 Class Struggle, the State and Medicine. New York: Prodist.

Ndetei, D. M.
1980 Psychiatry in Kenya. Acta Psychiatrica Scandinavica 62:201–211.

Neki, J. S.
1973 Psychiatry in South-East Asia. British Journal of Psychotherapy 123:257–269.

Ngubane, Harriet
1977 Body and Mind in Zulu Medicine: New York: Academic Press.

Nichter, Mark
1981 Idioms of Distress: Alternatives in the Expression of Psychosocial Distress. Culture, Medicine and Psychiatry 5(4):379–408.
1985 Clinical Anthropologist as Therapy Facilitator. Human Organization 44(1):72–80.

Nomura, Naoki
1987 Japanese Mental Hospitals and Elementary Schools: The Parallel in Social Interaction. Paper presented at the American Anthropological Association Annual Meeting. Chicago, IL. November.

Nuckolls, Charles, ed.
1992 The Cultural Construction of Psychiatric Classification. Social Science and Medicine Special Issue/Section. (In press)

Nyiro, Gyula
1968 The History of Hungarian Psychiatry: An Outline. In Psychiatry in the Communist World. Ari Kiev (ed.). New York: Science House.

Obeyesekere, Gananath
1976 Psychological Medicine in Ayurveda. In Asian Medical Systems. Charles Leslie (ed.). Berkeley: University of California Press.
1981 Medusa's Hair. Chicago: University of Chicago Press.
1985 Depression, Buddhism and the Work of Culture in Sri Lanka. In Culture and Depression. Arthur Kleinman and Byron Good (eds.). Berkeley: University of California Press.

O'Grady, John
1990 The Prevalence and Diagnostic Signs of Schneiderian First-Rank Symptoms in a Random Sample of Acute Psychotic In-patients. British Journal of Psychiatry 156:496–500.

Ohnuki-Tierney, Emiko
1984 Health and Illness in Contemporary Japan. Cambridge: Cambridge University Press.

Oltmanns, Thomas and Brendan Maher, eds.
1988 Delusions: Interdisciplinary Perspectives. New York: John Wiley.

O'Neil, J. D.
1986 Colonial Stress in the Canadian Arctic: An Ethnography of Young Adults Changing. In Anthropology and Epidemiology. C. Janes et al. (eds.). Dordrecht: D. Reidel.

O'Nell, Theresa D.
1989 Psychiatric Investigations Among American Indians and Alaska Natives: A Critical Review. Culture, Medicine and Psychiatry 13(1):51–87.

Ong, Aihwa
1988 The Production of Possession: Spirits and the Multinational Corporation in Malaysia. American Ethnologist 15(1):28–42

Opler, Marvin K.
1959 Culture and Mental Health. New York: The Macmillan Co.

Orley, J.
1970 Culture and Mental Illness: A Study from Uganda. Nairobi: East African Publishing House.

Orley, J. H. and J. K. Wing
1979 Psychiatric Disorders in Two African Villages. Archives of General Psychiatry 36:513–520.

Ozturk, Orhan
1964 Folk Treatment of Mental Illness in Turkey. In Magic, Faith and Healing. Ari Kiev (ed.). New York: Free Press.

Padilla, Amado
1980 Psychological Dimensions of the Acculturation Process. Boulder, CO: Westview.

Pandolfi, Mariella
1987 Psychothérapie et Milieu Rural en Itali. In Régards Anthropologiques en Psychiatrie. Montréal: Éditions du GIRAME.
1988 Refusing Knowledge, Embodying Emotions: Women in a Southern Italian Village. Paper presented at the Conference, Medical Anthropologies. University of Hamburg, Hamburg, Germany. December 4–8. Also, 1991. In Anthropoligies of Medicine. B. Pfleiderere and G. Bibeau (eds.). Wiesbaden: Vieweg.

Pang, Keum Y. C.
1990 *Hwabyung*: The Construction of a Korean Popular Illness Among Korean Elderly Immigrant Women in the U.S. Culture, Medicine and Psychiatry 14(4):495–512.

Papeschi, Raffaell
1985 The Denial of the Institution: A Critical Review of Franco Basaglia's Writings. British Journal of Psychiatry 146:247–254.

Parsons, Anne
1969 Belief, Magic and Anomie. New York: Free Press.

Parsons, Clare
1984 Idioms of Distress: Kinship and Sickness Among the People of the Kingdom of Tonga. Culture, Medicine and Psychiatry 8(1):71–93.

Payer, Lynn
1990 Borderline Cases: How Medical Practice Reflects National Culture. The Sciences 30(4):38–40.

Pelzer, Karl and Samuel M. Woldu
1990 The *Brain-Fag* Syndrome of French Nigerian Students and Gender Identity. Curare 13(3):141–146.

Petros, S. and E. Schier
1989 Traditional Attitudes Towards Mental Illness in Ethiopia. Curare 12(3/4): 161–167.

Philipe, J. and J. B. Romain
1979 *Indisposition* in Haïti. Social Science and Medicine 13B:129–133.

Pliskin, Karen
1987 Silent Boundaries. New Haven: Yale University Press.

Post, Stephen
1992 DSM-III-R: Psychiatry, Religion and Bias. In The Cultural Construction of Psychiatric Classification. C. Nuckolls (ed.). Social Science and Medicine Special Issue/Section. (In Press)

Prince, Raymond
1960 *Brainfag* Syndrome in Nigerian Students. Journal of Mental Science 106:559–570.
1964 Indigenous Yoruba Psychiatry. In Magic, Faith and Healing. Ari Kiev (ed.). New York: Free Press.
1985 The Concept of Culture-Bound Syndromes: *Anorexia Nervosa* and *Brain Fag*. Social Science and Medicine 21(2)197–204.
1988 Shamans and Endorphins. Curare 11(1):57–67.

Prince, Raymond and Françoise Tcheng-Laroche
1987 Culture-Bound Syndromes and International Classification of Diseases. Culture, Medicine, and Psychiatry 11(1):3–20.

Prokupek, Josef, Jaroslav Stuchlik and Stanislav Grof
1968 Czechoslovak Psychiatry. In Psychiatry in the Communist World. Ari Kiev (ed.). New York: Science House.

Provencher, R.
1984 'Mother Needles': Lessons of the Inter-Ethnic Psychiatry in Malaysian Society. Social Science and Medicine 18(2):139–146.

Racy, J.
1970 Psychiatry in the Arab East. Acta Psychiatrica Scandinavica Supplement 21:1–171.
1980 Somatization in Saudi Women. British Journal of Psychiatry 137:212–216.

Rakawy, Y.
1978 Psychiatry in Egypt Today. Egyptian Journal of Psychiatry 1(1):13–23.
1979 Psychiatry in Egypt Today; Part II. Egyptian Journal of Psychiatry 2(1):19–26.

Ratnavale, David N.
1973 Psychiatry in Shanghai, China: Observations in 1973. American Journal of Psychiatry 130(10):1082–1087.

Resner, J. and J. Hartog
1970 Concepts and Terminology of Mental Disorders Among Malays. Journal of Cross-Cultural Psychology 1:369–381.

Reynolds, David K.
1976 Morita Psychotherapy. Berkeley: University of California Press.
1980 The Quiet Therapies. Honolulu: University Press of Hawaii.
1983 Naikan Psychotherapy. Chicago: University of Chicago Press.

Rhodes, Lorna Amarasingham
1984 "This Will Clear Your Mind": The Use of Metaphors for Medicine in Psychiatric Settings. Culture, Medicine and Psychiatry 8(1):49–70.
1985 The Anthropologist as Institutional Analyst. Ethos 14(2):204–217.
1991 Emptying Beds. Berkeley: University of California Press.

Rich, Vera
1985 Soviet Psychiatry Aiming for Rehabilitation? Nature 17:467.

Ritchie, J. E.
1976 Cultural Time Out: Generalized Therapeutic Sociocultural Mechanisms Among the Maori. In Culture-Bound Syndromes, Ethnopsychiatry and Alternate Therapies. William Lebra (ed.). Honolulu: University Press of Hawaii.

Ritenberg, William and Ronald C. Simons
1985 Gentle Interrogation: Inquiry and Interaction in Brief Initial Psychiatric Evaluations. In Physicians of Western Medicine: Anthropological Approaches to Theory and Practice. Robert A. Hahn and Atwood D. Gaines (eds.). Dordrecht: D. Reidel.

Robins, Lee N. and Darrel A. Regier, eds.
1991 Psychiatric Disorders in America. New York: Free Press.

Rogler, L. H. and A. B. Hollingshead
1961 The Puerto Rican Spiritist as Psychiatrist. American Journal of Sociology 87(1):17–21.

Rogler, Lloyd, Robert Malgady and Orlando Rodrigues
1989 Hispanics and Mental Health: A Framework for Research. Malabar, Florida: Robert E. Krieger Publishing.

Roosens, E.
1979 Mental Patients in Town Life. Beverly Hills: Sage.

Rosenhahn, D.
1973 On Being Sane in Insane Places. Science 179:250–258.

Rubel, Arthur
1977 *Susto*: Epidemiology of a Folk Disorder. In Culture, Illness and Disease. D. Landy (ed.). New York: Macmillan.

Rubel, Arthur et al.
1984 *Susto*. Berkeley: University of California Press.

Saint-Gérard, Yves
1984 L'État de Mal en Haïti. Toulouse: Eche.

Salan, Rudy and Thomas Maretzki
1983 Mental Health Services and Traditional Healing in Indonesia: Are the Roles Compatible? Culture, Medicine and Psychiatry 7(4):377–412.

Sandner, Donald
1979 Navaho Symbols of Healing: New York: Harcourt Brace.

Sartorius, N. and A. Jablensky
1976 Transcultural Studies of Schizophrenia. WHO Chronicle 30:481–485.

Sartorius, N., A. Jablensky and R. Shapiro
1978 Cross-Cultural Differences in the Short-Term Prognosis of Schizophrenic Psychosis. Schizophrenia Bulletin 4(1):102–113.

Sartorius, Norman, et al.
1983 Depressive Disorders in Different Cultures. Geneva: WHO.
1986 Early Manifestation and First Contact Incidence of Schizophrenia. Psychological Medicine 16:909–928.

Scheff, Thomas
1966 Being Mentally Ill: A Sociological Theory. Chicago: Aldine.

Scheper-Hughes, Nancy
1979 Saints, Scholars and Schizophrenics. Berkeley: University of California Press.
1987 'Mental' in Southie. Culture, Medicine and Psychiatry 11(1):53–78.
1988 The Madness of Hunger. Culture, Medicine and Psychiatry 12(4):429–458.

Scheper-Hughes, Nancy and Margaret Lock
1988 The Mindful Body: A Prolegomenon to Future Work in Medical Anthropology. Medical Anthropology Quarterly *(n.s.)* 1(1):6–41.

Scheper-Hughes, Nancy and Anne Lovell, eds. and trans.
1987 Psychiatry Inside and Out: Selected Writings of Franco Basaglia. New York: Columbia University Press.

Schieffelin, Edward
1985 The Cultural Analysis of Depressive Affect: An Example from New Guinea. In Culture and Depression. A. Kleinman and B. Good (eds.). Berkeley: University of California Press.

Schulsinger, Fini and Assen Jablensky, eds.
1991 The National Mental Health Programme in the United Republic of Tanzania. Acta Psychiatrica Scandinavica 83; Supplement 364.

Segal, Boris M.
1975 The Theoretical Bases of Soviet Psychotherapy. American Journal of Psychotherapy 29:503–523.

Sethi, B. B.
1977 The Theory and Practice of Psychiatry in India. American Journal of Psychotherapy 31(1):43–65.

Seva-Diaz, A. et al.
1985 Sociocultural Studies of Mental Disorders in the Iberian Peninsula. Transcultural Psychiatric Research Review 22(4):225–236.

Sharp, Lesley
1990 Possessed and Dispossessed Youth: Spirit Possession of School Children in Northwest Madagascar. Culture, Medicine and Psychiatry 14(3):339–364.

Shweder, Richard and E. Bourne
1982 Do Conceptions of the Person Vary Cross Culturally? In Cultural Conceptions of Mental Health and Therapy. A. Marsella and G. White (eds.). Dordrecht: D. Reidel.

Sidel, Ruth
1973 The Role of Revolutionary Optimism in the Treatment of Mental Illness in the People's Republic of China. American Journal of Orthopsychiatry 43(5):732–736.

Simon, B.
1978 Mind and Madness in Ancient Greece: The Classical Roots of Modern Psychiatry. Ithaca: Cornell University Press.

Simons, Ronald C. and Charles Hughes, eds.
1985 Culture-Bound Syndromes. Dordrecht: D. Reidel.

Skultans, Vieda
1975 Madness and Morals. Ideas on Insanity in the Nineteenth Century. London: Routledge and Kegan Paul.
1979 English Madness: Ideas on Insanity, 1580–1890. London: Routledge and Kegan Paul.

Snow, Loudell
1977 Popular Medicine in a Black Neighborhood. In Ethnic Medicine in the Southwest. Edward Spicer (ed.). Tucson: University of Arizona Press.

Srinivasa, D. K. and S. Trivedi
1982 Knowledge and Attitude of Mental Disease in a Rural Community of South India. Social Science and Medicine 16:1635–1639.

Stevens, Rosemary
1966 Medical Practice in Modern England. New Haven: Yale University.

Stevenson, I. Neil
1977 *Colerina*: Reactions to Emotional Stress in the Peruvian Andes. Social Science and Medicine 11:303–307.

Sue, S. and J. Morishima
1982 The Mental Health of Asian Americans. San Francisco: Josey Bass.

Suzuki, T. and R. Suzuki
1977 Morita Therapy. In Psychosomatic Medicine. E. Wittkower and H. Warnes (eds.). New York: Harper and Row.

Swartz, Leslie
1985 Issues for Cross-Cultural Psychiatric Research in South Africa. Culture, Medicine and Psychiatry 9(1):59–74.
1986 Transcultural Psychiatry in South Africa Part I. Transcultural Psychiatric Research Review 23:273–303.
1987 Transcultural Psychiatry in South Africa. Part II. Transcultural Psychiatric Research Review 24:5–30.

Szasz, Thomas
1961 The Myth of Mental Illness. New York: Hoeber-Harper.

Talbot, John
1980 An In-Depth Look at DSM-III. Hospital and Community Psychiatry 31(1): 25–32.

Tanaka-Matsumi, J.
1979 *Taijin Kyofusho:* Diagnostic and Cultural Issues in Japanese Psychiatry. Culture, Medicine and Psychiatry 3(3):231–245.

Tanaka-Matsumi, J. and A. J. Marsella
1976 Cross-cultural Variations in the Phenomenological Experience of Depression. Journal of Cross-Cultural Psychology 7(4):379–396.

Tousignant, Michel
1984 *Pena* in the Ecuadorian Sierra. Culture, Medicine and Psychiatry 8(4): 381–398.

Townsend, J. M.
1975 Cultural Conceptions and Mental Illness: A Controlled Comparison of Germany and America. Journal of Nervous and Mental Disease 160:409–421.

1978 Cultural Conceptions and Mental Illness. Chicago: University of Chicago Press.
1979 Stereotypes and Mental Illness: A Comparison with Ethnic Stereotypes. Culture, Medicine and Psychiatry 3(3):205–230.

Trimble, J., S. Manson, N. Dinges and B. Medicine
1984 American Indian Concepts of Mental Health: Reflections and Directions. In Mental Health Services: The Cross-Cultural Context. P. Pederson et al. (eds.). Beverly Hills: Sage.

Trimble, Michael R.
1990 First-Rank Symptoms of Schneider: A New Perspective? British Journal of Psychiatry 156:195–200.

Tseng, Wen-Shing
1974 The Development of Psychiatric Concepts in Traditional Chinese Medicine. Archives of General Psychiatry 29:569–575.
1975 The Nature of Somatic Complaints Among Psychiatric Patients: The Chinese Case. Comprehensive Psychiatry 16(3):237–245.
1975 Traditional and Modern Psychiatric Care in Taiwan. In Medicine in Chinese Cultures. A. Kleinman et al. (eds.). Washington, DC: U.S.D.H.E.W. for the Fogerty Center.

Tseng, Wen-Shing, Hu Di, Keisuke Ebata, Jin Hsu and Cui Yuhua
1986 Diagnostic Pattern for Neuroses in China, Japan, and the United States. American Journal of Psychiatry 143(8):1010–1014.

Tseng, Wen-Shing and John McDermott
1981 Culture, Mind and Therapy. New York: Bruner/Mazel.

Tung, May
1984 Life Values, Psychotherapy and East-West Integration. Psychiatry 47:285–292.

Turkle, Sherry
1978 Psychoanalytic Politics: Freud's French Revolution. New York: Basic Books.

Turner, Bryan
1987 Medical Power and Social Knowledge. London: Sage.

Turner, Victor
1964 An Ndembu Doctor in Practice. In Magic, Faith and Healing. Ari Kiev (ed.). New York: Basic Books.

Valle, Ramón
1989 Outreach to Ethnic Minorities with Alzheimer's Disease. Health Matrix 6(4):13–27.

Van Moffaert, Myriam and André Vereecken
1989 Somatization of Psychiatric Illness in Mediterranean Immigrants in Belgium. Culture, Medicine and Psychiatry 13(3):297–313.

Verwey, Gerlof
1985 Psychiatry in its Anthropological and Historical Context. Dordrecht: D. Reidel.

Visher, John S. and Emily B. Visher
1979 Impressions of Psychiatric Problems and Their Management; China, 1977. American Journal of Psychiatry 136(1):28–32.

Waitzkin, Howard
1983 The Second Sickness: Contradictions of Capitalist Health Care. New York: Free Press.

Wallace, Anthony F. C.
1959 The Institutionalization of Cathartic and Control Strategies in Iroquois Religious Psychotherapy. In Culture and Mental Health. Marvin K. Opler (ed.). New York: Macmillan.
1961 Mental Illness, Biology and Culture. In Psychological Anthropology. F. L. K. Hsu (ed.). Homewood, IL: Dorsey Press.
1972 The Death and Rebirth of the Seneca. New York: Random House.

Walls, Philip D., Lichun Han Walls and Donald Langsley
1975 Psychiatric Training and Practice in the People's Republic of China. American Journal of Psychiatry 132(2):121–128.

Warner, R.
1985 Recovery From Schizophrenia: Psychiatry and Political Economy. London and New York: Routledge and Kegan Paul.

Watson-Gegeo, Karen Ann and David W. Gegeo
1990 Shaping the Mind and Straightening Out Conflicts: The Discourse of Kwara'ae Family Counseling. In Disentangling: Conflict Discourse in Pacific Societies. Karen Ann Watson-Gegeo and Geoffrey M. White (eds.). Stanford: Stanford University Press.

Watson-Gegeo, Karen Ann and Geoffrey M. White, eds.
1990 Disentangling: Conflict Discourse in Pacific Societies. Stanford: Stanford University Press.

Waxler, Nancy (aka Waxler-Morrison)
1974 Culture and Mental Illness. Journal of Nervous and Mental Disease 159(6):379–395.
1979 Is Outcome for Schizophrenia Better in Nonindustrial Countries? Journal of Nervous and Mental Disease 167(3):144–158.

Waxler-Morrison, Nancy et al.
1990 Cross-Cultural Caring. Vancouver, B.C.: University of British Colombia Press.

Weidman, Hazel
1969 Cultural Values, Concept of Self and Projection: The Burmese Case. In Mental Health Research in the Pacific. W. Caudill and T.-Y. Lin (eds.). Honolulu: East West Center Press.
1979 *Falling-Out*: A Diagnostic and Treatment Problem Viewed From a Transcultural Perspective. In Special Issue on the Transcultural Perspective in Health and Illness. H. Weidman (ed.). Social Science and Medicine B13(2):95–112.

Weidman, Hazel, et al.
1978 The Miami Health Ecology Project Report. Volume I: A Statement on Ethnicity and Health. Miami: University of Miami.

Weisberg, Daniel and Susan Long, eds.
1984 Biomedicine in Asia: Transformations and Variations. Culture, Medicine and Psychiatry Special Issue 8(2).

Weiss, Mitchell
1985 The Interrelationship of Tropical Disease and Mental Disorder: Malaria. Culture, Medicine and Psychiatry 9(2):121–200.

**Weiss, Mitchell, S. D. Sharma, R. K. Gaur, J.S . Sharma,
A. Desai and D. R. Doongaj**
1986 Traditional Concepts of Mental Disorder Among Indian Psychiatric Patients. Social Science and Medicine 23(4):379–386.

Wen, Jung-Kwang
1990 The Hall of the Dragon Metamorphoses. Culture, Medicine and Psychiatry 14(1):1–19.

Westermeyer, Joseph
1973 On the Epidemicity of *Amok* Violence. Archives of General Psychiatry 28:873–876.
1989 Psychiatric Care of Migrants: A Clinical Guide. Washington, D.C.: American Psychiatric Press, Inc.

Westermeyer, Joseph and Ronald Wintrob
1979 "Folk" Criteria for the Diagnosis of Mental Illness in Rural Laos: On Being Insane in Sane Places. American Journal of Psychiatry 136:755–761.

White, Geoffrey
1982 The Ethnographic Study of Cultural Knowledge of "Mental Disorder." In Cultural Conceptions of Mental Health and Therapy. A. Marsella and G. White (eds.). Dordrecht: D. Reidel.
1990 Emotion Talk and Social Inference: Disentangling in Santa Isabel, Solomon Islands. In Disentangling: Conflict Discourse in Pacific Societies. Karen Ann Watson-Gegeo and Geoffrey M. White (eds.). Stanford: Stanford University Press.

Wig, N. N.
1990 The Third World Perspective on Psychiatric Diagnosis and Classification. In Sources and Traditions of Classification in Psychiatry. N. Sartorius, R. Hirschfeld, A. Jablenski, D. Regier and J. Burke (eds.). Toronto: Hans Huber.

Wikan, Unni
1989 Illness from Fright and Soul Loss. Culture, Medicine and Psychiatry 13(1):25–50.

Women and Mental Health International Conference Committee
1991 Women and Mental Health. British Journal of Psychiatry 158; Supplement 10.

World Health Organization (WHO)
1973 The International Pilot Study of Schizophrenia. Geneva: WHO.
1979 Schizophrenia: An International Follow-Up Study. Chichester: John Wiley.

Wu, David
1982 Psychotherapy and Emotion in Traditional Chinese Medicine. In Cultural Conceptions of Mental Health and Therapy. A. Marsella and G. White (eds.). Dordrecht: D. Reidel.

Yap, Pow-Ming
1951 Mental Diseases Peculiar to Certain Cultures. Journal of Mental Science 97:313–32.

1965 *Koro*—A Culture-Bound Depersonalization Syndrome. British Journal of Psychiatry III: 43–50.

1969 The Culture-Bound Reactive Syndromes. In Mental Health Research in Asia and the Pacific. W. Caudill and T.-Y. Lin (eds.). Honolulu: East-West Center Press.

1974 Comparative Psychiatry: A Theoretical Framework. Toronto: University of Toronto Press.

Ying, Yu-Wen

1990 Explanatory Models of Major Depression and Implications for Help-Seeking Among Immigrant Chinese-American Women. Culture, Medicine and Psychiatry 14(3):393–408.

Young, Allan

1975 Why Amhara Get *Kurenya*: Sickness and Possession in an Ethiopian *Zar* Cult. American Ethnologist 2:567–584.

1980 The Discourse on Stress and the Reproduction of Conventional Knowledge. Social Science and Medicine 14B:133–146.

1988 Unpacking the Demoralization Thesis. Medical Anthropology Quarterly *(n.s.)* 2(1):3–16.

1990 Moral Conflicts in a Psychiatric Hospital Treating Combat-Related Posttraumatic Stress Disorder (PTSD). In Social Science Perspectives on Medical Ethics. George Weisz (ed.). Dordrecht: Kluwer Academic Publishers.

1991 Emil Kraepelin and the History of American Psychiatric Classification. In: Anthropologies of Medicine. Beatrix Pfleiderer and Gilles Bibeau (eds.). Wiesbaden: Vieweg Verlag.

Young, Derson and Mingyan Chang

1983 Psychiatry in the People's Republic of China. Comprehensive Psychiatry 24(5):431–438.

Ziferstein, Isidore

1972 Group Psychotherapy in the Soviet Union. American Journal of Psychiatry 129:107–112.

Zung, W. W.

1965 A Self-Rating Depression Scale. Archives of General Psychiatry 12:63–70.

List of Contributors

AMY V. BLUE, Ph.D. (Anthropology; Case Western Reserve*): Department of Behavioral Science, College of Medicine, University of Kentucky. Lexington, KY, United States.

THOMAS J. CSORDAS, Ph.D. (Anthropology; Duke): Department of Anthropology, Case Western Reserve University. Cleveland, OH, United States.

ELLEN DWYER, Ph.D. (History; Columbia): Department of Criminal Justice, Indiana University. Bloomington, IN, United States.

PAUL FARMER, M.D., Ph.D. (Anthropology; Harvard): Department of Social Medicine and Health Policy, Harvard University School of Medicine. Cambridge, MA, United States; Zanmi Lasante and Clinique Bon Sauveur. Port au-Prince, Haïti, West Indies.

ATWOOD D. GAINES, Ph.D. (Anthropology; UC Berkeley): M.P.H. (UC Berkeley School of Public Health): Department of Anthropology and Department of Psychiatry, Case Western Reserve University and School of Medicine. Cleveland, OH, United States.

HELENA JIA HERSHEL, Ph.D. (Sociology; UC Berkeley): M.A. (Counseling; Hayward State): California School of Professional Psychology, San Francisco, CA, and private practice. Berkeley and San Francisco, CA, United States.

JANIS HUNTER JENKINS, Ph.D. (Anthropology, UCLA): Department of Anthropology and Department of Psychiatry, Case Western Reserve University and School of Medicine. Cleveland, OH, United States.

PEARL KATZ, Ph.D. (Anthropology, SUNY Buffalo): Department of Psychiatry, The Johns Hopkins University Medical School; Department of Psychiatry, University of Maryland School of Medicine, Baltimore, MD; and Department of Psychiatry, Uniform Services University Medical School, Bethesda, MD, United States.

THOMAS W. MARETZKI, Ph.D. (Anthropology; Princeton): Department of Anthropology and Department of Allied Health Sciences, University of Hawaii and School of Medicine. Honolulu, HI, United States.

NAOKI NOMURA, Ph.D. (Anthropology; Stanford): Nagoya Women's Junior College of Commerce. Owari Asahi City, Japan.

*Field and school of academic degree(s).

CHARLES W. NUCKOLLS, Ph.D. (Anthropology; Chicago): Department of Anthropology. Emory University. Atlanta, GA, United States.

KATHRYN S. OTHS, Ph.D. (Anthropology; Case Western Reserve): Department of Anthropology and Department of Family Medicine, University of Alabama and School Of Medicine. Tuscaloosa, AL, United States.

LORNA AMARASINGHAM RHODES, Ph.D. (Anthropology; Cornell): Department of Anthropology and Department of Health Services, University of Washington. Seattle, WA, United States.

LESLIE SWARTZ, Ph.D. (Psychology; Cape Town): Department of Psychology, University of Cape Town. Cape Town, South Africa.

Name Index

Subject Index